Clinical Pediatric Surgery

Clinical Pediatric Surgery

Editor: Aden Breland

AMERICAN
MEDICAL PUBLISHERS
www.americanmedicalpublishers.com

AMERICAN
MEDICAL PUBLISHERS
www.americanmedicalpublishers.com

Cataloging-in-Publication Data

Clinical pediatric surgery / edited by Aden Breland.
p. cm.
Includes bibliographical references and index.
ISBN 979-8-88740-003-7
1. Children--Surgery. 2. Infants--Surgery. 3. Surgery, Operative.
4. Children--Diseases--Treatment. I. Breland, Aden.
RD137 .C55 2023
617.98--dc23

American Medical Publishers,
41 Flatbush Avenue,
1st Floor, New York,
NY 11217, USA

ISBN 979-8-88740-003-7 (Hardback)

Contents

Preface

Clinical pediatric surgery is a surgical sub-specialty that involves the diagnostic, operative and postoperative surgical care of children, infants, adolescents and young adults. It deals with conditions including congenital and acquired anomalies and diseases, as well as inflammatory, developmental, traumatic and neoplastic complications. Neonatal surgery and fetal surgery are the two major areas of clinical pediatric surgery. There are several types of diseases that are treated with the help of pediatric surgery. Some of these congenital conditions include pectus excavatum, hypertrophic pyloric stenosis, intestinal atresia, necrotizing enterocolitis, meconium plugs, Hirschsprung's disease, anorectal malformations, undescended testes, intestinal malrotation, and biliary atresia. Several childhood tumors like Wilms' tumor, neuroblastoma, rhabdomyosarcoma, liver tumors, ATRT, kidney tumors and teratomas are also treated through this area of surgery. This book is a practical guide to clinical pediatric surgery. From theories to research to practical applications, case studies related to all contemporary topics of relevance to this field have been included herein. This book will serve as a valuable source of reference to students and professionals associated with the field of pediatric surgery.

Significant researches are present in this book. Intensive efforts have been employed by authors to make this book an outstanding discourse. This book contains the enlightening chapters which have been written on the basis of significant researches done by the experts.

Finally, I would also like to thank all the members involved in this book for being a team and meeting all the deadlines for the submission of their respective works. I would also like to thank my friends and family for being supportive in my efforts.

Editor

Esophageal Perforation and EVAC in Pediatric Patients: A Case Series of Four Children

Laura Antonia Ritz[1†], *Mohammad Samer Hajji*[2†], *Tobias Schwerd*[2], *Sibylle Koletzko*[2], *Dietrich von Schweinitz*[1], *Eberhard Lurz*[2†] and *Jochen Hubertus*[1*†‡]

[1] Department of Pediatric Surgery, Dr. von Hauner Children's Hospital, Ludwig-Maximilian-University of Munich, Munich, Germany, [2] Department of Pediatric Gastroenterology, Dr. von Hauner Children's Hospital, Ludwig-Maximilian-University of Munich, Munich, Germany

***Correspondence:**
Jochen Hubertus
jochen.hubertus@
med.uni-muenchen.de

Introduction: In pediatric patients, esophageal perforation (EP) is rare but associated with significant morbidity and mortality rates of up to 20–30%. In addition to standard treatment options, endoscopic esophageal vacuum-assisted closure (EVAC) therapy has shown promising results, especially in adult patients. Thus far, the only data on technical success and effectiveness of EVAC in pediatric patients were published in 2018 by Manfredi et al. at Boston Children's Hospital. The sparse data on EVAC in children indicates that this promising technique has been barely utilized in pediatric patients. More data are needed to evaluate efficacy and outcomes of this technique in pediatric patients.

Method: We reviewed five cases of therapy using EVAC, ArgyleTM Replogle Suction Catheter (RSC), or both on pediatric patients with EP in our institution between October 2018 and April 2020.

Results: Five patients with EP (median 3.4 years; 2 males) were treated with EVAC, RSC, or a combination. Complete closure of EP was not achieved after EVAC alone, though patients' health stabilized and inflammation and size of EP decreased after EVAC. Four patients then were treated with RSC until the EP healed. One patient needed surgery as the recurrent fistula did not heal sufficiently after 3 weeks of EVAC therapy. Two patients developed stenosis and were successfully treated with dilatations. One patient treated with RSC alone showed persistent EP after 5 weeks.

Conclusion: EVAC in pediatric patients is technically feasible and a promising method to treat EP, regardless of the underlying cause. EVAC therapy can be terminated as soon as local inflammation and C-reactive protein levels decrease, even if the mucosa is not healed completely at that time. A promising subsequent treatment is RSC. An earlier switch to RSC can substantially reduce the need of anesthesia during subsequent treatments. Our findings indicate that EVAC is more effective than RSC alone. In some cases, EVAC can be used to improve the tissues condition in preparation for a re-do surgery. At 1 year after therapy, all but one patient demonstrated sufficient weight gain. Further prospective studies with a larger cohort are required to confirm our observations from this small case series.

Keywords: esophageal perforation, VAC, vacuum therapy, children, pediatric patients

INTRODUCTION

In pediatric patients, esophageal perforation (EP) is rare but associated with high morbidity rates of up to 20–30% (1). The most common cause for EP (75%) in children is dilatation of preexisting stenosis (2). The overall risk of perforation after dilatation is only 0.6% for all types of stenosis (3) but this risk increases up to 3.4–18% for congenital stenoses of the esophagus (4, 5). Other reasons for perforation can be foreign body ingestion or anastomotic leak after esophageal anastomosis (1, 2). In neonates, nasogastric tube insertions and attempted endotracheal intubation are main sources of EP (6). Interrupted continuity of the esophageal wall can cause saliva, bacteria, and digestive enzymes to migrate into the mediastinum, which can lead to empyema, abscess formation, and mediastinitis and potentially progress to sepsis and necrosis of pulmonary tissue (7).

The treatment for EP used to be primary repair (8–10) or stenting (11) for both pediatric and adult patients. Whereas, EP in adults commonly occurs with underlying pathology (1), thus favoring invasive approaches, EP in children mostly occurs in vital tissue with greater propensity to heal (1, 2), in which case non-operative treatments (e.g., parenteral nutrition and broad-spectrum antibiotics) may be preferred, as described by Van der Zee et al. (12).

Over the last several years, non-operative techniques have been introduced in adult patients. Among these, endoscopic esophageal vacuum-assisted closure (EVAC) therapy has shown promising results. This well-established technique originated as a treatment for infected wounds, burns, and ulcers (13–18). In 2011, Loske et al. (19) and Schorsch et al. (20) modified it for intraluminal use in adult patients with EP. Multiple studies have verified the success of EVAC (19–26) for this purpose and have shown that it is more effective than stents (27).

The only data on the technical success and effectiveness of EVAC among pediatric patients were published in 2018 by Manfredi et al. (28) from Boston Children's Hospital (29). This promising technique therefore needs further investigation in pediatric patients. We aim to describe our experience using a therapy combining EVAC with an Argyle™ Replogle Suction Catheter (RSC) in pediatric patients with EP.

In our hospital, stents are not used in the treatment of EP. The therapy used to be non-operative with parenteral nutrition and broad-spectrum antibiotics and was then extended by the additional use of EVAC.

In our patients EVAC was technically possible and effective. No patient experienced complete closure of EP after EVAC alone, though patients were subsequently treated with RSC until restitutio ad integrum.

MATERIALS AND METHODS

We performed an institutional review on all patients aged ≤18 years with EP who were treated with EVAC or RSC between October 2018 and April 2020. Indication for EVAC therapy was a radiologically and endoscopically proven perforation of the esophagus with saliva leaking into the mediastinum. Patients aged >18 years or those with perforation of the esophagus or fistulation into the trachea or bronchi were excluded.

The EVAC sponge was placed using a size-adapted gastroscope and inserted antegrade. Correct position was confirmed by a retrograde endoscopy over a gastrostomy, in analogy to Manfredi et al. (28). An Eso-SPONGE®-system (Braun, Melsungen, Germany) was cut to size according to the patient's size. If an extraluminal cavity was present, the sponge was initially placed in the cavity and retracted with every session. If there was no extraluminal cavity, the sponge was placed in the esophagus, overlapping the EP on both sides. The position of the sponge was secured by a holding thread which was passed out and secured over the gastrostomy. The tube was connected to a Medela Thopaz+® Digital Chest Drainage and Monitoring System (Medela, Baar, Switzerland). Negative pressure of −100 cm H_2O was applied. Blood inflammation levels, mainly C-reactive protein (CrP), were determined before and during treatment. Antibiotics were given in a weight-adjusted dosage according to the antibiotic susceptibility test results.

The correct position was confirmed using a flexible endoscope. In the first two patients, the sponge was initially changed every 3 days. To minimize the number of anesthesia, intervals were lengthened to 5 days for these and all patients thereafter. Prior to removal, the sponge was flushed with 10–20 ml of NaCl 0.9% to avoid mucosal defects. Removal was performed under the guidance of the holding thread. After several intervals of EVAC, the sponge was replaced by an ArgyleTM® Replogle Suction Catheter (RSC). The RSC was connected to a Medela Thopaz+® Digital Chest Drainage and Monitoring System using a negative pressure of −100 cm H_2O. The RSC was inserted endoscopically and placed at the level of the perforation. The correct position was checked radiologically. Patient 5 was treated with RSC alone.

The primary outcome was technical feasibility of EVAC in pediatric patients. The secondary outcome was the impact of an earlier switch to RSC on number of anesthesia. Finally, we assessed efficacy of RSC treatment alone and the medium-term outcome at 1 year after EVAC or RSC. Results are presented in a descriptive manner due to the size of our cohort.

Since this is a retrospective single-center study, data was collected prior to the study at our institution in the progress of treating the patients. As an inhouse-research, no approval of the ethics committee is needed.

RESULTS

Between October 2018 and April 2020, five pediatric patients (aged 7 months to 11.3 years, median 3.4 years; 2 males) with EP were treated with EVAC and/or RSC at our hospital. Patients 1 and 2 were born with esophageal atresia Gross type D and developed anastomotic leakage after failed primary repair and re-do surgery. Patient 3 was transferred to our hospital after iatrogenic EP post-dilatation of a congenital distal esophageal stenosis. Patient 4 suffered from anastomotic leakage after gastric transposition due to caustic injury at the age of 4 years. Gastric transposition was performed because of recurrent fistula

TABLE 1 | Patients treated with endoscopic esophageal vacuum-assisted closure (EVAC) between 2018 and 2020.

Patient	1	2	3	4	5
Age /month	41	7	30	136	24
Diagnosis	EA[1] Gross D	EA Gross D	CES[2]	Caustic injury	BA[3], liver Tx[4]
Reason for treatment	AL[5]	RF[6]	IP[7]	AL	EGF[8]
Position of EP[9]	T[10]3	T5/6	T11	T6/7	T11/12
EP distance to dental arch					
Lenght of EVAC[11]	30	21	11	12	24*
Sessions	8	6	2	3	4
Subsequent therapy	RSC[12]	Surgery	RSC	RSC	RSC
Days of treatment	45	21	26	23	38
Diet after 1 year	PEG[13]/SF[14]	Normal diet	Normal diet	Normal diet	PEG

For Patients 1 and 2, the sponge was changed every 3 days. For the other patients, it was changed every 5 to 6 days, and duration of EVAC therapy was reduced. The Replogle Suction Catheter (RSC) was continued until the esophageal perforation (EP) healed. Patient 5 was treated with RSC alone and had a persistent fistula at 5 weeks after treatment.
*[1]EA, Esophageal atresia; [2]CES, Congenital esophageal stenosis; [3]BA, Biliary atresia; [4]Tx, Transplantation; [5]AL, Anastomotic leak; [6]RF, Recurrent fistula; [7]IP, Iatrogenic perforation; [8]EGF, Esophagogastric fistula; [9]EP, Esophageal perforation; [10]Tx, Thoracic vertebral body; [11]EVAC, Endoluminal vacuum-assisted closure therapy; [12]RSC, Replogle suction catheter; [13]PEG, percutaneous endoscopic gastrostomy; [14]SF, Soft food; *RSC only.*

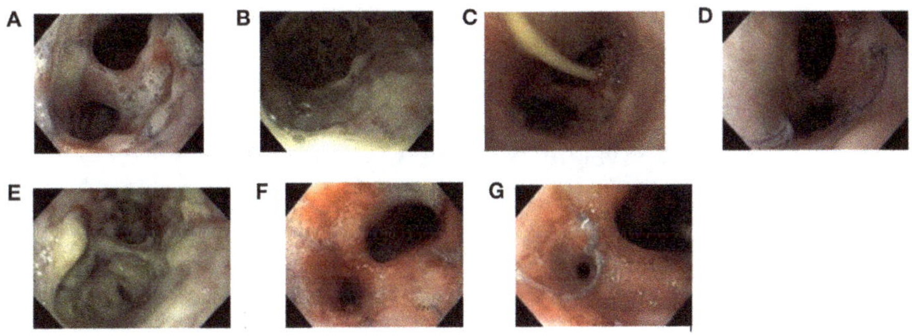

FIGURE 1 | Documentation of endoscopic findings during endoscopic esophageal vacuum-assisted closure (EVAC) and Replogle Suction Catheter (RSC) therapy (Patient 4). First impression of anastomotic insufficiency forming a second lumina into the mediastinum **(A)**, shown more closely **(B)**. Esophageal perforation after 4 days **(C)**, 8 days **(D)**, and 12 days **(E)** of EVAC therapy. After day 8, EVAC was replaced by an RSC **(F)**. Fully healed esophageal perforation 10 days after RSC **(G)**.

and refractory esophageal stenosis despite multiple dilatations. Patient 5 was born with biliary atresia and treated with a Kasai procedure (heopatoportoenterostomy) and liver transplantation. Over time, the patient developed esophageal varices. After massive bleeding with neurologic consequences, a nasogastric tube was blindly placed causing EP. Later, an esophagogastric fistula was detected endoscopically. **Table 1** summarizes the clinical data.

In Patients 1 and 2, the sponge was initially changed every 3 days, and EVAC therapy was administered for 21 and 30 days, respectively. In Patients 3 and 4, EVAC therapy was shortened to 11 and 12 days, respectively. None of these 4 patients experienced complete EP closure after EVAC alone (**Figure 1**). However, their health stabilized, EP size decreased, and initially high CrP-levels (as a marker of inflammation) normalized (**Figure 2**). All four patients were subsequently treated with RSC until their EP healed.

With increasing experience in EVAC therapy, time between EVAC sessions was prolonged from 3 to 5 to 6 days to minimize anesthesia. Learning from the experience of Patient 1 and 2, the RSC was placed as soon as CrP-levels began falling and when mucosal inflammation and size of EP macroscopically decreased (**Figure 1**). All patients were treated with antibiotics according to antibiotic susceptibility test results until the EP healed.

In Patient 2, recurrent fistula did not heal after 3 weeks (six sessions) of EVAC therapy, thus requiring surgery. But EVAC therapy reduced local inflammation in this patient, thereby reducing the risk of major or fatal complications during surgery. No other patient required surgery. Patient 1 and 3 developed stenosis after EVAC, and both were successfully treated with dilatations.

Based on shortening the duration of EVAC therapy from 21–30 days to 11–12 days, it was decided to completely dispense EVAC for Patient 5. The patient's EP was instead treated using an RSC and broad-spectrum antibiotics only. Despite normalizing

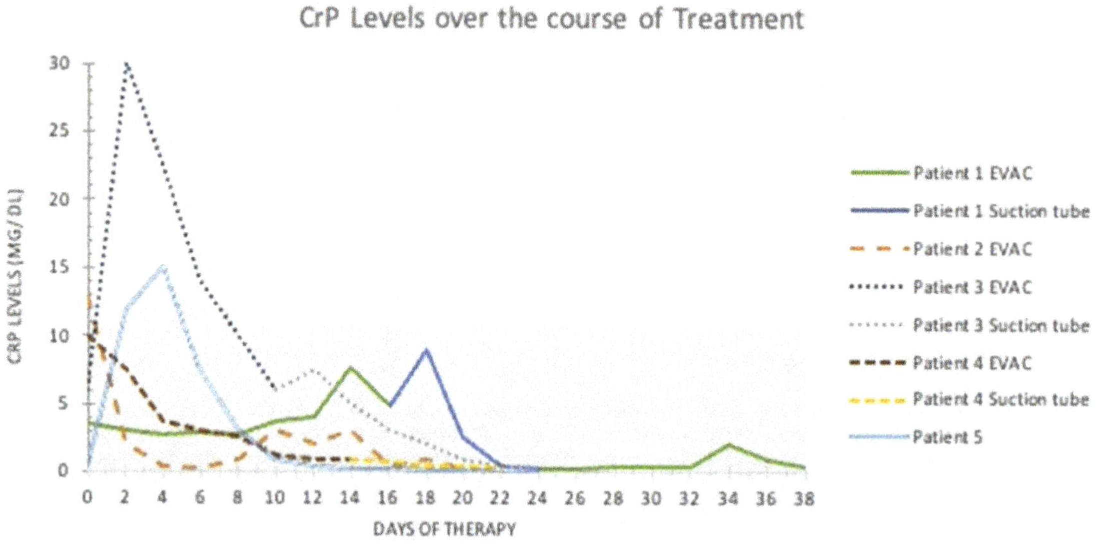

FIGURE 2 | C-reactive protein levels over time. The x- axis shows the duration of esophageal perforation therapy (in days). The y-axis shows the C-reactive protein levels in milligrams per deciliter (mg/dL). Values < 0.5 mg/dL are considered normal and without inflammation. EVAC, endoscopic esophageal vacuum-assisted closure; CRP, C-reactive protein.

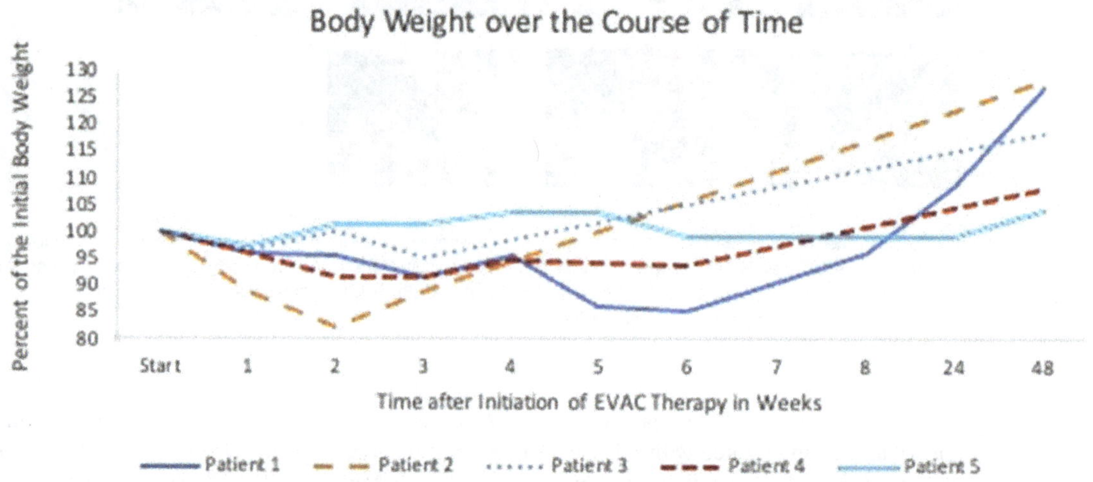

FIGURE 3 | This graph shows the course of body weight over the 1 year after treatment.

CrP levels, the EP persisted after 5 weeks. The patient continues to be fed via gastrostomy.

Oral feeding is not possible during EVAC therapy. Prior to the EP, Patients 1 and 4 were already partially fed via gastrostomy. Patient 2 received a gastrostomy with the first placement of EVAC. Whether patients were enterally fed through a gastrostomy or with parenteral nutrition alone during the 6 week study period, weight loss, in general, was <10% (**Figure 3**). Patient 2 experienced rapid weight loss due to the persistent EP, and the patient's weight returned to normal within 4 weeks after surgery. Enteral nutrition was initiated in all patients after fluoroscopy confirmed a closed EP. All but Patient 5 gained sufficient weight (30) at 1 year after EVAC therapy started.

DISCUSSION

Vacuum-assisted closure is a well-established technique of applying sub-atmospheric pressure to treat infected wounds, burns, or ulcers (13–18). The pressure is applied continuously or in alternating 5-min cycles with 2-min pauses (13). This technique helps remove bacteria and excess fluids to improve

blood flow and formation of granulation tissue (13, 17). Endoluminal vacuum-assisted closure was first described by Weidenhagen et al. o repair anastomotic leakage after anorectal surgery (31). In 2011, Loske et al. adapted this method for use in the upper gastro-intestinal tract (19). Since then, therapy of EP in adult patients has shifted from surgical repair (8, 10) or stenting (11) to conservative treatment (32).

The overall healing rate of EP treated with EVAC is reportedly between 70 and 100% (19–21, 23, 33–35), which is superior to that for stenting (28). Complete closure was not achieved in a single patient with EVAC alone. But the combination of EVAC and RSC was successful in 75%. Maybe the sponge was still too big, even after size adaption. Thus, the vulnerable tissue in children might be affected by the pressure of the sponge. Therefore, complete healing was only achieved by RSC as subsequent therapy.

All patients showed significant reduction in local and systematic inflammation, shortly after insertion of EVAC. Therefore, EVAC was helpful even in the one patient who needed re-do surgery in the end. In this case, local inflammation was reduced and operative field was well-prepared for the surgery. The results indicate that in some cases, EVAC facilitates improved outcomes in subsequent surgery even if the EVAC itself does not fully resolve the EP.

Finally, our results of a very small cohort showed a success rate of 75% for EVAC and RSC, which is similar to results of pediatric patients described by Manfredi et al. (28).

After treating the first two patients we learned that increasing the interval between EVAC sessions to 5 days was well tolerated by the patients, thus reducing the number of anesthesia. This approach was similarly described by Schorsch et al. (20) and Bludau et al. (34, 35).

Mean duration of EVAC therapy described in the first study was 17 days for adult patients (19). Later studies reported have a median duration of 11 to 12 days (20, 34, 35). In our cohort of four pediatric patients, the median EVAC duration was 18 days. When local inflammation and CrP levels decreased sufficiently in these patients, EVAC was replaced by RSC until the mucosa completely healed. The duration of EVAC therapy was shortened from initially 30 to 11 days in the last patient. RSC was installed earlier with good results. The space consuming effect of the sponge might have been a hindrance to a complete closure. Nevertheless, the sponge seems to be important for healing, as a complete omission of EVAC, as in Patient 5, did not yield a satisfactory result. Although only a single patient, this case nevertheless emphasizes the benefit EVAC therapy in treating EP.

The prolonged EVAC intervals and earlier use of RSC reduced anesthesia sessions significantly from 8 to 2 days.

All 5 patients were treated with antibiotics until the EP healed. As shown in the graph, it is worth assessing whether treatment with antibiotics should be terminated earlier due to rapidly falling CrP levels. EVAC was technically possible in four patients. Initially, removal was difficult due to the sponge being too dry. Flushing the sponge with 10–20 ml NaCl 0.9% solved the problem.

At our hospital, stents have not been used, therefore we have only little experience in this field. After our opinion, stents are not a save option in children as they tend to dislocate (36) and bear the risk of damaging the vulnerable tissue in children.

CONCLUSION

EVAC in pediatric patients is a technically feasible and promising method to treat EP, regardless of etiology. EVAC therapy can be terminated as soon as local inflammation and CrP levels decrease sufficiently, even if the mucosa is not yet healed. A promising subsequent therapy is use of an RSC. An early switch can decrease anesthesia time drastically. Overall, EVAC appeared to be more effective than RSC alone. We also observed that EVAC improved the tissue condition in preparation for re-do surgery. At 1 year after therapy, all patients but one gained sufficient weight. Further prospective studies with a larger cohort are required to confirm our experience from this small case series.

AUTHOR CONTRIBUTIONS

All authors listed have made a substantial, direct and intellectual contribution to the work, and approved it for publication.

REFERENCES

1. Rentea RM, St. Peter SD. Neonatal and pediatric esophageal perforation. *Semi Pediat Surg.* (2017) 26:87–94. doi: 10.1053/j.sempedsurg.2017.02.005
2. Garey CL, Laituri CA, Kaye AJ, Ostlie DJ, Snyder CL, Holcomb GW, et al. Esophageal perforation in children: a review of one institution's experience. *J Surg Res.* (2010) 164:13–7. doi: 10.1016/j.jss.2009.11.532
3. Fernandez FF, Richter A, Freudenberg S, Wendl K, Manegold BC. Treatment of endoscopic esophageal perforation. *Surg Endosc.* (1999) 13:962–6. doi: 10.1007/s004649901147
4. Mccann F, Michaud L, Aspirot A, Levesque D, Gottrand F, Faure C. Congenital esophageal stenosis associated with esophageal atresia. *Dis Esophagus.* (2015) 28:211–5. doi: 10.1111/dote.12176
5. Michaud L, Coutenier F, Podevin G, Bonnard A, Becmeur F, Khen-Dunlop N, et al. Characteristics and management of congenital esophageal stenosis: findings from a multicenter study. *Orphanet J Rare Dis.* (2013) 8:1–5. doi: 10.1186/1750-1172-8-186
6. Onwuka EA, Saadai P, Boomer LA, Nwomeh BC. Nonoperative management of esophageal perforations in the newborn. *J Surg Res.* (2016) 205:102–7. doi: 10.1016/j.jss.2016.06.027
7. Attar S, Hankins JR, Suter CM, Coughlin TR, Sequeira A, McLaughlin JS. Esophageal perforation: a therapeutic challenge. *Ann Thorac Surg.* (1990) 50:45–9. doi: 10.1016/0003-4975(90)90082-H
8. Goldstein LA, Thompson WR. Esophageal perforations: A 15 year experience. *Am J Surg.* (1982) 143:495–503. doi: 10.1016/0002-9610(82)90202-1
9. Richardson JD, Tobin GR. Closure of esophageal defects with muscle flaps. *Arch Surg.* (1994) 129:541–8. doi: 10.1001/archsurg.1994.01420290087013
10. Kaman L. Management of esophageal perforation in adults. *Gastroenterol Res.* (2011) 3:235. doi: 10.4021/gr263w
11. Dasari BVM, Neely D, Kennedy A, Spence G, Rice P, Mackle E, et al. The role of esophageal stents in the management of esophageal anastomotic leaks and benign esophageal perforations. *Ann Surg.* (2014) 259:852–60. doi: 10.1097/SLA.0000000000000564
12. Van der Zee DC, Festen C, Severijnen RSVM, Van der Staak FHJ. Management

of pediatric esophageal perforation. *J Thorac Cardiovasc Surg.* (1988) 95:692–5. doi: 10.1016/S0022-5223(19)35738-1
13. Venturi ML, Attinger CE, Mesbahi AN, Hess CL, Graw KS. Mechanisms and clinical applications of the vacuum-assisted closure (VAC) device: a review. *Am J Clin Dermatol.* (2005) 6:185–94. doi: 10.2165/00128071-200506030-00005
14. Braakenburg A, Obdeijn MC, Feitz R, Van Rooij IALM, Van Griethuysen AJ, Klinkenbijl JHG. The clinical efficacy and cost effectiveness of the vacuum-assisted closure technique in the management of acute and chronic wounds: a randomized controlled trial. *Plastic Reconstruct Surg.* (2006) 118:390–7. doi: 10.1097/01.prs.0000227675.63744.af
15. Schintler MV. Negative pressure therapy: theory and practice. *Diabetes Metab Res Rev.* (2012) 28 (Suppl. 1):72–7. doi: 10.1002/dmrr.2243
16. Schintler MV, Prandl EC. Vacuum-assisted closure - what is evidence based? *Euro Surg.* 40:11–8. (2008) doi: 10.1007/s10353-008-0381-5
17. Saziye K, Afksendiyos K. The vacuum-assisted closure (V.A.C®) system for surgical site infection with involved vascular grafts. *Vascular.* (2014), 23:144–50. doi: 10.1177/1708538114537488
18. Bütter A, Emran M, Al-Jazaeri A, Ouimet A. Vacuum-assisted closure for wound management in the pediatric population. *J Pediatr Surg.* (2006) 41:940–2. doi: 10.1016/j.jpedsurg.2006.01.061
19. Loske G, Schorsch T, Müller C. Intraluminal and intracavitary vacuum therapy for esophageal leakage: a new endoscopic minimally invasive approach. *Endoscopy.* (2011) 43:540–4. doi: 10.1055/s-0030-1256345
20. Schorsch T, Müller C, Loske G. Endoscopic vacuum therapy of anastomotic leakage and iatrogenic perforation in the esophagus. *Surg Endosc.* (2013) 27:2040–5. doi: 10.1007/s00464-012-2707-4
21. Loske G, Schorsch T, Dahm C, Martens E, Müller C. Iatrogenic perforation of esophagus successfully treated with endoscopic vacuum therapy (EVT). *Endosc Int Open.* (2015) 3:E547–51. doi: 10.1055/s-0034-1392566
22. Costa J, Gorenstein LA, D'Ovidio F. Novel treatment for anastomotic leak after ivor-lewis esophagectomy. *Ann Thorac Surg.* (2018) 106:e107–9. doi: 10.1016/j.athoracsur.2018.03.025
23. Kuehn F, Schiffmann L, Janisch F, Schwandner F, Alfsasser G, Gock M, et al. Surgical endoscopic vacuum therapy for defects of the upper gastrointestinal tract. *J Gastrointest Surg.* (2016) 20:237–43. doi: 10.1016/S0016-5085(15)33782-3
24. Jeon JH, Jang HJ, Han JE, Park YS, Seong YW, Cho S, et al. Endoscopic vacuum therapy in the management of postoperative leakage after esophagectomy. *World J Surg.* (2020) 44:179–85. doi: 10.1007/s00268-019-05228-z
25. Smallwood NR, Fleshman JW, Leeds SG, Burdick JS. The use of endoluminal vacuum (E-Vac) therapy in the management of upper gastrointestinal leaks and perforations. *Surg Endosc.* (2016) 30:2473–80. doi: 10.1007/s00464-015-4501-6
26. Hwang JJ, Jeong YS, Park YS, Yoon H, Shin CM, Kim N, et al. Comparison of endoscopic vacuum therapy and endoscopic stent implantation with self-expandable metal stent in treating postsurgical gastroesophageal leakage. *Medicine.* (2016) 95:e3416. doi: 10.1097/MD.0000000000003416
27. Mennigen R, Harting C, Lindner K, Vowinkel T, Rijcken E, Palmes D, et al. Comparison of endoscopic vacuum therapy versus stent for anastomotic leak after esophagectomy. *J Gastrointest Surg.* (2015) 19:1229–35. doi: 10.1007/s11605-015-2847-7
28. Manfredi MA, Clark SJ, Staffa SJ, Ngo PD, Smithers CJ, Hamilton TE, et al. Endoscopic esophageal vacuum therapy: a novel therapy for esophageal perforations in pediatric patients. *J Pediatr Gastroenterol Nutr.* (2018) 67:706–12. doi: 10.1097/MPG.0000000000002073
29. Fraga JC, Nunes DL, Andreolio C, Ferreira J, Holanda F, Isolan PS, et al. Endoscopic vacuum sponge therapy for an infant with an esophageal leak. *J Thorac Cardiovasc Surg.* (2018) 156:e193–5. doi: 10.1016/j.jtcvs.2018.04.061
30. MedlinePlus. *Normal Growth and Development.* MedlinePlus (2021).
31. Weidenhagen R, Gruetzner KU, Spelsberg F, Lang RA, Jauch K-W. A new method for sepsis control caused by anastomotic leakage in rectal surgery - the endo-vac®. *Shock.* (2004). 21:152. doi: 10.1097/00024382-200403001-00608
32. Vogel SB, Rout WR, Martin TD, Abbitt PL. Esophageal perforation in adults. *Ann Surg.* (2005) 24:1016–21. doi: 10.1097/01.sla.0000164183.91898.74
33. Kuehn F, Loske G, Schiffmann L, Gock M, Klar E. Endoscopic vacuum therapy for various defects of the upper gastrointestinal tract. *Surg Endosc.* (2017) 31:3449–58. doi: 10.1007/s00464-016-5404-x
34. Bludau M, Hölscher AH, Herbold T, Leers JM, Gutschow C, Fuchs H, et al. Management of upper intestinal leaks using an endoscopic vacuum-assisted closure system (E-VAC). *Surg Endosc.* (2014) 28:896–901. doi: 10.1007/s00464-013-3244-5
35. Bludau M, Fuchs HF, Herbold T, Maus MKH, Alakus H, Popp F, et al. Results of endoscopic vacuum-assisted closure device for treatment of upper GI leaks. *Surg Endosc.* (2018) 32:1906–14. doi: 10.1007/s00464-017-5883-4
36. Raum M, von Schweinitz D, Hubertus J. Surgical treatment of massive bleeding of a right aberrant subclavian artery after oesophageal stent removal. *J Pediatr Surg Case Rep.* (2018) 33:55–7. doi: 10.1016/j.epsc.2018.04.001

2

Medium-Term Pulmonary Function Test After Thoracoscopic Lobectomy and Segmentectomy for Congenital Lung Malformation: A Comparative Study with Normal Control

Jin-Xi Huang [1,2,3,4†], *Song-Ming Hong* [1,2,3,4†], *Jun-Jie Hong* [1,2,3,4], *Qiang Chen* [1,2,3,4] and *Hua Cao* [1,2,3,4*]

[1] *Department of Cardiothoracic Surgery, Fujian Branch of Shanghai Children's Medical Center, Fuzhou, China,* [2] *Fujian Children's Hospital, Fuzhou, China,* [3] *Fujian Maternity and Child Health Hospital, Affiliated Hospital of Fujian Medical University, Fuzhou, China,* [4] *Fujian Key Laboratory of Women and Children's Critical Diseases Research, Fujian Maternity and Child Health Hospital, Fuzhou, China*

***Correspondence:**
Hua Cao
caohua0791@163.com

Purpose: This study aimed to compare the outcomes and pulmonary function test (PFT) of thoracoscopic segmentectomy and lobectomy in infants with congenital lung malformation and study the result of PFT on a medium-term basis.

Methods: The clinical data of 19 infants with congenital lung malformation who underwent thoracoscopic surgery in our hospital from January 2018 to March 2019 were retrospectively studied; these infants were paired with another 19 infants who underwent thoracoscopic lobectomy during the same period using propensity score matching. Age-matched healthy individuals with similar body sizes were recruited for PFT as the control group. Patient characteristics, postoperative PFT, and outcomes were extracted for statistical analysis.

Results: The average length of hospital stay did not significantly differ between segmentectomy and lobectomy groups. The segmentectomy group had more chest tube drainage than the lobectomy group. PFT 1 month after the operation showed that the tidal volume of the lobectomy group was lower than that of the segmentectomy group. Time to peak expiratory flow/time of expiration and peak flow/terminal airway velocity (V25%) indicated small airway dysfunction in the lobectomy group, and no obvious abnormalities were found in "time of inspiratory/time of expiration" in either group. Reexamination of pulmonary function 2 years after the operation showed that the small airway function of the segmentectomy group returned to normal, and no significant difference in pulmonary function was noted among the three groups.

Conclusion: The short-term pulmonary function recovery was better after segmentectomy than after lobectomy. Patients who underwent thoracoscopic lobectomy and segmentectomy have normal lung function 2 years after the operation.

Keywords: congenital lung malformation, segmentectomy, lobectomy, pulmonary function test, thoracoscopy

INTRODUCTION

Congenital lung malformation (CLM) is an uncommon pathology that involves the proliferation of terminal respiratory bronchioles at the expense of alveoli, leading to cysts of various sizes. The incidence is ~9–13.6 per 100,000 (1). It is accepted that abnormal airway patterning and branching during lung morphogenesis results in the appearance of lung cysts (2). Giubergia et al. (3) proposed that the alteration is considered a hamartomatous abnormality of the bronchial tree by some authors, whereas others favor the etiology of an arrest in the development of the fetal bronchial tree with airway obstruction.

Most infants with CLM are asymptomatic at birth, and some of them experience symptomatic infections, pneumothorax, and respiratory distress during growth. The complication rate ranges from 12 to 47% (4). Wong (5) suggested that asymptomatic CLM patients would later develop symptoms and that early surgery might be beneficial to avoid complications. Regarding the necessity of surgical treatment, Pelizzo et al. (6) considered that the potential infection and risk of malignant transformation of CLM justified surgical resection within 1 year. A radionuclide imaging study of long-term lung function in children undergoing lobectomy by Komori (7) found that the optimal age of surgery for CLM appears to be younger than 1 year to allow sufficient time for lung regrowth. With advances in surgical technology, surgeons are now able to minimize the risk of thoracoscopic surgery (8). Many pediatric thoracic diseases, including CLM, can be treated by thoracoscopic surgery (9). Thoracoscopic surgery is widely used mainly because it has the advantages of short perioperative thoracic drainage time, short hospitalization time, and fewer chest wall deformities in the long term (10). Experienced surgeons can now perform thoracoscopic lobectomy in newborns. Our center also reported thoracoscopic lobectomy for a 4-day-old neonate with a large congenital pulmonary airway malformation (11). Although thoracoscopic surgery has become a conventional technique for the treatment of CLM (12), there are few reports on segmentectomy and the clinical comparison of lobectomy and segmentectomy for CLM. We compared the outcomes and mid-term follow-up of thoracoscopic segmentectomy and lobectomy for infants and evaluated the pulmonary function of CLM patients after thoracoscopic surgery on a medium-term basis.

PATIENTS AND METHODS

The present study was approved by the ethics committee of our hospital and adhered to the tenets of the Declaration of Helsinki. The written informed consent was obtained from the parents of the children.

Patients

From January 2018 to March 2019, we examined 19 consecutive infants who underwent thoracoscopic segmentectomy in our institution. These infants were paired with another 19 infants who underwent thoracoscopic lobectomy during the same period, based on their sex, age, weight, lesion location, and preoperative pulmonary function test (PFT), using propensity score matching. Our basic selection criteria for thoracoscopic segmentectomy was one of the following: (1) Patients with a peripheral small-sized lesion; (2) the lesion was localized to only one segment; (3) the lesions were located in two adjacent lung segments (excluding the middle lobe of the right lung). Exclusion criteria were patients with other preoperative complications such as congenital heart disease, immunocompromised state, or restrictive or obstructive chest wall disease. PFTs were carried out 1 month and 2 years after surgery.

Surgical Technique

The same thoracic surgery team consecutively operated on all patients. In the segmental approach, ultrasonic scalpel and LigaSure were used to divide the vessels individually. Segmental bronchi were clamped, as inflating the operative side of the lung, the line between inflation and deflation became clear (**Figure 1**). The segmental bronchi were ligated with Hem-o-Lok clips (Sinolinks Clips; Sinolinks Medical Innovation, Inc. Jiangsu, China) and resected after identifying the correct segment. The lung parenchyma was dissected from the hilum to the periphery with ultrasonic scalpel and LigaSure; intersegmental veins were preserved. For lobectomy, pulmonary arteries, veins, and bronchi were dissected one by one, and the incomplete fissure was cut off with an ultrasonic scalpel and LigaSure. After reinflation of the lung and if no air leakage was detected, a closed thoracic drainage tube was indwelled, and the thoracic cavity was closed. The chest tube was removed when there was no air leak, and the amount of daily drainage was <1 ml/kg. Patients were discharged 1 day after removal of the chest tube if the follow-up chest X-ray showed no signs of pneumothorax and no signs of complications.

Pulmonary Function Test

All patients received oral choral hydrate (0.5 ml/kg) to be kept asleep during PFTs, which were performed at least 4 h after feeding to avoid abdominal distension or vomiting. Temperature and humidity in the test room were maintained at 22°C and 40%. Infants laid flat on the testbed on their back; a face mask was attached to a face covering the nose and mouth to prevent air leakage and then connected to the MasterScreen PFT System (Jaeger, Germany). The PFTs were measured by a trained physician after smooth breathing had been established, and 15–20 cycles of tidal breathing were recorded, with five repeats. Age-matched healthy individuals with similar body sizes were recruited for PFT as the control group with informed consent obtained. Data analysis includes the following (13, 14):

① Tidal volume (VT): expressed in milliliters per kilogram.

② Tidal breath flow volume loop: The ratio of expiratory flow to inspiratory flow at 50% tidal volume (TEF50/TIF50), the ratio of the volume reaching the peak expiratory flow rate to the expiratory volume (VPEF/VE), the ratio of the time to peak expiratory flow to time of expiration (TPTEF/TE), the ratio of the peak flow to the terminal airway velocity (PF/V25%), and the ratio of the time of inspiratory to the time of expiration (TI/TE).

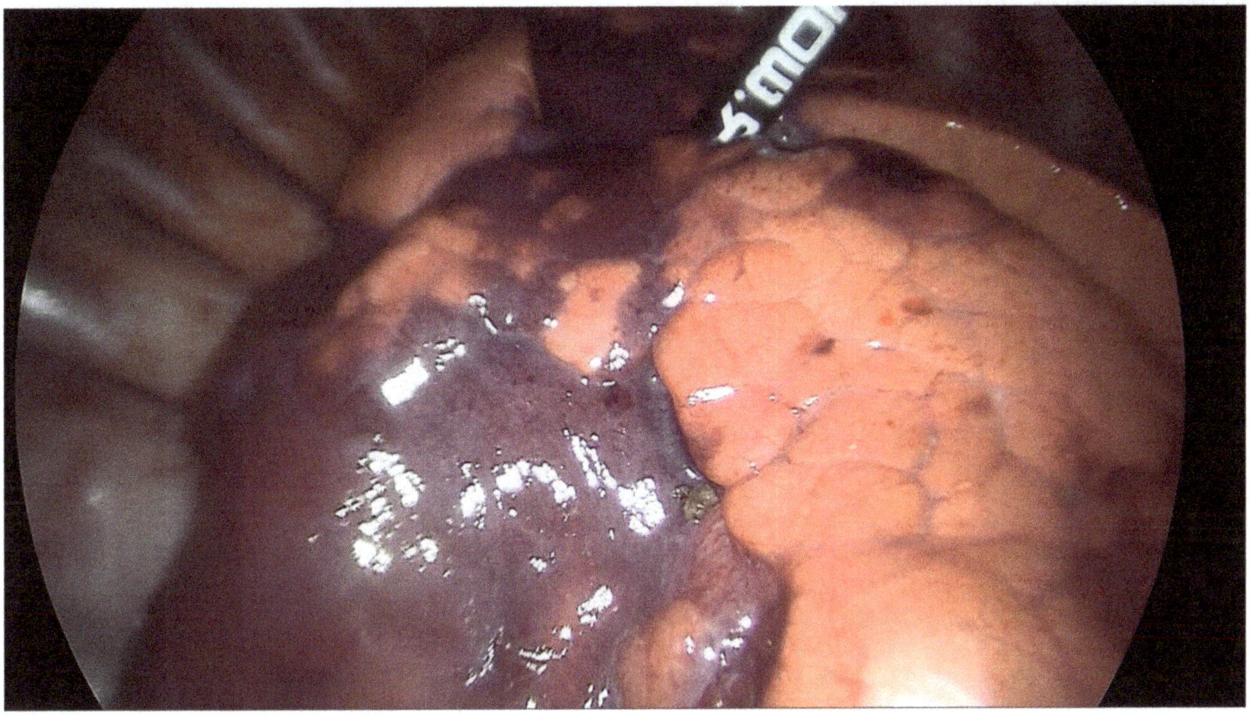

FIGURE 1 | The appearance of the line between inflation and deflation under both clamping the segmental bronchi (RS9+10) and inflating the lung.

Result Criterion

① Restricted lesion: VT per kilogram is less than normal (6–10 ml/kg).
② Small airway obstruction: TPTEF/TE. The normal range is 28–55%, mild obstruction 23–28%, moderate obstruction 15–22%, and severe obstruction <15%.
③ Large airway obstruction: TI/TE. The normal range is ≥80%, mild obstruction is 60–79%, moderate obstruction is 40–59%, and severe obstruction <40%.

Statistical Analysis

SPSS software (version 17; SPSS, Chicago, IL, USA) was used for statistical comparison between the two groups. Continuous variables were tested by Student's t-test, categorical variables were tested by the chi-square test, and one-way analysis of variance was used for statistical comparison among three groups. $P < 0.05$ was considered statistically significant.

RESULTS

The patient characteristics and the results of the overall operation are summarized in **Table 1**. The average operation time values were 86.631 ± 3.71 min in segmentectomy and 52.898 ± 0.74 min in a lobectomy. Although the volume of the chest tube in the segmentectomy group (53.162 ± 1.72 ml) was more than that in the lobectomy group (34.211 ± 0.29 ml), the length of the chest tube and the length of hospital stay were not statistically significant. Pathological examination confirmed the diagnosis of congenital pulmonary airway malformation for all cases.

All of the children received regular follow-up without loss. PFT was carried out 1 month and 2 years after surgery, and there was no statistically significant difference in the average weight of the children at the time of PFT. No current respiratory infections, chest wall deformity, or other factors that could impact lung function happened at the time of testing. **Table 2** shows that 1 month after the operation, the lobectomy group's VT (7.6333 ± 0.523 ml/kg) was lower than that of the segmentectomy group (8.4632 ± 0.614 ml/kg) (P < 0.01). Both TPTEF/TE and PF/V25% showed that the lobectomy group had small airway dysfunction 1 month after the operation. No significant abnormalities were observed in the large airway function (TI/TE) of the two groups (0.8280 ± 0.105 in the segmentectomy group and 0.8170 ± 0.150 in the lobectomy group). Two years after the operation, PFT showed that VT was improved in the lobectomy group. A group of 19 healthy individuals, age and body size-matched, were selected as a normal control for comparison. Statistical analysis showed that the age, sex ratio, and body weight were comparable between the three groups (**Table 3**), and the PFTs of the segmentectomy group and lobectomy group returned to normal (not significantly different from the normal control group) (**Table 4**). Examinations of chest computerized tomography (CT)

TABLE 1 | Patients' characteristics and outcomes.

		Segmentectomy group	Lobectomy group	p
Numbers		19	19	
Sex (male)		12 (63%)	12 (63%)	NS
Age (months)		4.39 ± 0.78	4.46 ± 0.91	0.790 (NS)
Body weight (kg)		7.78 ± 0.91	7.75 ± 0.88	0.900 (NS)
Location of CLM	Left	11 (57.9%)	11 (57.9%)	NS
	Right	8 (42.1%)	8 (42.1%)	NS
Duration of operation (min)		86.63 ± 13.71	52.89 ± 8.74	<0.01
Time of chest tube (days)		3.95 ± 0.85	3.74 ± 0.84	0.455 (NS)
Chest tube output (mL)		53.16 ± 21.72	34.21 ± 10.29	0.02
Postoperative Complications		3 (15.8%)	3 (15.8%)	NS
Pneumothorax		3	2	
Subcutaneous emphysema		0	1	
Length of hospital stay (days)		5.05 ± 0.78	4.79 ± 0.85	0.328 (NS)

Results are given as the number (%), average or as the mean ± standard error of mean.
NS indicates not significant.

TABLE 2 | Pulmonary function test results (1 month after surgery).

	Segmentectomy group	Lobectomy group	p
VT(ml/kg)	8.463 ± 2.614	7.633 ± 3.523	<0.01
TEF50/TIF50	0.842 ± 0.120	0.831 ± 0.144	0.797 (NS)
VPEF/VE	0.260 ± 0.030	0.254 ± 0.025	0.462 (NS)
TPTEF/TE	0.319 ± 0.053	0.255 ± 0.062	<0.01
PF/V25%	1.633 ± 0.143	2.038 ± 0.754	0.027
TI/TE	0.827 ± 0.079	0.817 ± 0.107	0.731 (NS)

Results are given as the mean ± standard error of mean.
NS indicates not significant.

TABLE 3 | Comparison of demographic data at PFT (2 years after surgery).

	Segmentectomy group	Lobectomy group	Control group	F	p
Numbers	19	19	19		NS
Sex (male)	12 (63%)	12 (63%)	12 (63%)		NS
Age (months)	28.37 ± 0.81	28.53 ± 1.09	28.11 ± 0.97	0.877	0.422 (NS)
Weight (kg)	13.67 ± 1.16	14.06 ± 1.52	14.29 ± 0.96	1.148	0.325 (NS)

Results are given as the mean ± standard error of mean.
NS indicates not significant.

TABLE 4 | Comparison of pulmonary function test results in segmentectomy group, lobectomy group and control group (2 years after surgery).

	Segmentectomy group	Lobectomy group	Control group	F	p
VT(ml/kg)	8.051 ± 0.423	8.114 ± 0.540	8.500 ± 0.863	2.772	0.071 (NS)
TEF50/TIF50	0.831 ± 0.144	0.836 ± 0.076	0.834 ± 0.091	0.014	0.987 (NS)
VPEF/VE	0.254 ± 0.025	0.254 ± 0.027	0.244 ± 0.028	0.839	0.438 (NS)
TPTEF/TE	0.255 ± 0.062	0.271 ± 0.081	0.270 ± 0.052	0.360	0.699 (NS)
PF/V25%	1.634 ± 0.165	1.595 ± 0.316	1.676 ± 0.235	0.517	0.599 (NS)
TI/TE	0.805 ± 0.076	0.817 ± 0.159	0.844 ± 0.100	0.567	0.570 (NS)

Results are given as the mean ± standard error of mean.
NS indicates not significant.

2 years after the operation showed that all children recovered well without residual lesion.

DISCUSSION

The dramatic growth of minimally invasive technology had allowed segmentectomy and lobectomy to be performed thoracoscopically. In our data, the operative time in the segmentectomy group was longer than that in the lobectomy group, which was considered due to more surgical procedures. We operate in an artery-oriented manner: open the sheath of the pulmonary artery and further dissect the corresponding segmental artery, whereas lobectomy only needs to dissect the pulmonary lobar artery without dissecting the pulmonary parenchyma. It is reassuring that there was no significant difference in length of hospital stay between the two groups.

Our study found that the segmentectomy group had a greater chest tube output than the lobectomy group. Thoracic drainage after surgery was associated with lymph node dissection in adult non-small cell lung tumors (15), and thoracic drainage after thoracoscopic surgery in children was mainly derived from the exudation of intersegmental and perihilar wounds. The lung parenchyma was dissected from the lung hilum to the periphery by ultrasonic scalpel and LigaSure in the segmentectomy group, which resulted in much more intersegmental wounds and thermal damage than the lobectomy group. Another reason may be that the operation time and one-lung ventilation time of the segmentectomy group are inevitably longer than that of the lobectomy group due to the increase of operation procedure, which may lead to more pulmonary edema and pulmonary exudation (16, 17).

Pneumothorax (air-leakage >2 days) after thoracic surgery is mainly derived from the leakage of the lung parenchyma, which is related to the operation mode (18). We observed three cases of asymptomatic pneumothorax in the segmentectomy group and two cases in the lobectomy group. However, by increasing the thoracic closed drainage time, these cases were cured, and no invasive operation or secondary surgery was performed again.

Postoperative recovery of pulmonary function is another focus. The assessment of pulmonary function in children is indeed a vexing problem. The regrowth of the lung after pulmonary resection is still debated. Komori (7) tried a radionuclide CT scan and found that alveolar multiplication of the remaining lung occurs after lobectomy in patients. However, as imaging studies are difficult to quantify the extent of compensatory emphysema and increase the radiation exposure of children, they are difficult to be widely accepted by parents. Tocchioni (19) considers that the long-term prognosis after lobectomy is good for the majority of patients. For asymptomatic patients, surgery before the age of 1 year ensures optimal catch-up of pulmonary function. Lau CT's researches showed that CLM patients have normal lung function after thoracoscopic lobectomy at medium and long-term (20, 21). Those are basically consistent with our research, but there are some peculiarities to our data. In our study, 1 month after surgery, the PFT results showed that the VT of the lobectomy group was 8.4632 ± 0.614 ml/kg, which was lower than that of the segmentectomy group (7.6333 ± 0.523 ml/kg) ($P < 0.01$). In small airway functions, we found that the TPTEF/TE of the lobectomy group was 0.2550 ± 0.092 and that of the segmentectomy group was 0.3050 ± 0.060 1 month after the operation ($P < 0.01$), indicating that the lobectomy group had increased small airway dysfunction, which was also verified in the PF/V25% results. In the comparison of large airway function data, no significant differences in TEF50/TIF50 and TI/TE were noted between the two groups. We reviewed the postoperative chest radiographs of the two groups and found that the lobectomy group presented increased lung transparency and a slightly elevated diaphragmatic surface on the affected side, which was more significant than that in the segmentectomy group. We considered that the lobectomy group had more compensatory emphysema after surgery, suggesting compensatory dilation of the respiratory bronchioles and alveoli, which may have led to increased small airway dysfunction. This compensatory dilatation was still present 1 month after surgery (22). It is reassuring that we found no statistically significant differences in TPTEF/TE, PF/V25%, TEF50/TIF50, and TI/TE between the two groups 2 years after the operation. We consider that increased pulmonary parenchyma leads to improved airway function over a 2-year period of compensatory lung growth. Further prospective studies are needed to confirm the effect of short-term small airway dysfunction on the quality of life of infants.

However, there are still many limitations in our study. First, the lack of PFT data on older CLM children in our center makes it impossible to know how the compensatory growth potential changes with age. Second, obviously, the wide range of CLM is too extensive to justify segmentectomy in most cases at present. In our entire series, segmentectomy was chosen in <13% of cases. We recognized the importance of postoperative multidisciplinary follow-up, and we will also continue to observe the recovery of pulmonary function with more cases to obtain more comprehensive data and long-term follow-up outcomes.

CONCLUSIONS

The thoracoscopic approach in infants with CLM does not interfere with normal lung function and represents a safe procedure in pediatric age. Thoracoscopic segmentectomy makes better short-term pulmonary function recovery than lobectomy. Children who underwent thoracoscopic lobectomy and segmentectomy have normal pulmonary function 2 years after the operation.

AUTHOR CONTRIBUTIONS

J-XH and HC made a significant contribution to the conception and design of the work. J-XH and S-MH drafted the work and revised it critically for important intellectual content. QC and J-XH are responsible for all aspects of the work and ensure that questions related to the accuracy or integrity of any part of the work are appropriately investigated and resolved. All authors read and approved the final manuscript.

ACKNOWLEDGMENTS

We thank all doctors in our center for their fruitful advice and discussions.

REFERENCES

1. Gornall AS, Budd JL, Draper ES, Konje JC, Kurinczuk JJ. Congenital cystic adenomatoid malformation: accuracy of prenatal diagnosis, prevalence and outcome in a general population. *Prenat Diagn.* (2003) 23:997-1002. doi: 10.1002/pd.739
2. David M, Lamas-Pinheiro R, Henriques-Coelho T. Prenatal and Postnatal Management of Congenital Pulmonary Airway Malformation. *Neonatology.* (2016) 110(2): p. 101-15. doi: 10.1159/000440894
3. Giubergia V, Barrenechea M, Siminovich M, Pena HG, Murtagh P. Congenital cystic adenomatoid malformation: clinical features, pathological concepts and management in 172 cases. *J Pediatr (Rio J).* (2012) 88:143–8. doi: 10.2223/JPED.2177
4. Downard CD, Calkins CM, Williams RF, Renaud EJ, Jancelewicz T, Grabowski J, et al. Treatment of congenital pulmonary airway malformations: a systematic review from the APSA outcomes and evidence based practice committee. *Pediatr Surg Int.* (2017) 33:939–53. doi: 10.1007/s00383-017-4098-z
5. Wong A, Vieten D, Singh S, Harvey JG, Holland AJ. Long-term outcome of asymptomatic patients with congenital cystic adenomatoid malformation. *Pediatr Surg Int.* (2009) 25:479–85. doi: 10.1007/s00383-009-2371-5
6. Pelizzo G, Costanzo F, Andreatta E, Calcaterra V. Congenital pulmonary airway malformations: from prenatal diagnosis to postnatal outcome. *Minerva Pediatr.* (2016) 68:299–311.
7. Komori K, Kamagata S, Hirobe S, Toma M, Okumura K, Muto M, et al. Radionuclide imaging study of long-term pulmonary function after lobectomy in children with congenital cystic lung disease. *J Pediatr Surg.* (2009) 44:2096–100. doi: 10.1016/j.jpedsurg.2009.04.033
8. Mattioli G, Pio L, Disma NM, Torre M, Sacco O, Pistorio A, et al. Congenital lung malformations: shifting from open to thoracoscopic surgery. *Pediatr Neonatol.* (2016) 57:463–6. doi: 10.1016/j.pedneo.2015.10.009
9. Zoeller C, Ure BM, Dingemann J. Perioperative complications of video-assisted thoracoscopic pulmonary procedures in neonates and infants. *Eur J Pediatr Surg.* (2018) 28:163–70. doi: 10.1055/s-0038-1636917
10. Kiblawi R, Zoeller C, Zanini A, Ure BM, Dingemann J, Kuebler JF, et al. Video-assisted thoracoscopic or conventional thoracic surgery in infants and children: current evidence. *Eur J Pediatr Surg.* (2020) 31:54–64. doi: 10.1055/s-0040-1716878
11. Huang J, Zhou C, Chen Q, Wu D, Hong J, Hong S, Thoracoscopic lobectomy for a 4-day-old neonate with a large congenital pulmonary airway malformation: a case report. *J Cardiothorac Surg.* (2020) 15:159. doi: 10.1186/s13019-020-01174-3
12. Ganarin A, Sgro A, Garcia MM, Volpe A, Tognon C, Gamba, P, Thoracoscopy versus thoracotomy for congenital lung malformations treatment: A single center experience. *Pediatr Pulmonol.* (2021) 56:196–202. doi: 10.1002/ppul.25138
13. Fuchs O, Latzin P, Thamrin C, Stern G, Frischknecht P, Singer F, et al. Normative data for lung function and exhaled nitric oxide in unsedated healthy infants. *Eur Respir J.* (2011) 37:1208–16. doi: 10.1183/09031936.00125510
14. Nguyen TT, Hoo AF, Lum S, Wade A, Thia LP, Stocks, J, New reference equations to improve interpretation of infant lung function. *Pediatr Pulmonol.* (2013) 48:370–80. doi: 10.1002/ppul.22656
15. Zhao W, Chen T, Feng J, Gu Z, Wang Z, Ji C, et al. Comparison of lymph node dissection and lymph node sampling for non-small cell lung cancers by video-assisted thoracoscopic surgery. *J Thorac Dis.* (2019) 11:505–13. doi: 10.21037/jtd.2019.01.39
16. Sivrikoz MC, Tuncozgur B, Cekmen M, Bakir K, Meram I, Kocer E, et al. The role of tissue reperfusion in the reexpansion injury of the lungs. *Eur J Cardiothorac Surg.* (2002) 22:721–7. doi: 10.1016/S1010-7940(02)00447-5
17. Jordan S, Mitchell JA, Quinlan GJ, Goldstraw P, Evans TW. The pathogenesis of lung injury following pulmonary resection. *Eur Respir J.* (2000) 15:790–9. doi: 10.1034/j.1399-3003.2000.15d26.x
18. Yoo A, Ghosh SK, Danker W, Kassis E, Kalsekar I. Burden of air leak complications in thoracic surgery estimated using a national hospital billing database. *Clinicoecon Outcomes Res.* (2017) 9:373–83. doi: 10.2147/CEOR.S133830
19. Tocchioni F, Lombardi E, Ghionzoli M, Ciardini E, Noccioli B, Messineo A, Long-term lung function in children following lobectomy for congenital lung malformation. *J Pediatr Surg.* (2017) 52:1891–7. doi: 10.1016/j.jpedsurg.2017.08.059
20. Lau CT, Wong KKY, Tam P. Medium term pulmonary function test after Thoracoscopic lobectomy for congenital pulmonary airway malformation: a com- parative study with normal control. *J Laparoendosc Adv Surg Tech A.* (2018) 28:595–8. doi: 10.1089/lap.2017.0276
21. Lau CT, Wong K. Long-term pulmonary function after lobectomy for congenital pulmonary airway malformation: is thoracoscopic approach really better than open? *J Pediatr Surg.* (2018) 53:2383–5. doi: 10.1016/j.jpedsurg.2018.08.029
22. Gurney JW. The pathophysiology of airways disease. *J Thorac Imaging.* (1995) 10:227–35. doi: 10.1097/00005382-199524000-00001

3

Amputation Predisposes to Higher Cancer-Specific Mortality than Limb Salvage Surgery in Pediatric Patients with Osteosarcoma of the Limbs

Jinkui Wang[1]*, Jie Tang*[2]*, Xiaojun Tan*[1]*, Chenghao Zhanghuang*[1]*, Liming Jin*[1]*, Mujie Li*[1]*, Zhaoxia Zhang*[1]*, Tao Mi*[1] *and Dawei He*[1*]

[1] Department of Urology, Chongqing Key Laboratory of Children Urogenital Development and Tissue Engineering, Chongqing Key Laboratory of Pediatrics, Ministry of Education Key Laboratory of Child Development and Disorders, National Clinical Research Center for Child Health and Disorders, China International Science and Technology Cooperation Base of Child Development and Critical Disorders, Children's Hospital of Chongqing Medical University, Chongqing, China, [2] *Department of Epidemiology, Public Health School, Shenyang Medical College, Shenyang, China*

***Correspondence:**
Dawei He
hedawei@hospital.cqmu.edu.cn

Objective: With the devolopment of osteosarcoma treatment, limb salvage surgery is gradually replacing amputation as the primary surgical option. Most pediatric osteosarcomas of the limbs undergo limb-salvage surgery. We aimed to use propensity score matching (PSM) analysis test the difference in cancer-specific mortality (CSM) between amputation and limb-salvage surgery in pediatric patients with Osteosarcoma of the limbs. PSM is a statistical method used to deal with data from an Observational Study. The PSM method is designed to reduce the influence of biases and confounding variables to make a more reasonable comparison betwoon experimental and control groups.

Methods: Patient information was downloaded from the SEER (surveillance, epidemiology, and End Results) database from 2004 to 2018. We included all primary pediatric osteosarcoma patients who underwent limb salvage or amputation. Multivariate logistic regression models were used to explore the factors influencing patient choice of amputation. Differences in CSM and other causes of mortality (OSM) between limb salvage and amputation were analyzed using cumulative incidence plots and competitive risk regression tests after 1:1 proportional propensity score matching.

Results: A total of 1,058 pediatric patients with limbs Osteosarcoma were included. Patients who underwent amputations were more likely to be male (OR 1.4, $P = 0.024$) and more likely to have distant metastasis (OR 2.1, $P < 0.001$). Before propensity matching, CSM was 1.4 times higher in patients undergoing amputation than in patients undergoing limb salvage ($P = 0.017$) and 3.4 times higher in OSM ($P = 0.007$). After adjustment for propensity matching, CSM was 1.5 times higher in patients undergoing amputation than in patients undergoing limb salvage ($P = 0.028$), but there was no significant difference in OSM (HR 3.2, $P = 0.078$).

Conclusions: Our results suggested that amputation is associated with a 1.5-fold increase in CSM in pediatric patients with limbs Osteosarcoma. Therefore, in the surgical selection of pediatric patients with Osteosarcoma, limb salvage surgery should be the first choice in the absence of other contraindications.

Keywords: Osteosarcoma, limbs, amputation, limb salvage, mortality

INTRODUCTION

Osteosarcoma is the most common bone malignancy in children and young adults (1). Previous studies have shown that the incidence varies with age, with an annual incidence of 1.7 per 100,000 children under ten years of age and 8.2 per 100,000 between 10 and 19 years of age (2). Another study found Osteosarcoma in 2–3 per million in all populations and 8–11 per million in people aged 15–19 years (3). Osteosarcomas peak mainly during adolescence between the ages of 10 and 14, with another peak after 80 (4). Osteosarcomas often occur in the metaphysis of long bones, mainly in the lower limbs. Progression of Osteosarcoma is associated with rapid bone growth during adolescence (5). The etiology of Osteosarcoma includes a variety of factors; currently recognized risk factors include ionizing radiation, alkylation agents, chromosomal abnormalities, hereditary retinoblastoma and Paget's disease (6). Current treatment strategies include neoadjuvant chemotherapy, surgical resection of primary tumors and metastases, and additional adjuvant chemotherapy after surgery (7). The treatment of Osteosarcoma has improved over the past 20 years, including neoadjuvant chemotherapy and radiotherapy, but the overall prognosis of Osteosarcoma remains poor (8–10). Osteosarcoma is one of the health hazards in children, accounting for 8.9% of childhood cancer-related deaths. The 5-year survival rate for Osteosarcoma without distant metastasis is 65 to 70% (11), but only 19 to 30% for Osteosarcoma with distant metastasis (12).

Surgery has been recognized as treating primary and recurrent or metastatic Osteosarcoma (13). In the past 30 years, with the development of neoadjuvant chemotherapy, limb salvage therapy has become one of the standard treatment methods for limb osteosarcoma, 90% of patients can be treated with limb salvage therapy, and the success rate of limb salvage is 60~80% (14, 15). Limb salvage surgery can improve patients' quality of life and health psychology, and more than 80% of patients are willing to accept limb salvage surgery (16). However, sometimes amputation is necessary, such as Osteosarcoma of the distal tibia, which is challenging to achieve a negative margin (17). At present, the survival outcome of amputation and limb-salvage surgery is still controversial. Some studies have shown no significant difference in survival rates between amputation and amputation (15, 18), while others have shown significantly higher survival rates for amputation (18, 19). However, the sample size of these articles is small, and there are many selection biases. Although there have been meta-analyses comparing survival rates for amputations and limb salvage, the heterogeneity of the articles makes the results less convincing (20, 21). Therefore, patients from the National Cancer Institute's Surveillance, Epidemiology, and End Results (SEER) program were used for analysis. We performed a propensity score analysis to reduce selection bias and the effect of confounding factors. We created a matched cohort to analyze the difference in survival rates between amputation and salvage surgery for pediatric limb osteosarcoma. Most of the previous studies were single-center studies with fewer patients. In addition, meta-analysis is a synthesis of the results of multiple studies, which has great heterogeneity. Therefore, we used big data analysis to compare survival differences between amputation and limb salvage in children with limb osteosarcoma.

METHODS

Data Source and Study Population

The patient information was downloaded from the SEER Database, the leading cancer database in the United States, collecting data from 18 cancer registries and covering approximately 28% of the US population (22). The SEER database is public, and patient information is anonymous, so our study does not require ethical approval and informed consent from patients. Our methodology follows the guidelines of the SEER database.

We collected clinicopathological information from all pediatric osteosarcoma patients from 2004 to 2018. Inclusion criteria: (1) Pathological diagnosis of Osteosarcoma (ICD-O-3 histological codes: 9180-9187 and 9192-9194); (2) The primary site is limb (ICD-O-3 anatomical code: 400-409); (3) The patient was younger than or equal to 18 years old. Exclusion criteria were: (1) tumor size was unknown; (2) the cause of death was not clear; (3) survival time < 1 month; (4) TNM staging was unknown. The screening flow chart of all patients is shown in **Figure 1.**

Study Variables

In this study, the clinicopathological information of patients was collected. Demographic characteristics include age, sex, race and year of diagnosis; basic tumor information including the pathological grade of tumor, TNM stage of tumor and tumor size; treatment information including surgery, radiotherapy and chemotherapy. To see if the year of diagnosis affected mortality, we divided the patient's years of diagnosis into two categories: 2004-2011 and 2012-2018. Patients were grouped into three racial groups: white, black, and other races (American Indian /AK Indian, Asian/Pacific Islander). There were four tumor grades: grade I (highly differentiated), grade II (moderately differentiated), grade III (poorly differentiated) and grade IV

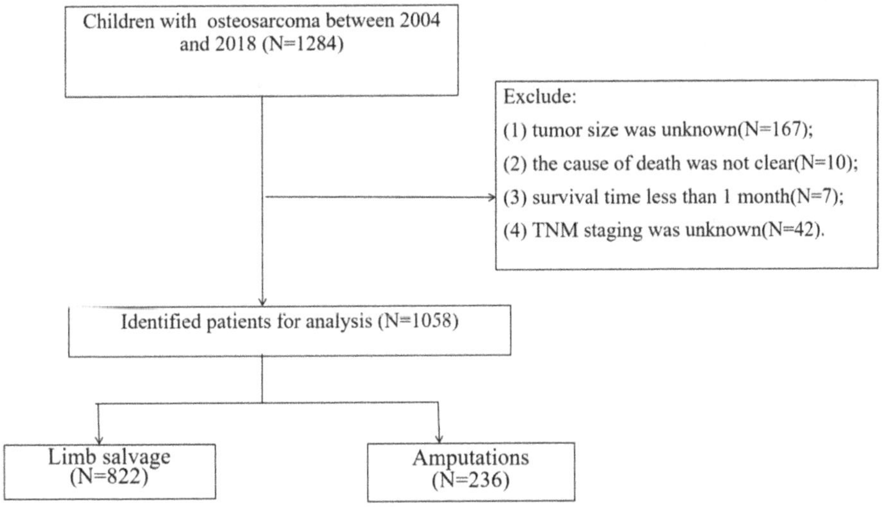

FIGURE 1 | CONSORT (Consolidated Standards of Reporting Trials) diagram of study inclusion criteria.

(undifferentiated). Surgical methods include limb salvage and amputation. According to the SEER definition of death, patients die from cancer (CSM) or other causes (OSM). CSM is the death of a patient from cancer, including cancer recurrence and metastasis. OCM is the death of a patient from causes other than cancer, mainly cardiovascular disease, lung disease, etc.

Statistical Analyses

Categorical variables were described using frequency and proportion, and Continuous variables are described using mean and standard deviation. The proportion difference of categorical variables was analyzed by chi-square test, and the contrast of median was analyzed by *T*-test and Kruskal-Wallis test.

In a cohort of all patients, we used a multivariable logistic regression model to analyze the predictors of choice for amputation and limb-salvage surgery. Variables included age (continuous), gender (male vs. female), race (White vs. black vs. other), year of diagnosis (2004-2011 vs. 2012-2018), laterality (left vs. right), T staging (T1 vs. T2 vs. T3), N staging (N0 vs. N1), M staging (M0 vs. M1), tumor size (continuous).

We used nearest neighbor 1:1 matching in the primary study cohort, which makes the comparison cohort more reliable. The propensity-matched cohort was balanced by age, sex, race, year of diagnosis, tumor grade, laterality, tumor size, TNM stage, chemotherapy, and radiation. Finally, we examined the effects of limb salvage surgery and amputation on CSM and OCM using cumulative incidence plots and multivariable competitive risk regression (CRR) models (23). Competitive risk is that more than one type of event may occur in some cases. The occurrence of one type of event may hinder the observation or change the probability of other kinds of events being observed. The incident prevented another incident under investigation or fundamentally changed the likelihood of that other incident (23). In other words, we used a multivariate CRR model to explore independent risk factors for CSM and OCM in patients. We also compared patient's CSM and OCM differences between amputations and limb salvage under the CRR model.

Then, we performed three sensitivity analyses to optimize the matching results and ensure that our conclusions were reliable. (1) We compared the risk of CSM between amputation and limb salvage using a CRR model in the original cohort. (2) We used a 1:2 and 1:4 propensity match to compare CSM with amputation and limb salvage. (3) We compared the CSM of limb amputation and limb salvage in patients with complete tumor grade information. (4) After inverse probability of treatment weighting, we compared CSM and OCM in patients with amputation and limb salvage.

All statistical analyses were performed using R version 3.4.1 (http://www.r-project.org/) and SPSS software (version 23.0, SPSS, Chicago, IL, USA). We used "Matching," "nonrandom," "reshape2," and "survey" R software packages to create matched sample. We used "foreign," "survival," "cmprsk." and "rms" R software packages to construct a competitive risk model. *P*-values < 0.05 were considered statistically significant.

RESULTS

Clinical Features

A total of 1,058 patients were enrolled, with 822 patients undergoing limb salvage and 236 patients undergoing amputation. The basic information and clinicopathological features of patients are shown in **Table 1**. Compared with patients undergoing limb salvage surgery, more patients with amputation were male (61.9% vs. 54.1, $P = 0.042$), with higher T stage (T2-T3, 72.5% vs. 63.7, $P = 0.034$), with distant metastasis (28.8% vs. 15.5, $P < 0.001$), larger tumors (median size 103 vs. 90 mm).

TABLE 1 | Sociodemographic and clinical characteristics of patients receiving limb salvage vs. amputation in pediatric osteosarcoma patients.

	Unmatched					Matched				
	Overall N = 1,058	Limb salvage N = 822	Amputation N = 236	p-value	SMD	Overall N = 472	Limb salvage N = 236	Amputation N = 236	p-value	SMD
Age [mean (SD)]	12.751 (3.377)	12.809 (3.264)	12.551 (3.745)	0.3009	0.073	12.449 (3.529)	12.347 (3.304)	12.551 (3.745)	0.5319	0.058
Sex				0.042	0.157				0.638	0.052
Male	591 (55.9%)	445 (54.1%)	146 (61.9%)			286 (60.6%)	140 (59.3%)	146 (61.9%)		
Female	467 (44.1%)	377 (45.9%)	90 (38.1%)			186 (39.4%)	96 (40.7%)	90 (38.1%)		
Year of diagnosis				0.289	0.084				0.051	0.189
2004-2011	517 (48.9%)	394 (47.9%)	123 (52.1%)			268 (56.8%)	145 (61.4%)	123 (52.1%)		
2012-2018	541 (51.1%)	428 (52.1%)	113 (47.9%)			204 (43.2%)	91 (38.6%)	113 (47.9%)		
Race				0.054	0.181				0.205	0.165
white	788 (74.5%)	610 (74.2%)	178 (75.4%)			347 (73.5%)	169 (71.6%)	178 (75.4%)		
black	154 (14.6%)	129 (15.7%)	25 (10.6%)			63 (13.3%)	38 (16.1%)	25 (10.6%)		
other	116 (11.0%)	83 (10.1%)	33 (14.0%)			62 (13.1%)	29 (12.3%)	33 (14.0%)		
Grade				0.847	0.092				0.871	0.104
I	17 (1.61%)	14 (1.70%)	3 (1.27%)			7 (1.48%)	4 (1.69%)	3 (1.27%)		
II	28 (2.65%)	22 (2.68%)	6 (2.54%)			13 (2.75%)	7 (2.97%)	6 (2.54%)		
III	247 (23.3%)	198 (24.1%)	49 (20.8%)			106 (22.5%)	57 (24.2%)	49 (20.8%)		
IV	497 (47.0%)	382 (46.5%)	115 (48.7%)			220 (46.6%)	105 (44.5%)	115 (48.7%)		
Unknown	269 (25.4%)	206 (25.1%)	63 (26.7%)			126 (26.7%)	63 (26.7%)	63 (26.7%)		
Laterality				0.996	0.006				1.000	0.008
Left	558 (52.7%)	433 (52.7%)	125 (53.0%)			249 (52.8%)	124 (52.5%)	125 (53.0%)		
Right	500 (47.3%)	389 (47.3%)	111 (47.0%)			223 (47.2%)	112 (47.5%)	111 (47.0%)		
T				0.034	0.195				0.511	0.107
T1	363 (34.3%)	298 (36.3%)	65 (27.5%)			140 (29.7%)	75 (31.8%)	65 (27.5%)		
T2	658 (62.2%)	498 (60.6%)	160 (67.8%)			313 (66.3%)	153 (64.8%)	160 (67.8%)		
T3	37 (3.50%)	26 (3.16%)	11 (4.66%)			19 (4.03%)	8 (3.39%)	11 (4.66%)		
N				0.438	0.049				1.000	0.028
N0	1037 (98.0%)	807 (98.2%)	230 (97.5%)			461 (97.7%)	231 (97.9%)	230 (97.5%)		
N1	21 (1.98%)	15 (1.82%)	6 (2.54%)			11 (2.33%)	5 (2.12%)	6 (2.54%)		
M				<0.001	0.326				0.681	0.047
M0	863 (81.6%)	695 (84.5%)	168 (71.2%)			341 (72.2%)	173 (73.3%)	168 (71.2%)		
M1	195 (18.4%)	127 (15.5%)	68 (28.8%)			131 (27.8%)	63 (26.7%)	68 (28.8%)		
Radiation				0.121	-				0.5738	-
No/Unknown	1036 (97.9%)	808 (98.3%)	228 (96.6%)			459 (97.25)	231 (97.88)	228 (96.61)		
Yes	22 (2.08%)	14 (1.70%)	8 (3.39%)			13 (2.75)	5 (2.12)	8 (3.39)		
Chemotherapy				0.238	-				0.0925	-
No/Unknown	38 (3.59%)	33 (4.01%)	5 (2.12%)			18 (3.81)	13 (5.51)	5 (2.12)		
Yes	1020 (96.4%)	789 (96.0%)	231 (97.9%)			454 (96.19)	223 (94.49)	231 (97.88)		
Tumor.size [mean (SD)]	107.319 (60.855)	105.439 (62.501)	113.869 (54.354)	0.0607	0.144	111.750 (61.667)	109.631 (68.252)	113.869 (54.354)	0.456	0.069

Original Study Cohort Multivariate Logistic Regression Analysis

In the original cohort of propensity score matching, multivariate Logistic regression analysis was performed on all patients to identify the factors contributing to selecting reasons for limb salvage or amputation. We found that the predictors of patient choice for amputation were male (OR 1.4, $P = 0.024$), other races (OR 1.4, $P = 0.047$), and distant metastasis (OR 2.1, $P < 0.001$). The results of multivariate logistic regression are shown in **Table 2**.

Multivariate Competitive Risk Regression Model After Propensity Score Matching

In the original cohort before matching, the CSM of amputation was significantly higher than that of limb salvage ($P = 0.017$). At the same time, the OSM of amputation was also higher than that of limb salvage ($P = 0.007$) (**Figure 2**). After 1:1 propensity matching, 236 children underwent amputation, and 236 children underwent limb salvage surgery, allowing for subsequent statistical analysis. The propensity score density before and after matching was shown in **Figure 3**. The patient's

TABLE 2 | Multivariate Logistic regression model to predict limb salvage surgery or amputation in pediatric osteosarcoma patients.

	OR	(5–95% CI)		*p*-value
Age	0.965	0.923	1.009	0.12
Sex				
Male	Reference			
Female	0.703	0.517	0.955	0.024
Year of diagnosis				
2004–2011	Reference			
2012–2018	0.765	0.566	1.032	0.08
Race				0.047
white	Reference			
black	0.64	0.4	1.023	0.062
other	1.365	0.871	2.139	0.175
Laterality				
Left	Reference			
Right	0.963	0.715	1.297	0.804
T				0.351
T1	Reference			
T2	1.322	0.892	1.959	0.165
T3	1.46	0.645	3.304	0.364
N				
N0	Reference			
N1	1.083	0.394	2.977	0.877
M				
M0	Reference			
M1	2.111	1.474	3.023	<0.001
Tumor size	1	0.997	1.003	0.826

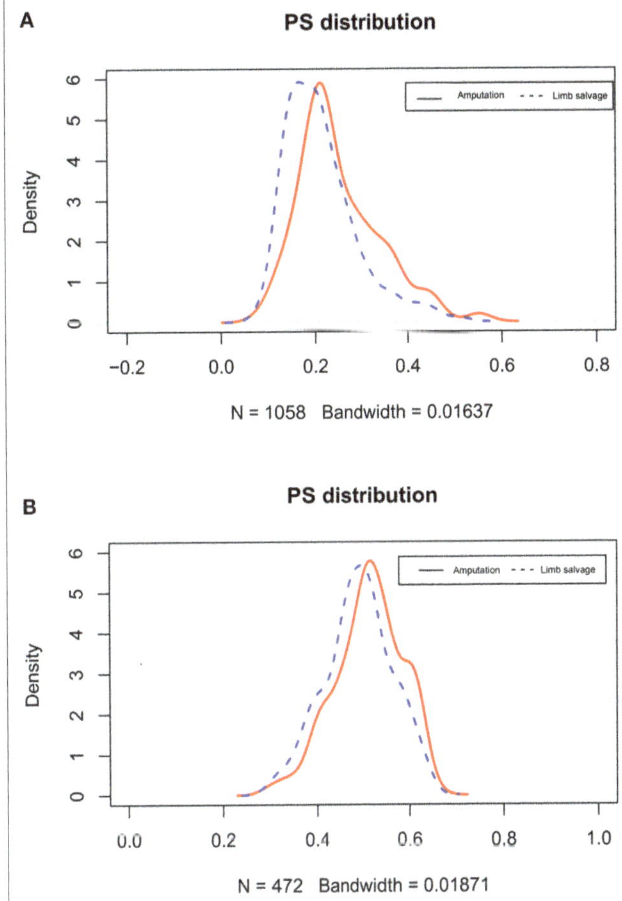

FIGURE 2 | Density plots of propensity score before **(A)** and after matching **(B)**.

information in the two groups was shown in **Table 1**, and there was no statistical difference in clinicopathological details between the two groups. In the 1:1 propensity matching cohort, the cumulative incidence plot showed a significant difference in CSM between limb salvage surgery and amputation ($P = 0.028$), but no significant difference in OSM ($P = 0.078$) (**Figure 4**). After propensity matching, multivariable CRR model analysis showed higher CSM in amputation than limb salvage (HR 1.49, $P = 0.028$), but no significant difference in OCM (HR 3.17, $P = 0.078$). Finally, CSM and OSM were analyzed using the multivariate Cox regression model, demonstrating the risk of amputation (**Table 3**).

Sensitivity Analyses

After an optimized propensity matching analysis, a multivariable CRR model was used to compare CSM between limb salvage and amputation. (1) In the original cohort, amputation had a higher CSM than limb salvage (HR 1.4, $P = 0.017$); (2) There was no significant difference in CSM between amputation and limb salvage in the 1:2 cohort (HR 1.3, $P = 0.065$); but amputations still had higher CSM in the 1:4 cohort (HR 1.4, $P = 0.017$). (3) Patients who retained complete tumor grade information had higher CSM after amputation (HR1.4, $P = 0.019$). (4) We used inverse probability of treatment Weighting to match patients (**Figure 5**). After the inverse probability of treatment weighting, the Kaplan-Meier curve showed that patients who received amputation had a lower survival rate than those who had limb salvage (**Figure 6**).

DISCUSSION

In this study, amputation was found to have a higher CSM rate than limb salvage in children with limb osteosarcoma, similar to previous studies. However, compared with previous studies, this study included more patients and used PSM analysis to exclude confounding factors, resulting in more accurate results. The comparison between amputation and limb-salvage surgery was first studied by Simon et al. on 227 patients with Osteosarcoma and found that limb salvage surgery did not significantly improve the survival rate of patients (24). A subsequent analysis of 227 patients with Osteosarcoma at 26 institutions by Rougraff et al. (25) found the same results. The findings of Bacci et al. (26) also support the appellate results. However, with the development of multidisciplinary treatment and the maturity of prosthesis technology, the proportion of

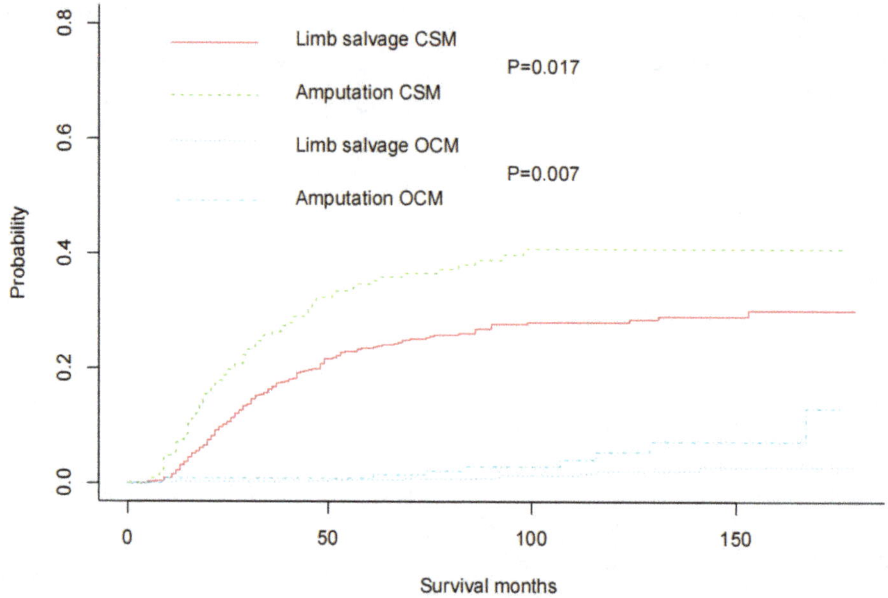

FIGURE 3 | Cumulative incidence plots in the original cohort showed CSM and OCM rates in pediatric patients with Osteosarcoma of the limbs.

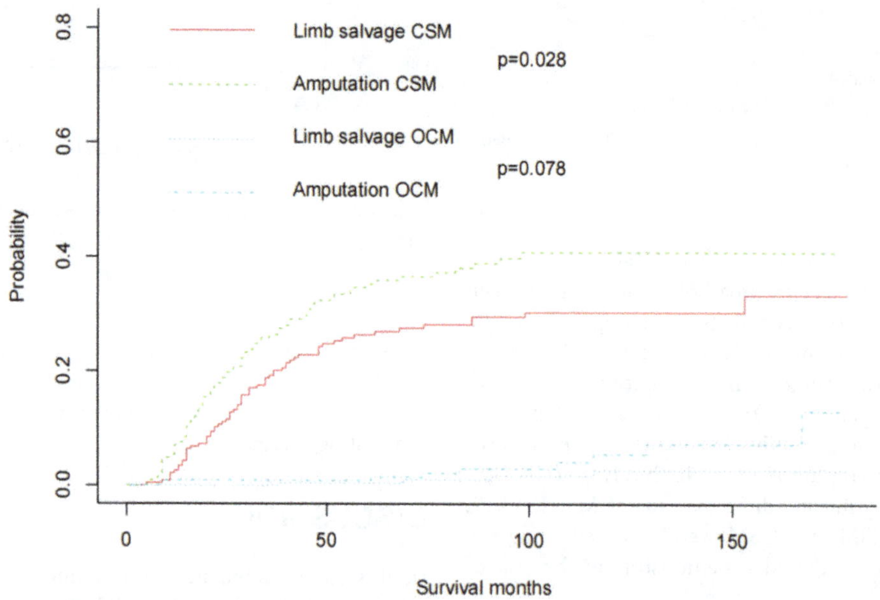

FIGURE 4 | After 1:1 propensity score matching, Cumulative incidence plots showed CSM and OCM rates in pediatric patients with Osteosarcoma of the limbs.

limb salvage surgery has been increasing (27). Recent studies have shown that limb salvage surgery significantly improves patient survival compared with amputation in patients with osteosarcoma (28–30). Although current osteosarcoma surgery tends to be limb salvage, previous studies have been small sample sizes and single-center studies, and few studies have specifically addressed pediatric Osteosarcoma. And the conclusions of previous studies may be influenced by confounding factors. Han et al. (20) conducted a meta-analysis showing that patients who underwent amputation had significantly lower survival rates than those who had limb preservation. But the heterogeneity between studies also leads to inevitable bias.

Moreover, there is another important outcome that we need to keep an eye on. Local recurrence of the tumor also puts the patient at risk for a second operation or amputation. Local recurrence is related to the tumor response

TABLE 3 | Propensity score-adjusted multivariate Cox regression models predict cancer-specific mortality and other causes mortality in pediatric osteosarcoma patients.

	Cancer-specific mortality			Other cause mortality		
	HR	**(5–95% CI)**	***p*-value**	**HR**	**(5–95% CI)**	***p*-value**
Age	1.028	0.979–1.08	0.272	1.004	0.864–1.167	0.957
Sex				1.132	0.366–3.503	0.83
Male	Reference			Reference		
Female	0.932	0.661–1.312	0.685	1.132	0.366–3.503	0.83
Year of diagnosis						
2004–2011	Reference			Reference		
2012–2018	1.071	0.746–1.537	0.709	0.411	0.043–3.917	0.44
Race						
white	Reference			Reference		
black	0.843	0.506–1.403	0.511	0.899	0.184–4.384	0.895
other	1.3	0.807–2.092	0.28	0.645	0.079–5.297	0.683
Grade						
I	Reference			Reference		
II	0.843	0.506–1.403	0.511	0.882	0-1.82E+143	0.999
III	1.3	0.807–2.092	0.28	2071.991	0-7.63E+120	0.956
IV	0.843	0.506–1.403	0.511	3033.215	0-1.11E+121	0.954
Unknown	1.3	0.807–2.092	0.28	3850.809	0-1.42E+121	0.952
Laterality						
Left	Reference			Reference		
Right	0.804	0.571–1.132	0.212	0.683	0.221-2.112	0.508
T						
T1	Reference			Reference		
T2	0.942	0.589–1.506	0.802	0.446	0.103-1.921	0.278
T3	1.291	0.581–2.868	0.53	0	0-3.58E+78	0.924
N						
N0	Reference			Reference		
N1	1.422	0.601–3.364	0.423	0	0-3.53E+114	0.954
M						
M0	Reference			Reference		
M1	3.347	2.34–4.786	<0.001	2.689	0.602–12.021	0.195
Surgery						
Limb salvage	Reference			Reference		
Amputation	1.525	1.097–2.121	0.012	3.171	0.972–10.342	0.056
Tumor size	1.003	1–1.005	0.037	1.001	0.99–1.012	0.839

to chemotherapy and the surgical margin, not the surgical method itself. Although limb salvage surgery has a higher survival rate, surgeons still prefer amputation for larger or more aggressive tumors. Still, some studies offer exciting news. Reddy et al. (15) analyzed 360 patients with Osteosarcoma and found that the survival rate of the second amputation after local tumor recurrence was similar to that of the first amputation. Grimer et al. (31) have also shown that patients with locally recurrent tumors can be cured by reoperation or amputation and radiotherapy. Therefore, limb salvage surgery remains the surgical option for pediatric osteosarcoma patients. However, amputation is still appropriate for stage IIB tumors that do not respond to chemotherapy, significant vascular and nerve tract involvement, and lack of bone or soft tissue reconstruction opportunities.

In this study, we focused on pediatric patients with Osteosarcoma, using the SEER database for a series of analyses. We used rigorous statistical methods, including propensity score matching and competitive risk models, to compare mortality differences between limb salvage surgery and amputation. Our study showed that girls are more likely to opt for limb salvage surgery, similar to a previous study (32). Previous studies have shown that tumor stage, tumor grade, and tumor size are all risk factors for the prognosis of Osteosarcoma and factors affecting surgical decision-making (30, 33). Limb salvage surgery has a higher survival rate than amputation, but this may be due to selection bias due to more aggressive tumors, such as neurovascular wrapping, poor response to chemotherapy, and tumor metastasis. In this study, the 5-year survival rate was 65.1% for patients with amputation and 76.5% for patients

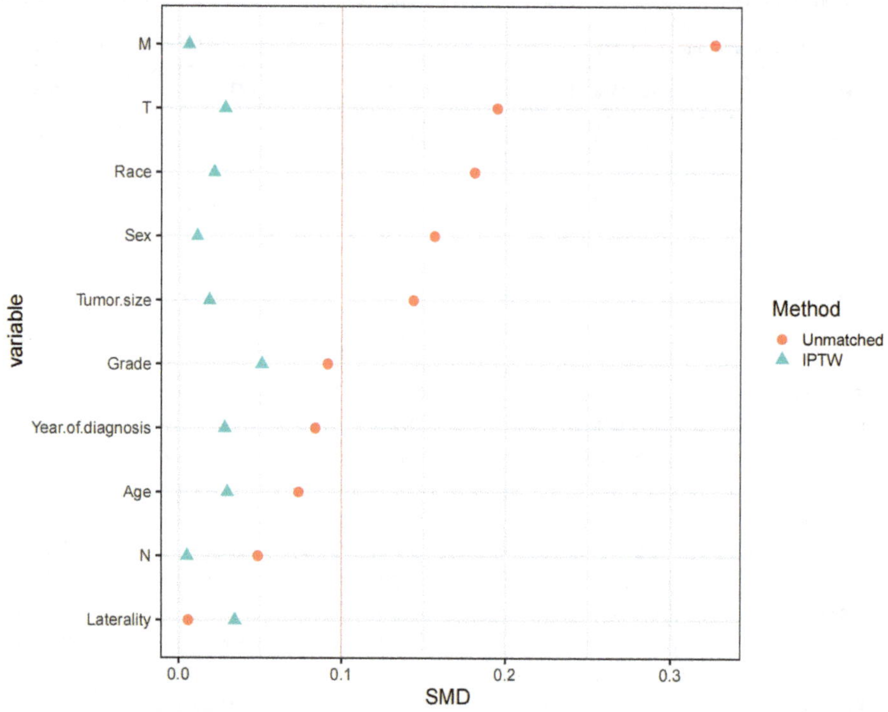

FIGURE 5 | Standardized mean difference distribution of patients after the inverse probability of treatment weighting matching.

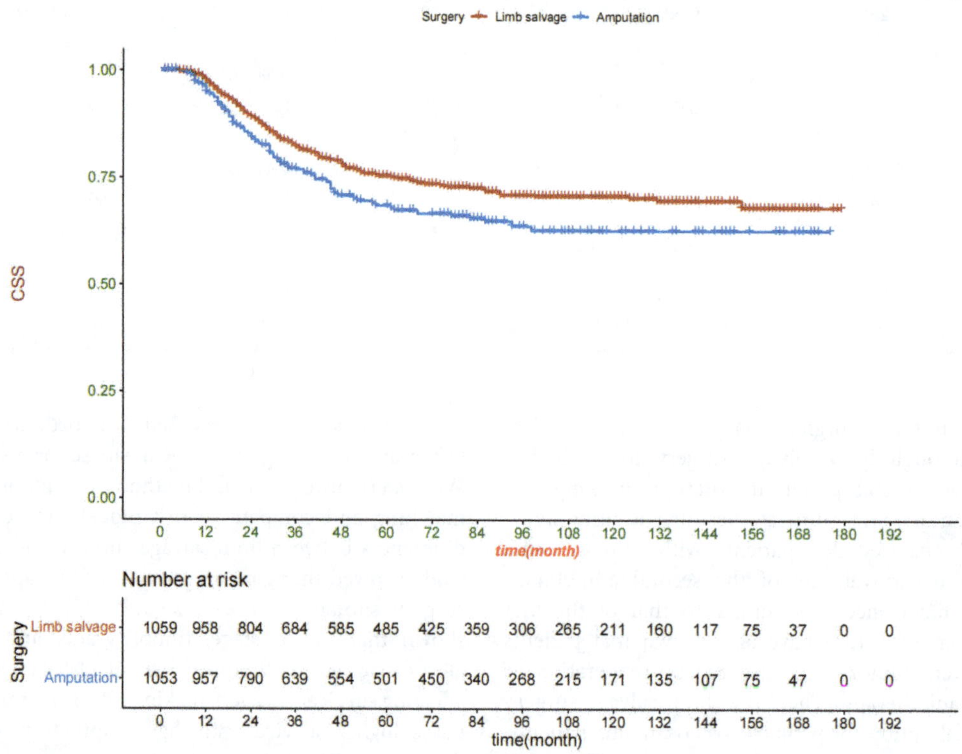

FIGURE 6 | Kaplan-meier curve of patients receiving amputation and limb salvage after the inverse probability of treatment weighting matching.

with limb salvage. However, these data have not been well recorded in the SEER database, and propensity matching cannot exclude confounding factors. Therefore, amputation is still recommended for highly invasive tumors.

In addition, the final endpoint of the patients was CSM. According to the SEER database, amputation has a higher CSM than limb salvage, and our results confirmed that patients with amputation have a 1.5-fold increase in CSM compared with patients with limb salvage. Further, we used various statistical methods to eliminate the differences caused by confounding factors. This included detailed adjustments for the patient's demographic information and underlying tumor characteristics using propensity matching. A competitive risk model was also used to adjust for the potential bias caused by OCM. We looked at the risk of death from amputation primarily in the 1:1 propensity matching cohort, and the same phenomenon was observed in the 1:4 matched cohort and the original cohort. In the end, the same results were found when unknown tumor grades were removed, confirming our concerns. Thus, amputation does indeed have a higher risk of death than limb salvage in pediatric osteosarcoma patients. Besides, we focused on OCM. Before matching, amputation had a higher OCM than limb salvage (HR3.4, $P = 0.007$), and there was no significant difference in survival between amputation and limb salvage after matching (HR3.2, $P = 0.056$). Thus, OCM was evenly distributed between amputees and patients with limb salvage, excluding differences in other causes of death. Since our study was a retrospective observational study, there were many data biases and confounding variables due to various reasons. We used PSM to reduce the impact of these biases and confounding variables.

Although our study used rigorous statistical methods, there are some limitations. First, this study was still retrospective, with no standardized specimen handling, lack of central pathological review, and no data on local recurrence and disease-free survival. Second, we also lack the patient's comorbidities information, cannot adjust the patient's other comorbidities. Although propensity score matching and the use of OCM to exclude comorbidities were performed to minimize bias, this is not equivalent to a prospective clinical randomized controlled trial. Finally, the SEER database does not contain information about the hospital, such as the level and capacity of the hospital. It does not include information about repeated treatments, such as surgery or radiotherapy after recurrence.

CONCLUSIONS

Our results suggested that amputation is associated with a 1.5-fold increase in CSM in pediatric patients with limbs Osteosarcoma. Therefore, in the surgical selection of pediatric patients with Osteosarcoma, limb salvage surgery should be the first choice.

AUTHOR CONTRIBUTIONS

JT, DH, and JW contributed to the conception, design, contributed to manuscript writing, and revision. CZ, JW, XT, TM, and JT collected and analyzed the data. ZZ, ML, XT, LJ, JW, and JT drew the figures and tables. JT and JW wrote the draft. All authors approved the final manuscript.

REFERENCES

1. Moore DD, Luu HH. Osteosarcoma. *Cancer Treat Res.* (2014) 162:65–92. doi: 10.1007/978-3-319-07323-1_4
2. Nagarajan R, Weigel BJ, Thompson RC, Perentesis JP. Osteosarcoma in the first decade of life. *Med Pediatr Oncol.* (2003) 41:480–3. doi: 10.1002/mpo.10403
3. Qureshi A, Ahmad Z, Azam M, Idrees R. Epidemiological data for common bone sarcomas. *Asian Pac J Cancer Prev.* (2010) 11:393–5.
4. Mirabello L, Troisi RJ, Savage SA. Osteosarcoma incidence and survival rates from 1973 to 2004: data from the surveillance, epidemiology, and end results program. *Cancer.* (2009) 115:1531–43. doi: 10.1002/cncr.24121
5. Schiller AL. Orthopaedic pathology. *Semin Diagn Pathol.* (2011) 28:1–3. doi: 10.1053/j.semdp.2011.02.003
6. Martin JW, Squire JA, Zielenska M. The genetics of osteosarcoma. *Sarcoma.* (2012) 2012:627254. doi: 10.1155/2012/627254
7. Isakoff MS, Bielack SS, Meltzer P, Gorlick R. Osteosarcoma: current treatment and a collaborative pathway to success. *J Clin Oncol.* (2015) 33:3029–35. doi: 10.1200/JCO.2014.59.4895
8. Marina NM, Smeland S, Bielack SS, Bernstein M, Jovic G, Krailo MD, et al. Comparison of MAPIE versus MAP in patients with a poor response to preoperative chemotherapy for newly diagnosed high-grade osteosarcoma (EURAMOS-1): an open-label, international, randomized controlled trial. *Lancet Oncol.* (2016) 17:1396–408. doi: 10.1016/S1470-2045(16)30214-5
9. Martin-Broto J, Redondo A, Valverde C, Vaz MA, Mora J, Muro XGD, et al. Gemcitabine plus sirolimus for relapsed and progressing osteosarcoma patients after standard chemotherapy: a multicenter, single-arm phase II trial of Spanish group for research on sarcoma (GEIS). *Ann Oncol.* (2017) 28:2994–9. doi: 10.1093/annonc/mdx536
10. Smrke A, Anderson PM, Gulia A, Gennatas S, Huang PH, Jones RL. Future directions in the treatment of osteosarcoma. *Cells.* (2021) 10:172. doi: 10.3390/cells10010172
11. Meyers PA, Schwartz CL, Krailo M, Kleinerman ES, Betcher D, Bernstein ML, et al. Osteosarcoma: a randomized, prospective trial of the addition of ifosfamide and/or muramyl tripeptide to cisplatin, doxorubicin, and high-dose methotrexate. *J Clin Oncol.* (2005) 23:2004–11. doi: 10.1200/JCO.2005.06.031
12. Jafari F, Javdansirat S, Sanaie S, Naseri A, Shamekh A, Rostamzadeh D, et al. Osteosarcoma: a comprehensive review of management and treatment strategies. *Ann Diagn Pathol.* (2020) 49:151654. doi: 10.1016/j.anndiagpath.2020.151654
13. Jackson TM, Bittman M, Granowetter L. Pediatric malignant bone tumors: a review and update on current challenges, and emerging drug targets. *Curr Probl Pediatr Adolesc Health Care.* (2016) 46:213–28. doi: 10.1016/j.cppeds.2016.04.002
14. Bernthal NM, Federman N, Eilber FR, Nelson SD, Eckardt JJ, Eilber FC, et al. Long-term results (>25 years) of a randomized, prospective clinical trial evaluating chemotherapy in patients with high-grade, operable Osteosarcoma. *Cancer.* (2012) 118:5888–93. doi: 10.1002/cncr.27651

14. Bernthal NM, Federman N, Eilber FR, Nelson SD, Eckardt JJ, Eilber FC, et al. Long-term results (>25 years) of a randomized, prospective clinical trial evaluating chemotherapy in patients with high-grade, operable Osteosarcoma. *Cancer.* (2012) 118:5888–93. doi: 10.1002/cncr.27651
15. Reddy KI, Wafa H, Gaston CL, Grimer RJ, Abudu AT, Jeys LM, et al. Does amputation offer any survival benefit over limb salvage in osteosarcoma patients with poor chemonecrosis and close margins? *Bone Joint J.* (2015) 97-B:115–20. doi: 10.1302/0301-620X.97B1.33924
16. Yang Y, Han L, He Z, Li X, Yang S, Yang J, et al. Advances in limb salvage treatment of Osteosarcoma. *J Bone Oncol.* (2017) 10:36–40. doi: 10.1016/j.jbo.2017.11.005
17. Han K, Dang P, Bian N, Chen X, Yang T, Fan QY, et al. Is limb salvage with microwave-induced hyperthermia better than amputation for osteosarcoma of the distal tibia? *Clin Orthop Relat Res.* (2017) 475:1668–77. doi: 10.1007/s11999-017-5273-1
18. Xu S, Yu X, Xu M, Fu Z, Chen Y, Sun Y, et al. Limb function and quality of life after various reconstruction methods according to tumor location following resection of Osteosarcoma in distal femur. *BMC Musculoskelet Disord.* (2014) 15:453. doi: 10.1186/1471-2474-15-453
19. Weeden S, Grimer RJ, Cannon SR, Taminiau AH, Uscinska BM, European Osteosarcoma Intergroup. The effect of local recurrence on survival in resected Osteosarcoma. *Eur J Cancer.* (2001) 37:39–46. doi: 10.1016/S0959-8049(00)00362-2
20. Han G, Bi WZ, Xu M, Jia JP, Wang Y. Amputation versus limb-salvage surgery in patients with osteosarcoma: a meta-analysis. *World J Surg.* (2016) 40:2016–27. doi: 10.1007/s00268-016-3500-7
21. Jauregui JJ, Nadarajah V, Munn J, Pivec R, Kapadia BH, Lerman DM, et al. Limb salvage versus amputation in conventional appendicular osteosarcoma: a systematic review. *Indian J Surg Oncol.* (2018) 9:232–40. doi: 10.1007/s13193-018-0725-y
22. Hankey BF, Ries LA, Edwards BK. The surveillance, epidemiology, and end results program: a national resource. *Cancer Epidemiol Biomarkers Prev.* (1999) 8:1117–21.
23. Austin PC, Lee DS, Fine JP. Introduction to the analysis of survival data in the presence of competing risks. *Circulation.* (2016) 133:601–9. doi: 10.1161/CIRCULATIONAHA.115.017719
24. Simon MA, Aschliman MA, Thomas N, Mankin HJ. Limb-salvage treatment versus amputation for osteosarcoma of the distal end of the femur. *J Bone Joint Surg Am.* (1986) 68:1331–7. doi: 10.2106/00004623-198668090-00005
25. Rougraff BT, Simon MA, Kneisl JS, Greenberg DB, Mankin HJ. Limb salvage compared with amputation for osteosarcoma of the distal end of the femur. a long-term oncological, functional, and quality-of-life study. *J Bone Joint Surg Am.* (1994) 76:649–56. doi: 10.2106/00004623-199405000-00004
26. Bacci G, Ferrari S, Lari S, Mercuri M, Donati DM, Longhi A, et al. Osteosarcoma of the limb. amputation or limb salvage in patients treated by neoadjuvant chemotherapy. *J Bone Joint Surg Br.* (2002) 84:88–92. doi: 10.1302/0301-620X.84B1.0840088
27. Anderson ME. Update on survival in osteosarcoma. *Orthop Clin North Am.* (2016) 47:283–92. doi: 10.1016/j.ocl.2015.08.022
28. Bacci G, Longhi A, Fagioli F, Briccoli A, Versari M, Picci P. Adjuvant and neoadjuvant chemotherapy for osteosarcoma of the extremities: 27 year experience at rizzoli institute, Italy. *Eur J Cancer.* (2005) 41:2836–45. doi: 10.1016/j.ejca.2005.08.026
29. Ayerza MA, Farfalli GL, Aponte-Tinao L, Muscolo DL. Does increased rate of limb-sparing surgery affect survival in osteosarcoma? *Clin Orthop Relat Res.* (2010) 468:2854–9. doi: 10.1007/s11999-010-1423-4
30. Kamal AF, Widyawarman H, Husodo K, Hutagalung EU, Rajabto W. Clinical outcome and survival of osteosarcoma patients in cipto mangunkusumo hospital: limb salvage surgery versus amputation. *Acta Med Indones.* (2016) 48:175–83.
31. Grimer RJ, Sommerville S, Warnock D, Carter S, Tillman R, Abudu A, et al. Management and outcome after local recurrence of osteosarcoma. *Eur J Cancer.* (2005) 41:578–83. doi: 10.1016/j.ejca.2004.11.012
32. Schrager J, Patzer RE, Mink PJ, Ward KC, Goodman M. Survival outcomes of pediatric osteosarcoma and ewing's sarcoma: a comparison of surgery type within the SEER database, 1988-2007. *J Registry Manag.* (2011) 38:153–61.
33. Miller BJ, Cram P, Lynch CF, Buckwalter JA. Risk factors for metastatic disease at presentation with Osteosarcoma: an analysis of the SEER database. *J Bone Joint Surg Am.* (2013) 95:e89. doi: 10.2106/JBJS.L.01189

4

The Role of ICG Angiography in Decision Making About Skin-Sparing in Pediatric Acute Trauma

*Tao Han, Buhao Sun, Weidong Wang, Jie Cui and Weimin Shen**

Department of Burns and Plastic Surgery, Children's Hospital of Nanjing Medical University, Nanjing, China

Correspondence:
Weimin Shen
swmswmswm@sina.com

Background: Indocyanine green (ICG) angiography has proven useful in assessing skin flap perfusion in plastic and reconstructive surgeries. This research aimed to explore its role in decision making about skin-sparing in children's acute trauma.

Methods: A total of 19 patients suffering with acute trauma from January 2019 to September 2021 were retrospectively assessed. Both ICG angiography and clinical judgment were performed to evaluate skin tissue viability. The intraoperative decisions for each case depended on the specific condition of the traumatic wound, including tissue perfusion, skin defect area, and location of the wound. Postoperative vascular imaging software was used to quantify the tissue perfusion, and the duration of postoperative follow-up was from 6 to 18 months.

Results: Among them, 18 (94.7%) patients experienced treatments according to ICG angiography and did not develop postoperative necrosis. One case with right forearm trauma suffered from partial necrosis. Hypertrophic scar and local infection were the independent complications, which were managed by symptomatic treatment.

Conclusion: ICG angiography may reduce the risk of postoperative necrosis and renders a promising adjunctive technique for surgeons to make reasonable decisions in skin sparing in acute pediatric trauma.

Keywords: indocyanine green angiography, trauma, necrosis, perfusion, children

INTRODUCTION

The evaluation of skin tissue viability is the key to the management of children's acute trauma and is generally associated with the prognosis of local appearance or function (1, 2). An appropriate debridement of skin tissues with hypoperfusion, which can remarkably reduce the occurrence of postoperative necrosis, however, is mainly based on subjective experience. Therefore, decision making about skin sparing is a test for young surgeons, especially in cases of laceration or avulsion injury, that create a state of vasoconstriction intraoperatively (3, 4). Due to inaccurate judgment and individual differences, local necrosis often occurs after operation, resulting in surgical complications, such as scar hyperplasia, delayed wound healing, and infection.

Intraoperative indocyanine green (ICG) angiography has been widely used in assessing skin flap perfusion in various kinds of plastic and reconstructive surgeries (5–8). It can be an efficient adjuvant to enhance the surgeon's judgment of skin tissue viability and significantly decrease the odds of local necrosis after flap surgery. Moreover, an increasing amount of research focuses on the application of ICG angiography in both burn depth estimation and precise marking for burn excision (9–11). However, the current clinical study of ICG angiography on acute trauma surgery is extremely limited. Therefore, this study aimed to characterize the efficacy and safety of ICG angiography in decision making about skin sparing in children's acute trauma.

PATIENTS AND METHODS

We retrospectively assessed the clinical features, management, and follow-up of 19 patients suffering with acute trauma. All of the included cases were treated in our center between January 2019 and September 2021. Skin tissue viability was evaluated by both ICG angiography and clinical judgment (capillary refill, skin color, and bleeding of wound margin). Inclusion criteria included (1) hypoperfusion by clinical judgment, (2) the traumatic wound involving only skin and soft tissue, and (3) more than 6 months of follow-up. Exclusion criteria included (1) patients having undergone previous intervention and (2) a history of iodine allergy.

Under general anesthesia, 2.0–4.0 ml ICG (concentration: 2.5 mg/ml, Dandong Yichuang, China) was applied intravenously in 10 s followed by a 10-mL saline bolus injection. The maximum dose of ICG was 0.5 mg/kg per session. It took 20–30 s to observe the full effect of fluorescence, and then the area of skin tissue perfusion was visualized by using a fluorescence imaging system (Mingde Medical Diagnosis Inc., Langfang, China). Subsequently, real-time ICG angiography was continuously conducted for 5–10 min. The percentage of wound skin viability was estimated by viable skin area/total trauma area (cm^2). The interval should be more than 20 min if repeated ICG angiography is required. The intraoperative decisions for each case depended on the specific condition of the traumatic wound, including tissue perfusion, skin defect area, and location of the wound. Tissue with hypoperfusion was excised when identified by ICG results.

Moreover, postoperative vascular imaging software (Version 1.0, Mingde Medical Diagnosis Inc., Langfang, China) was used to quantify the tissue perfusion at a random point (**Figure 1**). A perfusion intensity of <33% of maximal perfusion in the trauma site was regarded as an indicator of hypoperfusion (7, 12). For all cases enrolled in this study, the duration of postoperative follow-up was from 6 to 18 months.

RESULTS

In this study, the male:female ratio was 13:6 with an age range of 2–10 years. The vast majority (14 cases, 73.7%) suffered with craniofacial trauma. Time to intraoperative ICG perfusion was from 15 to 75 s. A summary of clinical features of this study population is shown in **Table 1**. Precise marking for tissue with hypoperfusion was shown by excision ICG angiography. In 12 of 19 cases (63.2%), the skin viable portion judged by clinical finding was larger than that detected by ICG angiography (**Figure 2**). ICG angiography indicated acceptable perfusion in three cases (15.8%), which were determined to be an at-risk area by clinical judgment (**Figure 3**). Besides this, clinical findings were in accordance with ICG angiography in four cases (21.1%).

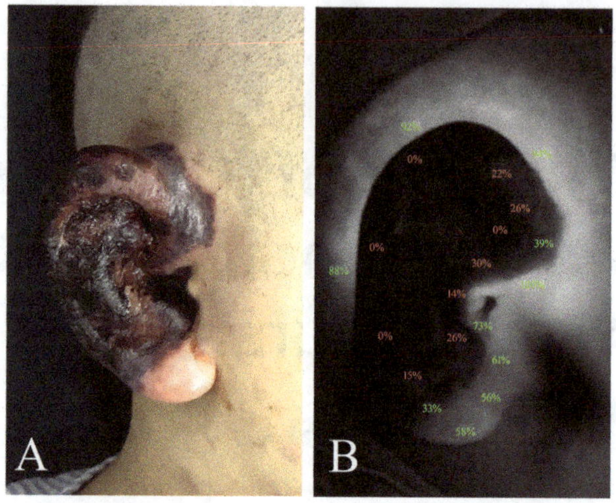

FIGURE 1 | The intraoperative perfusion area was assessed by ICG angiography, and postoperative vascular imaging software was used to quantify the tissue perfusion at random points. **(A)** Clinical appearance of right ear with crush injury. **(B)** The percentage in the image represented tissue perfusion compared with the maximal area of perfusion, which was set as 100%. A perfusion intensity of <33% of maximal perfusion in the trauma site was regarded as an indicator of hypoperfusion. ICG, indocyanine green.

Notably, 18 (94.7%) patients experienced appropriate treatment according to ICG angiography and did not develop postoperative necrosis. The case with partial necrosis was a fat boy. Part of the wound tissue with pale color and poor capillary refill was observed from clinical manifestation, and we performed resection of the tissue with hypoperfusion according to ICG assessments. A local skin flap with a thick fat layer was used to cover the defect of the wound, and postoperative skin necrosis was shown in the distal edge of the flap.

All cases underwent this investigation without any reports of allergic reactions, nausea, hematoma, or ICG-related pigmentation. Some minor complications were observed in this cohort, including two cases of hypertrophic scar and one case of local infection, which were managed by symptomatic treatment.

DISCUSSION

Characteristics owned uniquely by children make management of acute trauma more challenging. Distinguished from adults, children have less soft tissue to absorb the transmission of traumatic energy, leading to deeper injury and a larger extent of skin involvement (13, 14). Inaccurate acquisition of history and incompliant physical examination interfere with the surgeon's estimation of injury severity. Moreover, severe pain and crying may induce vasospasm and poor perfusion in the wound. For young surgeons, one of the major problems is how to determine the accurate extent and perfusion of involved skin tissue. As a result, optimizing the decision on skin sparing in acute trauma surgery to minimize any negative impact on postoperative appearance is becoming increasingly important.

TABLE 1 | Clinical features of 19 cases with acute trauma.

Caes No.	Gender	Age (yr)	Location of trauma	Skin viable portion (%)		Treatment	Postoperative necrosis	Follow-up (month)
				Clinical judgment	ICG angiography			
1	M	2	Nose	85	100	Suture *in situ* with skin-sparing	None	12
2	F	5	Left face	100	100	Suture *in situ* with skin-sparing	None	6
3	F	6	Left calf	90	82	Suture *in situ* after partial resection	None	12
4	M	3	Scalp	100	91	Suture *in situ* after partial resection	None	18
5	M	4	Left forehead	94	82	Local flap after partial resection	None	10
6	M	4	Bilateral upper eyelid	100	100	Suture *in situ* with skin-sparing	None	18
7	M	7	Lower lip	100	92	Local flap after partial resection	None	10
8	F	6	Right middle finger	85	80	Skin graft after partial resection	None	14
9	F	7	Upper lip	95	90	Suture *in situ* after partial resection	None	12
10	M	10	Left eyebrow	100	100	Suture *in situ* with skin-sparing	None	6
11	M	8	Right forearm	93	85	Local flap after partial resection	Partial necrosis	12
12	F	9	Right ear	35	20	Subtotal resection	None	12
13	M	3	Right ring finger	82	100	Skin graft after partial resection	None	18
14	M	6	Nose	100	95	Local flap after partial resection	None	18
15	M	7	Left upper arm	85	100	Suture *in situ* after partial resection	None	12
16	M	8	Neck	100	100	Suture *in situ* with skin-sparing	None	10
17	M	9	Left index finger	100	91	Distal-based thenar flap after partial resection	None	14
18	F	5	Right face	96	90	Local flap after partial resection	None	10
19	M	3	Right forehead	95	87	Suture *in situ* after partial resection	None	8

ICG, indocyanine green; M, male; F, female.

Some non-invasive techniques are reported in wound management for the estimation of depth and severity, including infrared thermography, laser doppler imaging, and ICG angiography. Infrared thermography is easily operated and permits accurate evaluation of wound viability much earlier than clinical judgment (15–17). However, due to its high sensitivity to the surrounding environment, small changes in room temperature may remarkably affect the infrared thermography signal from the wound (18). Laser doppler with low-resolution fast scan is reported to be more accurate and effective than clinical judgment alone in predicting burn wound outcome. The laser light in wound tissue exhibits a frequency change, which is correlated with the amount of tissue perfusion (19–21). It is worth noting that the high cost of the laser doppler imaging device hinders its wide clinical application. Besides this, any body movement during the scanning could result in inaccurate imaging (22).

ICG angiography, as a widely applied fluorescence imaging technique, can provide confirmatory information of tissue perfusion in various kinds of flap surgery and affect decision making about skin sparing to minimize the potential of necrosis. Driessen et al. (23) studied female patients undergoing mastectomies with or without immediate reconstruction and revealed a substantial decrease in skin necrosis with the use of ICG angiography. Kawamoto et al. (24) report that, compared with thermography, ICG angiography could confirm variation in perfusion of the intercostal muscle flap and make it possible for reducing bronchopleural fistula development. Abdelwahab et al. (25) notes that ICG angiography is an effective method to qualify and quantify neovascularization perfusion of forehead flaps, and time between stages and cartilage graft use were significantly associated with perfusion measures. However, the application of ICG on the prediction of extent and perfusion of traumatic wounds is still lacking.

To our knowledge, this study is the first clinical research to demonstrate a decreased risk of trauma-related necrosis after ICG angiography evaluation in children. Our analysis showed that 15 cases (78.9%) experienced inconsistent judgment on skin perfusion by both clinical findings and ICG angiography. All intraoperative decisions in skin sparing were based on ICG results, and no postoperative necrosis was observed in 18 cases (94.7%). This could provide surgeons with objective evidence, which was beneficial for judgment on perfusion, the surgical plan, and prediction of prognosis. Furthermore, postoperative imaging software was performed to quantify tissue perfusion as a percentage, which helped to objectively manifest the distribution of blood supply in the traumatic wound. By studying the comparison between clinical appearance and postoperative software results, it can facilitate a surgeon's ability to judge intraoperative skin sparing in the future. Due to the short plasma

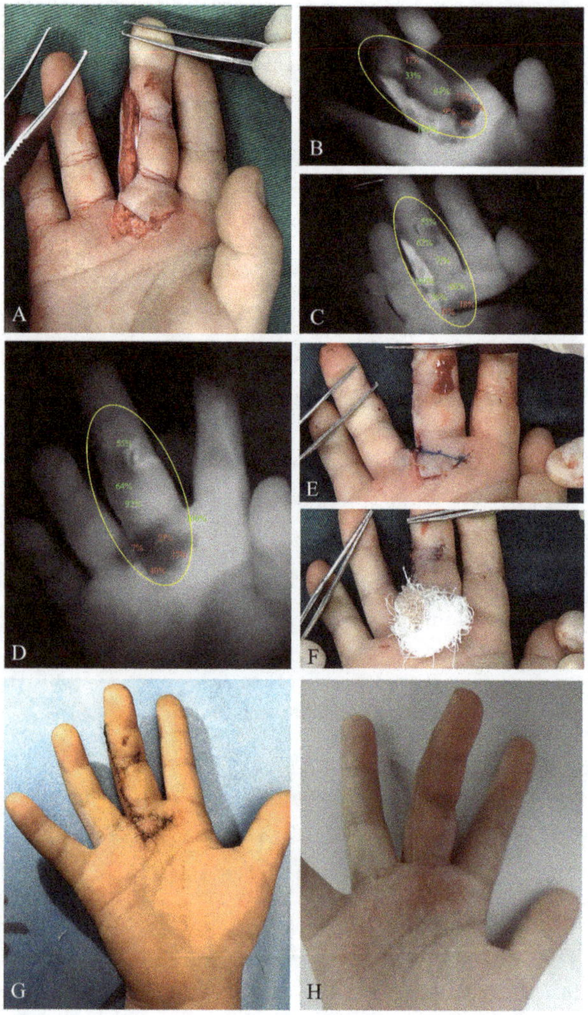

FIGURE 2 | A 6-year-old female patient suffered with a cut of right middle finger caused by an electric fan. **(A)** Clinical appearance of the right middle finger with retrograde skin avulsion injury. **(B)** Immediate ICG angiography indicated diminished ICG uptake of proximal wound portion. **(C)** After 5-min observation, hypoperfusion of the proximal wound edge was still detected. **(D)** With the wound closure, ICG angiography was performed again to evaluate the skin perfusion, demonstrating persistent hypoperfusion of the proximal wound portion. **(E)** The proximal wound portion with poor capillary refill was marked under angiography. **(F)** With resection of the poorly perfused tissue, a reverse full-thickness skin graft was performed in this area. **(G)** Fourteen days postoperatively, ideal skin survival was obtained. **(H)** Clinical appearance at the third month postoperatively. *Yellow circle,* region of trauma. ICG, indocyanine green.

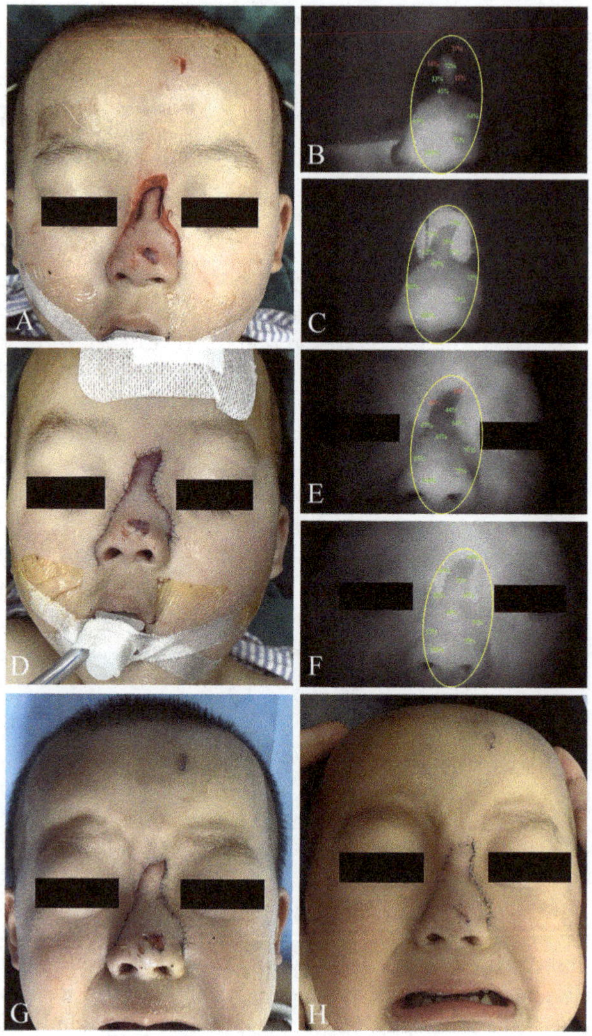

FIGURE 3 | A 2-year-old male patient suffered with nose trauma caused by running against a glass door. **(A)** Clinical appearance of the distal wound edge with unhealthy color and poor capillary refill. **(B)** Immediate ICG angiography indicated diminished ICG uptake of the distal wound edge, which was consistent with clinical finding. **(C)** With 5-min continuous observation, improved perfusion of the distal wound was demonstrated by ICG angiography. **(D)** According to ICG findings, suture *in situ* with skin sparing was chosen to perform for the wound. **(E)** The wound was sutured in place, and ICG angiography was repeated immediately, demonstrating hypoperfusion again of the distal wound portion. **(F)** An acceptable perfusion was achieved after 5-min observation. **(G)** Four days postoperatively, clinical appearance with uneventful healing was obtained. **(H)** Clinical appearance at the 10th day postoperatively. *Yellow circle,* region of trauma. ICG, indocyanine green.

half-life time of ICG, intraoperative ICG angiography with a 20-min interval could be repeated if necessary, and no ICG-related side effect was observed in this study.

The weaknesses of this research includes its small sample size and lack of prospective control study. Due to incompliant physical examination of children, ICG angiography can only be performed under general anesthesia. In addition, perfusion of deep tissue cannot be assumed by ICG angiography (limited to 10 mm for visualization), and thus, postoperative hypoperfusion of deep fat tissue might be the cause of one case with partial necrosis. Besides this, given that randomness of acute trauma (e.g., location, cause, extent, type), the control group without ICG evaluation was not included in our research.

In conclusion, our findings support the likelihood that ICG angiography renders a promising adjunctive technique for surgeons to make reasonable decisions in skin sparing in pediatric acute trauma.

ETHICS STATEMENT

The studies involving human participants were reviewed and approved by Ethics Committee of the Children's Hospital of Nanjing Medical University. Written informed consent to participate in this study was provided by the participants' legal guardian/next of kin. Written informed consent was obtained from the individual(s), and minor(s)' legal guardian/next of kin, for the publication of any potentially identifiable images or data included in this article.

AUTHOR CONTRIBUTIONS

WS revised the manuscript and approved the final manuscript as submitted. JC performed the surgery and conducted the data analyses. BS and WW performed postoperative follow-up and analyzed the data. TH wrote a draft of the article and edited the figures. All authors contributed to the article and approved the submitted version.

REFERENCES

1. Broussard KC, Powers JG. Wound dressings: selecting the most appropriate type. *Am J Clin Dermatol.* (2013) 14:449–59. doi: 10.1007/s40257-013-0046-4
2. Abbott PV. Diagnosis and management of transverse root fractures. *Dent Traumatol.* (2019) 35:333–47. doi: 10.1111/edt.12482
3. Muntean MV, Ardelean F, Strilciuc S, Pestean C, Georgescu AV, Muntean V. Flap warming improves intraoperative indocyanine green angiography (ICGA) assessment of perfusion. An experimental study. *J Plast Reconstr Aesthet Surg.* (2019) 72:1150–56. doi: 10.1016/j.bjps.2019.03.014
4. Beckler AD, Ezzat WH, Seth R, Nabili V, Blackwell KE. Assessment of fibula flap skin perfusion in patients undergoing oromandibular reconstruction: comparison of clinical findings, fluorescein, and indocyanine green angiography. *JAMA Facial Plast Surg.* (2015) 17:422–6. doi: 10.1001/jamafacial.2015.0961
5. Duggal CS, Madni T, Losken A. An outcome analysis of intraoperative angiography for postmastectomy breast reconstruction. *Aesthet Surg J.* (2014) 34:61–5. doi: 10.1177/1090820X13514995
6. Casey WJ, 3rd, Connolly KA, Nanda A, Rebecca AM, Perdikis G, Smith AA. Indocyanine green laser angiography improves deep inferior epigastric perforator flap outcomes following abdominal suction lipectomy. *Plast Reconstr Surg.* (2015) 135:491–97e. doi: 10.1097/PRS.0000000000000964
7. Moyer HR, Losken A. Predicting mastectomy skin flap necrosis with indocyanine green angiography: the gray area defined. *Plast Reconstr Surg.* (2012) 129:1043–8. doi: 10.1097/PRS.0b013e31824a2b02
8. Bigdeli AK, Thomas B, Falkner F, Gazyakan E, Hirche C, Kneser U. The impact of indocyanine-green fluorescence angiography on intraoperative decision-making and postoperative outcome in free flap surgery. *J Reconstr Microsurg.* (2020) 36:556–66. doi: 10.1055/s-0040-1710552
9. Wongkietkachorn A, Surakunprapha P, Jenwitheesuk K, Eua-Angkanakul K, Winaikosol K, Punyavong P, et al. Indocyanine green angiography precise marking for indeterminate burn excision: a prospective, multi-centered, double-blinded study. *Plast Reconstr Surg Glob Open.* (2021) 9:e3538. doi: 10.1097/GOX.0000000000003538
10. Wongkietkachorn A, Surakunprapha P, Winaikosol K, Eua-Angkanakul K, Wongkietkachorn N, Punyavong P, et al. Quantitative burn depth analysis using indocyanine green angiography. *J Burn Care Res.* (2019) 40:725. doi: 10.1093/jbcr/irz090
11. Wongkietkachorn A, Surakunprapha P, Jenwitheesuk K, Eua-Angkanakul K, Winaikosol K, Punyavong P, et al. An inconvenient truth of clinical assessment and indocyanine green angiography precise marking for indeterminate burn excision. *Plast Reconstr Surg Glob Open.* (2021) 9:e3497. doi: 10.1097/GOX.0000000000003497
12. Wongkietkachorn A, Surakunprapha P, Winaikosol K, Waraasawapati S, Chaiwiriyakul S, Eua-Angkanakul K, et al. Indocyanine green dye angiography as an adjunct to assess indeterminate burn wounds: a prospective, multicentered, triple-blinded study. *J Trauma Acute Care Surg.* (2019) 86:823–28. doi: 10.1097/TA.0000000000002179
13. Gaines BA. Intra-abdominal solid organ injury in children: diagnosis and treatment. *J Trauma.* (2009) 67:S135–9. doi: 10.1097/TA.0b013e3181adc17a
14. Sharp NE, Holcomb GW III. The role of minimally invasive surgery in pediatric trauma: a collective review. *Pediatr Surg Int.* (2013) 29:1013–8. doi: 10.1007/s00383-013-3401-x
15. Carriere ME, de Haas LEM, Pijpe A, Meij-de Vries A, Gardien KLM, van Zuijlen PPM, et al. Validity of thermography for measuring burn wound healing potential. *Wound Repair Regen.* (2020) 28:347–54. doi: 10.1111/wrr.12786
16. Bilska A, Stangret A, Pyzlak M, Wojdasiewicz P, Szukiewicz D. Skin surface infrared thermography in pressure ulcer outcome prognosis. *J Wound Care.* (2020) 29:707–18. doi: 10.12968/jowc.2020.29.12.707
17. Dang J, Lin M, Tan C, Pham CH, Huang S, Hulsebos IF, et al. Use of infrared thermography for assessment of burn depth and healing potential: a systematic review. *J Burn Care Res.* (2021). doi: 10.1093/jbcr/irab108. [Epub ahead of print].
18. Simmons JD, Kahn SA, Vickers AL, Crockett ES, Whitehead JD, Krecker AK, et al. Early assessment of burn depth with far infrared time-lapse thermography. *J Am Coll Surg.* (2018) 226:687–93. doi: 10.1016/j.jamcollsurg.2017.12.051
19. Nguyen K, Ward D, Lam L, Holland AJ. Laser Doppler Imaging prediction of burn wound outcome in children: is it possible before 48 h? *Burns.* (2010) 36:793–8. doi: 10.1016/j.burns.2009.11.016
20. Mill J, Cuttle L, Harkin DG, Kravchuk O, Kimble RM. Laser Doppler imaging in a paediatric burns population. *Burns.* (2009) 35:824–31. doi: 10.1016/j.burns.2008.11.016
21. La Hei ER, Holland AJ, Martin HC. Laser Doppler imaging of paediatric burns: burn wound outcome can be predicted independent of clinical examination. *Burns.* (2006) 32:550–3. doi: 10.1016/j.burns.2005.11.014
22. Jaspers ME, Maltha I, Klaessens JH, de Vet HC, Verdaasdonk RM, van Zuijlen PP. Insights into the use of thermography to assess burn wound healing potential: a reliable and valid technique when compared to laser Doppler imaging. *J Biomed Opt.* (2016) 21:96006. doi: 10.1117/1.JBO.21.9.096006
23. Driessen C, Arnardottir TH, Lorenzo AR, Mani MR. How should indocyanine green dye angiography be assessed to best predict mastectomy skin flap necrosis? A systematic review. *J Plast Reconstr Aesthet Surg.* (2020) 73:1031–42. doi: 10.1016/j.bjps.2020.02.025
24. Kawamoto N, Anayama T, Okada H, Hirohashi K, Miyazaki R, Yamamoto M, et al. Indocyanine green fluorescence/thermography evaluation of intercostal muscle flap vascularization. *Thorac Cancer.* (2018) 9:1631–7. doi: 10.1111/1759-7714.12871
25. Abdelwahab M, Kandathil CK, Most SP, Spataro EA. Utility of indocyanine green angiography to identify clinical factors associated with perfusion of paramedian forehead flaps during nasal reconstruction surgery. *JAMA Facial Plast Surg.* (2019) 21:206–12. doi: 10.1001/jamafacial.2018.1829

5

Super-Selective Partial Splenic Embolization for Hereditary Spherocytosis in Children

Rui-jue Wang [1†], Li Xiao [2†], Xi-ming Xu [2], Ming-man Zhang [1] and Qiang Xiong [1]*

[1] Chongqing Key Laboratory of Pediatrics, Department of Hepatobiliary Surgery, Children's Hospital of Chongqing Medical University, National Clinical Research Center for Child Health and Disorders, Ministry of Education Key Laboratory of Child Development and Disorders, Chongqing, China, [2] Department of Medical Record Statistics, Children's Hospital of Chongqing Medical University, National Clinical Research Center for Child Health and Disorders, Chongqing Higher Institution Engineering Research Center of Children's Medical Big Data Intelligent Application, Ministry of Education Key Laboratory of Child Development and Disorders, Chongqing, China

***Correspondence:**
Qiang Xiong
xiong537@163.com

Background: Hereditary spherocytosis (HS) is the most common hemolytic anemia due to erythrocyte membrane defects. Total splenectomy is the most effective treatment for moderate or severe HS. As a conservative alternative, partial splenic embolization (PSE) can preserve part of the spleen's function, thus reducing the risk of overwhelming post-splenectomy infection (OPSI) or sepsis, especially for pediatric patients. However, it is not easy to precisely control the scope of interventional embolization, limiting PSE applications. The present study aims to optimize the PSE procedure on smaller, which is named super-selective PSE (SPSE), to improve the controllability and assess the feasibility and effectiveness of SPSE.

Results: This study was conducted by retrospectively reviewing clinical data from HS patients treated by surgical treatments, which were diagnosed at the children's hospital of Chongqing medical university from January 2015 to December 2019. Patients were divided into two groups according to their treatment preference: SPSE (16 patients) group and total splenectomy (41 patients) group. The mean proportion range of splenic embolism by SPSE was 82.4%, close to the expected value (70–85%). The average hemoglobin value was increased significantly from 6.85 (5.6–8.0) g/dl before SPSE to 12.4 (10.4–13.3) g/dl after SPSE ($p < 0.001$). All children after SPSE suffered mild post-embolization syndrome, such as pain, fever, and vomiting, which could easily be controlled with appropriate supportive therapy.

Conclusions: Super-selective partial splenic embolization is a safe and effective treatment for moderate or severe HS in children. However, with a longer follow-up, more patients further assess the value of SPSE.

Keywords: hereditary spherocytosis, super-selective partial splenic embolization, children, interventional therapy, surgery therapy

INTRODUCTION

Hereditary spherocytosis (HS) is hemolytic anemia of varying severity caused by red blood cell membrane defects. Defects in the erythrocyte membrane and selective destruction of defective erythrocytes by the spleen are two critical factors in the pathophysiological process of HS. The destruction of the red blood cells by the spleen can lead to proliferative enlargement of the spleen, which leads to increased red blood cell accumulation, increased hemolysis, or both, thus creating a vicious cycle (1).

The treatment of HS aims to minimize the complications of chronic hemolysis and anemia. In addition to symptomatic treatment and blood transfusion, current guidelines recommend splenectomy if the patient has severe anemia complications or is transfusion-dependent (1–3). Since the spleen is a lymphoid organ, the overwhelming post-splenectomy infection (OPSI) is the most severe post-operative complication, especially in children. In addition to surgical risks, splenic resection is also prone to severe surgical complications, such as venous thromboembolism (VTE), pulmonary arthritis after splenectomy (4). Patients who have indications for splenectomy but were unwilling to undergo surgery, or who have contraindications to surgery, have been reported to be treated with relatively conservative surgery, such as partial splenectomy, partial splenic embolization (PSE), and partial splenic artery ligation, which exhibited better outcomes and fewer surgical complications due to residual partial splenic immunity (5, 6). However, PSE had not been widely studied and applied in pediatric HS patients due to the poor controllability of the embolic range.

Our study aims to accurately predict the extent of splenic embolism by further improving and optimizing PSE for super-selective cannulation of the splenic artery. The present study reports on the feasibility and efficacy of super-selective partial splenic embolization (SPSE) in a cohort of 16 children with HS.

STUDY PATIENTS

This study was conducted by retrospectively reviewing clinical data from 58 children patients with HS diagnosed at the Children's Hospital of Chongqing Medical University from January 2015 to December 2020, and the last follow-up visit was October 2021. The Children' s Hospital approved our study of Chongqing Medical University (No: 2020-288), and informed consent was obtained to review patients' medical records. We excluded one patient with splenectomy because follow-up data were lacking, leaving 57 patients for the study. All eligible patients were assessed according to the BCSH 2011 guidelines and European Hematology Association 2017 guidelines (2, 3), while only patients with moderate, severe HS, or impact daily life were operated on. Grouping was based on the treatment intention, 41 patients had undergone total splenectomy (median age 9, range 2–17 years), and 16 patients had undergone SPSE (median age 7 years, range 5–11 years). Before receiving the surgery, all patients and guardians were provided with two surgical consent forms for splenectomy and SPES surgery. The consent forms consist of detailed explanations on the two surgical treatment options to ensure that each patient and guardian fully understood the advantages and disadvantages of both surgical options before making their decision (for details, see Appendix).

SPSE SURGERY PROCEDURE

We performed super-selective embolization of the middle and lower parts of the spleen using splenic artery trunk angiography to analyze the distribution of splenic segmental arteries. The expected embolism range was 70–85%. The specific surgical procedure was as follows:

First, splenic arteriogram procedure: The patients were placed in the supine position, a 4Fr introducer sheath (RS*A40G07SQ, TERUMO) was inserted through the right common femoral artery by using the Seldinger technique, and a 4Fr catheter (RF*ZB54110, TERUMO) was passed through the main trunk of the splenic artery for imaging. Based on the visualization of the splenic vessels, adopting splenic segmental arteries in the lower and middle spleen as the target vessel, the arterial embolization, which was confirmed, by contrast, was performed by a 2.7 Fr microcatheter (MC-PE27131, TERUMO) to super-select the splenic segmental arteries.

Secondly, the configuration of embolic agents: Mixing polyvinyl alcohol granules (PVA-500, COOK) 1 g and lodixanol 320 (GE Healthcare Ireland) 5 ml thoroughly, extract 2 ml of suspension and add 0.25 g of triple cephalosporin, then add the appropriate amount of contrast agent to make a total of 15 ml of the embolic agent.

Third, embolization procedure: The embolization area was mainly in the middle and lower spleen, preserving most of the upper spleen and the splenic hilum. At the same time, the degree of embolization was judged by the intraoperative flow velocity of the embolized artery. The degree of embolization was determined according to a slight slowing of the flow as 30–40%, a marked slowing as 50–60%, a peristaltic advance after briefly stopped as 70–80%, a significant regurgitation as 90% and above. The extent of splenic embolism was predicted by the above two aspects. After completing embolization, the degree of embolization was determined again by imaging the main trunk of the splenic artery. If the embolic scope is insufficient, additional embolization operations can be performed until the embolic scope reaches 70–85%. Sterile gauze and pressure were applied to the puncture site for hemostasis, followed by bandaging and braking for 6–8 h. The operation time only requires 30 min maximum. The patency of splenic vein flow was detected by vascular ultrasound 3 days after surgery, and third-generation cephalosporin was applied by intravenous prophylactic in 48 h after surgery.

DATA COLLECTION AND FOLLOW-UP

We collected pre- and post-operative examination data of patients who underwent total splenectomy and SPSE, with a minimum 12-months follow-up. The last follow-up was in September 2020. The patients underwent CT scan using a 64-channel multidetector CT system (Lig_x0002_htspeed VCT, GE Medical Systems, USA). The Volume Rendering function analyzed splenic volumes with the Philips intellispace portal software platform, version 6.0.1.20700.

STATISTICAL METHODS

Statistical analyses were performed using the SPSS software version 22.0. Measurement data were expressed as mean ± SD and analyzed by Student's t-test. Enumeration data were expressed as a rate (%), and a Chi-square test was adopted. Comparison of laboratory parameters after splenic artery embolization was carried out using the paired t-test, the Wilcoxon signed ranks test, the Mann–Whitney U-test, or the chi-square test. Statistical significance was defined as $p < 0.05$.

RESULTS

No cases of serious post-operative complications or post-splenectomy infections were found in either group within 6 months after surgery during the follow-up period. There was no statistical difference in the pre-operative condition of the two groups (**Table 1**), and hemolysis was significantly improved in both groups. The average hemoglobin value was increased significantly from 7.4 g/dl before total splenectomy to 11.7 g/dl after total splenectomy ($p < 0.001$). The average hemoglobin value was increased significantly from 6.97 g/dl before SPSE to 12.2 g/dl after SPSE ($p < 0.001$).

The surgical results are in **Table 2**. Before and after embolization, the arterial phase showed the branches and

TABLE 1 | Comparison of clinical characteristics of patients undergoing total splenectomy and super-selective partial splenic embolization (SPSE).

	total splenectomy		SPSE		chi-square value /Z value	P
	$N = 41$	median (range)	$N = 16$	median (range)		
male (%)		53.7%		37.5%	1.202	0.273
Mean age at surgery, y		9 (2–17)		7 (5–11)	−1.563	0.118
Mean hemoglobin before surgery, g/L		74 (18–95)		68.5 (56–80)	−0.275	0.783
Mean hemoglobin after surgery, g/L		117 (97–175)		124 (104–133)	−0.703	0.482
Mean free bilirubin before surgery, μmol/L		109.45 (21.80–237.80)		61.4 (16.0–146.0)	−0.071	0.943
Mean free bilirubin after surgery, μmol/L		42.87 (2.80–66.80)		13.35 (7.00–86.00)	−1.633	0.102
Mean platelet count beforesurgery, $\times 10^9$/L		188 (27–364)		121 (77–333)	−1.368	0.171
Mean platelet count after surgery, $\times 10^9$/L		418 (165–1416)		442 (311–643)	−2.246	0.025
Mean white blood cell count before surgery, $\times 10^9$/L		5.57 (3.28–25.06)		7.37 (5.27–18.00)	−0.906	0.365
Mean white blood cell count after surgery, $\times 10^9$/L		7.09 (3.68–13.12)		10.11 (3.40–15.70)	−2.790	0.005

TABLE 2 | General conditions and surgical results in children with partial splenic artery embolization.

NO	Age at diagnosis (y)	Age at surgery, (y)	Estimated embolism range (%)	preoperative spleen volume (cm^3)	Postoperative spleen volume[a] (cm^3)	Actual embolism range (%)	Duration of postoperative abdominal pain (d)	Duration of postoperative fever (d)	Number of postoperative vomiting
1	1	5	75	NA	NA	NA	7	6	0
2	4	5	85	NA	NA	NA	6	5	1
3	1	6	80	NA	NA	NA	8	0	0
4	1	7	75	NA	NA	NA	9	0	0
5	2	7	85	NA	NA	NA	6	0	0
6	6	11	85	254.9	30.0	88.2	5	0	1
7	1	7	75	534.0	98.5	81.6	3	0	3
8	6	7	80	545.3	135.0	75.2	7	0	0
9	4	6	75	292.8	78.5	73.2	0	0	0
10	2	7	90	826.8	90.3	89.1	6	0	0
11	5	6	80	263.9	60.9	76.9	5	2	0
12	10	11	90	679.0	112.2	83.5	8	0	2
13	3	8	80	719.5	88.1	87.8	3	0	0
14	3	9	85	598.6	153.9	74.3	6	0	0
15	7	8	85	346.1	48.5	86.0	0	0	1
16	1	5	80	651.2	190.7	70.7	3	1	0

[a] *CT scan was arranged 6–9 days after SPSE.*

distribution of the splenic arteries, and the equilibrium phase showed the distribution of the parenchymal blood supply to the spleen (**Figure 1**).

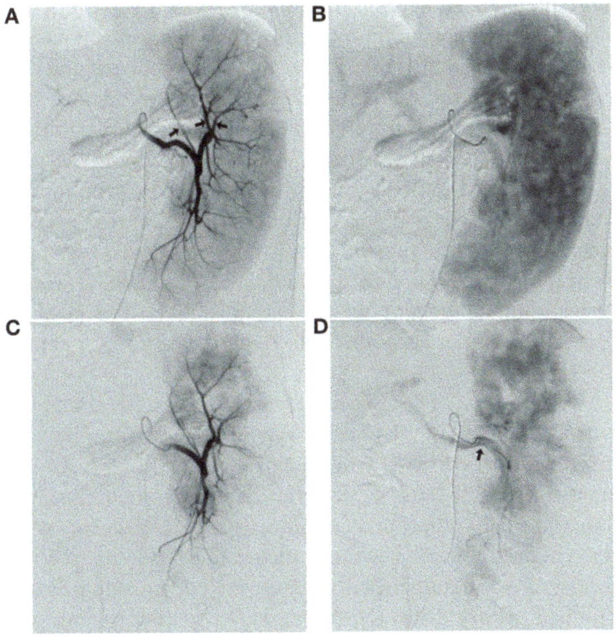

FIGURE 1 | (A) Image of the splenic segment arteries in arterial phase, with the planned preservation of the superior pole splenic segment artery shown by the arrow; **(B)** Image of the spleen in the equilibrium phase, showing the full projected area of the spleen; **(C)** Image of splenic segment artery after super-selective partial splenic embolization (SPSE) with preserved superior pole splenic segment artery; image of the spleen in equilibrium after SPSE with the area of residual spleen projection, with estimated embolization extent of up to 90% compared to **(B)**; **(D)** Splenic vein imaging.

The 16 children underwent embolization of the middle and lower pole of the spleen, and the expected intraoperative embolization extent was 75–90%. Pre-embolization and post-embolization (7–9 days) CT examinations were completed in 11 patients. The pre- and post-embolization spleen volumes were calculated, and the actual splenic embolic extent was 73.2–89.1% (**Figure 2**). The difference between the pre-assessed embolic extent and the actual post-operative embolic extent was not statistically significant. This result suggests that SPSE can accurately determine the extent of splenic embolization intraoperatively.

All patients treated with SPSE had no serious complications (**Table 2**) but experienced a milder post-embolization syndrome. Approximately 87.5% (14/16) of children presented with mild abdominal pain with median abdominal pain duration of 6 days (range 0–9 days), which could easily be controlled with appropriate supportive therapy. Post-operative fever and vomiting occurred in 25.0% (4/16) and 31.3% (5/16) of the children, both of which resolved rapidly on autonomy. No other serious complications, such as splenic abscess, portal vein embolism, pancreatitis, and pulmonary atelectasis, occurred.

The median follow-up time for this group of patients was 26 months (19–41 months), all children showed significant improvement in hemolysis, and no patient underwent transfusion for hemolysis during the follow-up period. Notably, there were no significant abnormalities in the common immune indicators before and after surgery, suggesting that the patient retained splenic immune function after surgery (**Table 3**).

DISCUSSION

Total splenectomy is a proven and effective method for treating patients with moderate to severe HS (3). The spleen is the largest peripheral lymphoid organ in the body, and it is an

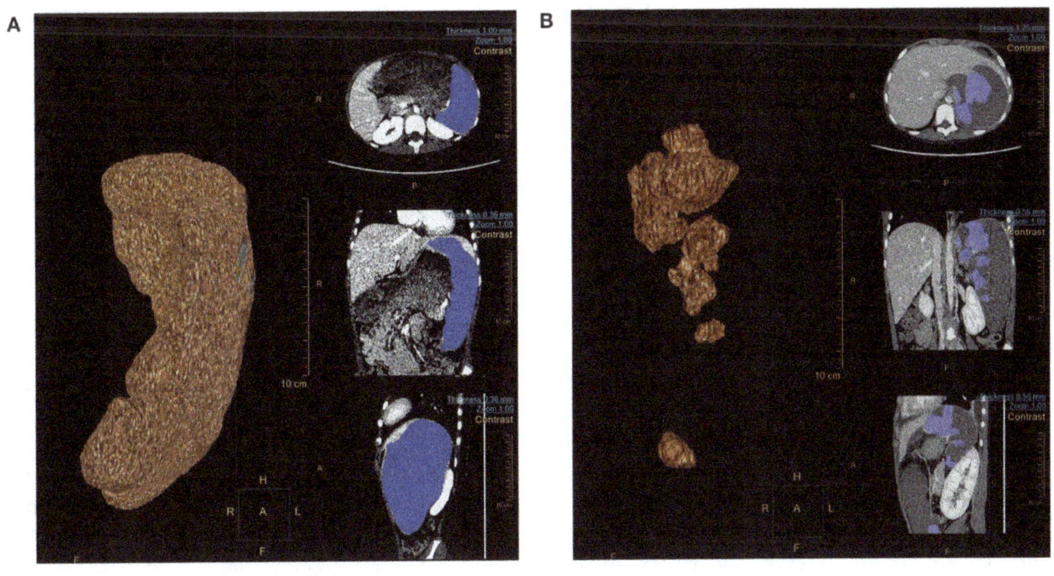

FIGURE 2 | (A) Spleen volume (679.0 cm^3) before embolization; **(B)** Spleen volume (112.2 cm^3) 1 week after embolization.

TABLE 3 | Comparison of clinical indicators before and after surgery in patients undergoing SPSE.

	preoperative	Postoperative [a]	t/Z	P
Spleen volume (cm^3)	545.72 ± 190.97	105.66 ± 45	7.90	<0.001
white blood cell count before surgery, $\times 10^9$/L	8.38 ± 3.05	9.78 ± 1.91	−1.59	0.132
hemoglobin before surgery	69.73 ± 6.88	122.13 ± 9.86	−16.19	<0.001
platelet count, $\times 10^9$/L	220.19 ± 60.90	425.20 ± 70.72	−11.64	<0.001
free bilirubin, µmol/L	61.40 (16–146)	13.35 (7.00–86.00)	−3.52	<0.001
IgG, g/L	11.51 ± 2.81	12.21 ± 3.84	−0.99	0.336
IgA, g/L	1.97 ± 0.81	2.17 ± 0.83	−1.30	0.214
IgE, g/L	10.3 (0.6–152)	12.55 (2.6–202)	−1.24	0.211
IgM, g/L	1.32 ± 0.53	1.28 ± 0.52	0.38	0.711
Complement C3, g/L	0.57 ± 0.08	0.82 ± 0.21	−5.90	<0.001
Complement C4, g/L	0.15 ± 0.04	0.20 ± 0.05	−4.75	<0.001

[a]*6 months after SPSE.*

indispensable immune barrier when the body receives external viruses and bacteria. The absence of a spleen might lead to an infection outbreak. For pediatric patients, possible post-operative aggressive complications, such as OPSI and surgical trauma, have been a long-term problem for physicians and patients. In 1973, Maddison (7) proposed splenic artery embolization as a minimally invasive procedure for treating hypersplenism that solves the problem of severe trauma. Spigos et al. (8) developed transcatheter PSE in adult HS to preserve the immune function of the spleen (5, 6). However, PSE has not been widely promoted in pediatric patients because of the poor controllability of the extent of PSE embolization. Later, conservative surgical options (such as partial splenectomy and partial splenic artery ligation) were considered viable options for HS because they preserved sufficient splenic tissue and relieving anemia, but neither could avoid the trauma of laparotomy.

In our study, based on the unique anatomy of the spleen and splenic artery, selective embolization of splenic segmental arteries branches was performed in the spleen by intraoperative angiography. We measured the embolic artery blood flow velocity and performed a comprehensive re-evaluation of the extent of splenic embolization to predict splenic embolic volume accurately. The extent of spleen volume examined by CT before and after embolization was 70–85%, consistent with the pre-evaluation results. Therefore, we believe SPSE can precisely control the degree of splenic embolization to achieve a therapeutic effect of reducing hemolysis. In this study, all the patients had moderate or severe HS. Post-operative hemolysis was significantly improved; no further transfusions were performed in our patients. Previous studies had shown that PSE effectively reduced the degree of hemolysis while maintaining the phagocytic function of the splenic remnant and the selective destruction of the spleen to defective red blood cells (5).

As with partial splenic artery resection and partial splenic artery ligation, this study was also effective in reducing the volume of the spleen and maintaining the immune function of the splenic to some extent (9). Compared to the preoperative period, the mild elevation of the complement system was considered an effect possibly related to surgical embolization (10, 11). The complement system exerts innate immune by lysing or killing bacteria, modulating phagocytosis, or participating in antibody-mediated specific immune responses. Our study also showed that all splenic immune functions were maintained in the normal range after SPSE and no surgery-related infection of SPSE during the follow-up period. Thus, we demonstrated that SPSE substantially improved in maintaining normal immune function than total splenectomy. We are aware that the younger the patients with HS diagnosis, the severer the symptoms of hemolytic anemia may have. Considering the risk of post-splenectomy fulminant infection, many patients with total splenectomy were significantly older. We believe SPSE preserves normal immune function while treating HS offers the possibility of surgery at earlier ages, and reduces complications for patients with HS.

These study's post-embolization syndromes are minor and controllable, mainly manifested by abdominal pain, fever, and vomiting. Most patients' symptoms resolve within 1 week after surgery. 87.5% (14/16) of children had mild abdominal pain with a median duration of 6 days (range 0–9 days), which most children tolerated without medication, and children with more severe abdominal pain were given 1–2 oral nonsteroidal antiinflammatory drugs (NSAIDs) daily (e.g., ibuprofen), post-operative fever lasting 1–6 days was observed in 25.0% (4/16) of the children, who also received ibuprofen orally and had a rapid decrease in temperature to normal, without recurrent daily fever and signs of infection. 31.3% (5/16) of the children had post-operative vomiting lasting 1–3 days, 1–2 times daily, and the vomitus was all gastric juice. All SPSE-treated patients did not develop other serious complications, such as splenic abscess, portal vein embolism, pancreatitis, or pulmonary atelectasis, during the follow-up time. All children treated with splenectomy had wound pain lasting 3–5 days, which most children tolerated without medication, and the more severe children were given oral NSAIDs (e.g., ibuprofen) 1–2 times daily for 2–3 days, all tolerating the pain. All children had fasted for 1–3 days after surgery. 7.3% (3/41) of the children had electrolyte disturbance after surgery, corrected with intravenous rehydration, and recovered. 7.3% (3/41) of the children had severe infections after surgery. On the fourth day after surgery, one case had severe pneumonia and respiratory failure. It was treated with a ventilator in ICU, and one case had pneumonia and atelectasis on the right side 5 days after surgery, which was treated with fiberoptic bronchoscopy and improved. One case developed abdominal infection 33 months after surgery and improved after reoperation. A child with splenectomy was found to have partial portal vein thrombosis during follow-up and improved after anticoagulation.

The previous studies have shown that common complications of total splenectomy include postoperative infection, OPSI, surgical bleeding, injury of adjacent organs, and VTE (2, 12, 13). The most severe complications of PSE are abdominal infection and spleen abscess formation, which is deadly for patients in severe cases (14). The cause of spleen abscess formation includes excessive embolization, which leads to liquefied necrosis of a large amount of spleen tissue and secondary bacterial infection. There are two possible sources of bacteria; one of them is interventional contamination. The other is that the enteric-derived bacteria retained in the portal venous system reverse into the spleen since the slow flow speed in the splenic vein after massive embolization of the splenic parenchyma (15). However, no patient had a splenic abscess in this study. The reason to do this study is as follows. Firstly, the number of patients is still small. Secondly, SPSE achieved the purpose of accurate embolization by the accurate selection of secondary arteries and narrowing the possibility of infection caused by stagnation of splenic vein blood flow, which is the result of over embolization of splenic artery trunk. Thirdly, the minified dosage of embolic agent during treatment also indirectly diminishes the risk of contamination. There is no exposure of significant flow stagnation or reflux in the splenic artery angiogram after SPSE had been confirmed by the color ultrasonography of the blood flow of the splenic vein 3 days after the procedure. In addition, triple cephalosporin was intravenously applied within 48 h postoperatively. Since these preventative anti-infection actions were actively performed, the risk of splenic infection was minimized by avoiding possible intraoperative contamination and post-operative entheogenic infection to the greatest extent.

A few reports of the previous study showed the growth of residual accessory spleen after total splenectomy (16), or growth of residual spleen after partial splenectomy trigger recurrence of anemia which requires secondary surgery (17, 18). In a long-term follow-up study of partial splenectomy (19), mild and moderate hemolysis may be a long-term symptom after partial splenectomy, and a small number of patients may be at risk of secondary gallstones and hemolytic anemia. In our observed SPSE patients with a median follow-up time of 22 months, there are no cases of hemolytic anemia which requires transfusion therapy, only a few children have mild hemolysis, and all patients with SPSE recovered well after surgery. We believe that the better results were mainly because the accurate control of embolization preserved only a tiny portion of the upper splenic (10–25%); moreover, the growth of the normal residual spleen was effectively limited by the blockage of the diaphragm and embolized spleen. Since we preserved the splenic artery trunk upfront, there is an opportunity to do another embolization as a re-intervention if symptomatic recurrence of anemia appeared at a later stage. The shortage of this study is the short follow-up period. Hence, long-term follow-up should be applied to clarify the dynamic changes of spleen volume and hemolysis after embolization. We considered modified super selective partial splenic artery embolization as a conservative surgical treatment for posterior globules.

The current study focuses on the safety of SPSE, so the initial case selection tends to be for the traditional splenectomy indication. We suggest splenectomy for children with HS who remain transfusion-dependent or have severe symptoms related to anemia after 1 year of age. If necessary, a total splenectomy can be postponed until after 6 years of age. Our current study follows the willingness of the child's guardian to treat the choice of surgical approach after detailed knowledge of the advantages and disadvantages of both surgical options, so the fact that the children treated with SPES were above 5 years of age is related to the small sample size. SPES is technically feasible for children with HS at 5 years or even younger. We have treated a 1-year-old child with Wiskott–Aldrich syndrome, and after a multidisciplinary assessment that splenectomy may pose a high risk of death, we successfully managed the symptoms and safely treated the child with SPES until he was treated with a hematopoietic stem cell transplant.

In conclusion, SPSE is a reliable, safe, and effective alternative to splenectomy for childhood HS, which resolved the disadvantage of difficulty in estimating the volume of splenic artery embolization and avoided the trauma of partial splenectomy and partial splenic artery ligation. SPSE may have more tremendous advantages on expanding the age range of surgery, reducing the severity of surgical trauma, and minimizing the possibility of infection. However, a more extended follow-up period, a larger sample size, and applying other indications, such as hypersplenism, are mandatory for the further assessment of SPSE.

ETHICS STATEMENT

The studies involving human participants were reviewed and approved by ethical approval for this study was provided by the Institutional Review Board of CHCMU and registered at No: 2020-288. Written informed consent to participate in this study was provided by the participants' legal guardian/next of kin. Written informed consent was obtained from the minor(s)' legal guardian/next of kin for the publication of any potentially identifiable images or data included in this article.

AUTHOR CONTRIBUTIONS

QX and M-mZ conceived the study and are the principal investigator. QX and R-jW initially designed the study protocol and wrote the first draft of this manuscript. M-mZ coordinated the doctors and nurses. At the same time, QX, R-jW, and M-mZ mainly provided clinical support and led the surgery. LX, X-mX, and R-jW collected and analyzed the data. R-jW and LX revised this manuscript. All authors contributed to subsequent drafts and approved the final manuscript.

ACKNOWLEDGMENTS

The authors would like to thank all families who generously accept participating in this study. The authors would like to thank the doctors and nurses of CHCMU for their facilitation of patients for the study. The authors also gratefully thank Xiao Li for their outstanding work in language editing.

REFERENCES

1. Perrotta S, Gallagher PG, Mohandas N. Hereditary spherocytosis. *Lancet.* (2008) 372:1411–26. doi: 10.1016/S0140-6736(08)61588-3
2. Iolascon A, Andolfo I, Barcellini W, Corcione F, Garçon L, De Franceschi L, et al. Recommendations regarding splenectomy in hereditary hemolytic anemias. *Haematologica.* (2017) 102:1304–13. doi: 10.3324/haematol.2016.161166
3. Bolton-Maggs PH, Langer JC, Iolascon A, Tittensor P, King MJ, General Haematology Task Force of the British Committee for Standards in Haematology. Guidelines for the diagnosis and management of hereditary spherocytosis—2011 update. *Br J Haematol.* (2012) 156:37–49. doi: 10.1111/j.1365-2141.2011.08921.x
4. Smedema JP, Louw VJ. Pulmonary arterial hypertension after splenectomy for hereditary spherocytosis. *Cardiovasc J Afr.* (2007) 18:84–9. doi: 10.10520/EJC24181
5. Pratl B, Benesch M, Lackner H, Portugaller HR, Pusswald B, Sovinz P, et al. Partial splenic embolization in children with hereditary spherocytosis. *Eur J Haematol.* (2008) 80:76–80. doi: 10.1111/j.1600-0609.2007.00979.x
6. Kimura F, Ito H, Shimizu H, Togawa A, Otsuka M, Yoshidome H, et al. Partial splenic embolization for the treatment of hereditary spherocytosis. *AJR Am J Roentgenol.* (2003) 181:1021–4. doi: 10.2214/ajr.181.4.1811021
7. Maddison FE. Embolic Therapy of Hypersplenism. *Invest Radiol.* (1973) 8:280–1. doi: 10.1097/00004424-197307000-00054
8. Spigos DG, Jonasson O, Mozes M, Capek V. Partial splenic embolization in the treatment of hypersplenism. *AJR Am J Roentgenol.* (1979) 132:777–82. doi: 10.2214/ajr.132.5.777
9. Balaphas A, Buchs NC, Meyer J, Hagen ME, Morel P. Partial splenectomy in the era of minimally invasive surgery: the current laparoscopic and robotic experiences. *Surg Endosc.* (2015) 29:3618–27. doi: 10.1007/s00464-015-4118-9
10. Walport MJ. Complement. *First of two parts N Engl J Med.* (2001) 344:1058–66. doi: 10.1056/NEJM200104053441406
11. Walport MJ. Advances in immunology: Complement (second of two parts). *N Engl J Med.* (2001) 344:1140. doi: 10.1056/NEJM200104123441506
12. Perkins LA, Jones SF, Bhargava RS. Dural venous thrombosis following splenectomy in a patient with hereditary spherocytosis. *South Med J.* (2009) 102:542–5. doi: 10.1097/SMJ.0b013e31819e90b5
13. Davidsen C, Larsen TH, Gerdts E, Lønnebakken MT. Giant right ventricular outflow tract thrombus in hereditary spherocytosis: a case report. *Thromb J.* (2016) 14:9. doi: 10.1186/s12959-016-0083-3
14. Cai M, Huang W, Lin C, Li Z, Qian J, Huang M, et al. Partial splenic embolization for thrombocytopenia in liver cirrhosis: predictive factors for platelet increment and risk factors for major complications. *Eur Radiol.* (2016) 26:370–80. doi: 10.1007/s00330-015-3839-4
15. Masada T, Tanaka T, Sakaguchi H, Nakagomi M, Miura Y, Hidaka T, et al. Coils versus gelatin particles with or without intraarterial antibiotics for partial splenic embolization: a comparative evaluation. *J Vasc Interv Radiol.* (2014) 25:852–8. doi: 10.1016/j.jvir.2013.12.563
16. MACKENZIE AE ELLIOT DH, EASTCOTT HH HUGHESJONES NC, BARKHAN P, MOLLISON PL. Relapse in hereditary spherocytosis with proven splenunculus. *Lancet.* (1962) 1:1102–4. doi: 10.1016/S0140-6736(62)92084-6
17. de Buys Roessingh AS, de Lagausie P, Rohrlich P, Berrebi D, Aigrain Y. Follow-up of partial splenectomy in children with hereditary spherocytosis. *J Pediatr Surg.* (2002) 37:1459–63. doi: 10.1053/jpsu.2002.35412
18. Rice HE, Oldham KT, Hillery CA, Skinner MA, O'Hara SM, Ware RE. Clinical and hematologic benefits of partial splenectomy for congenital hemolytic anemias in children. *Ann Surg.* (2003) 237:281–8. doi: 10.1097/01.SLA.0000048453.61168.8F
19. Bader-Meunier B, Gauthier F, Archambaud F, Cynober T, Miélot F, Dommergues JP, et al. Long-term evaluation of the beneficial effect of subtotal splenectomy for management of hereditary spherocytosis. *Blood.* (2001) 97:399–403. doi: 10.1182/blood.V97.2.399

6

Super-Minimal Incision Technique in Pediatric Kidney Transplantation: A Paired Kidney Analysis

*Junxiang Wang, Lixiang Zhao, Guiwen Feng and Wenjun Shang**

The Department of Kidney Transplantation, The First Affiliated Hospital of Zhengzhou University, Zhengzhou, China

Correspondence:
Wenjun Shang
fccshangwj@zzu.edu.cn

Background: Recently, the demand for minimally invasive techniques in kidney transplantation (MIKT) has increased. However, there is only a limited number of studies on MIKT, especially in pediatric kidney transplants. Hence, we evaluated whether there is a difference between the super-minimal incision technique in pediatric kidney transplantation (SMIPKT) and conventional kidney transplantation (CKT).

Methods: Between December 2018 and November 2021, 34 patients who underwent pediatric kidney transplantation with a follow-up of 1 month were enrolled. A paired kidney analysis was performed to minimize donor variability and bias. The SMIPKT and CKT groups included 17 patients.

Results: There was no difference in baseline clinical characteristics, including age, sex, the donor/ recipient weight ratio (DRWR), choice of dialysis modality, pretransplant dialysis time, BMI, renal artery number, cause of ESRD, DGF, length of the kidney and cold ischemic time, tacrolimus concentration at 3 and 7 days, serum creatinine at 1 month and postoperative complication rate between the SMIPKT and CKT groups (all $P > 0.05$). However, the length of the incision, operation time, intraoperative bleeding, postoperative drainage volume within 24 h and Vancouver scar scale at 1 month were statistically significant (all $P < 0.05$).

Conclusion: Compared with CKT, our results indicated that SMIPKT showed more satisfactory cosmetic results, shorter SMIPKT operating time, and reduced intraoperative bleeding and postoperative drainage volume within 24 h. There were also no statistical differences in postoperative complications. Hence, we suggest that SMIPKT is an appropriate method for pediatric kidney transplantation.

Keywords: pediatric kidney transplantation, super-minimal incision, conventional kidney transplantation, postoperative complications, cosmetic result

INTRODUCTION

Minimally invasive surgery (MIS) in laparoscopic living donor nephrectomy has become an optimal choice for many transplant centers (1, 2). Compared with open, conventional operations in living donor nephrectomy, the advantages of MIS include reduced tissue trauma and postoperative pain, and pleasing cosmetic results (3, 4). However, in the past few years, there have only been limited reports of minimally invasive techniques for adult kidney transplantation (MIKT) (5, 6), but few publications on pediatric kidney transplantation (PKT). Considering the potential advantages of reducing incision/tissue trauma in immunosuppressed pediatric kidney transplant recipients, a super-minimal incision technique (~4–6 cm) in pediatric kidney transplantation (SMIPKT) was evaluated in our transplant center. Therefore, the aim of the present study was to evaluate whether there is a difference between SMIPKT and conventional kidney transplantation (CKT) and the effectiveness of SMIPKT in pediatric recipients.

MATERIALS AND METHODS

Experimental Design

This was a single-center retrospective study. A paired kidney analysis was performed to minimize donor variability and bias. Thirty-four grafts from 17 pediatric donors after cardiac death were distributed to our transplant center using China's organ distribution system. Pediatric recipients from the same pediatric donor were divided into the SMIPKT and CKT groups, depending on whether the incision was minimal or not. All surgeons have been performing kidney transplantation for over 10 years.

Inclusion and Exclusion Criteria

The inclusion criteria were <18 years, first kidney transplantation, and no previous surgery at the transplant site.

The exclusion criteria were older than 18 years, more than two kidney grafts, En bloc or dual kidney transplantation, or only one kidney was distributed to our transplant center by China's organ distribution system.

Surgical Technique

SMIPKT

Before transplantation, we performed a careful back-table kidney preparation (**Figures 1A,B**). In SMIPKT, we used an incision starting 2–3 cm below the umbilicus and extending 4–6 cm along the outer edge of the rectus abdominis (**Figures 2A,B**). The length of the incision was selected based on the size of the graft. Only the "conjoined tendon" and hardly any muscular tissue were divided. The inferior abdominal vessels, spermatic cord, or ovoid ligament need not be dissected. The origin of the internal iliac artery and its terminal branches, the external iliac vein, and the bladder can be fully exposed and dissected in a minimalistic fashion (**Figures 2C, 3A,B**). After the back-table preparation of the kidney was completed, the renal graft was wrapped with gauze, leaving only vessels for anastomosis, and then placed into a custom-made ice bag wrapped with ice sludge for cooling. The graft vein was anastomosed to the external iliac vein (end-to-side), and the graft artery was anastomosed to the internal iliac artery (end-to-end). A continuous suture with 6-0 SurgiPro was used for both vascular anastomoses (**Figure 3C**). Following anastomosis, intraluminal air was thoroughly excluded by infusing heparin saline. The graft blood flow was then opened (**Figures 3D,E**). The graft ureter was anastomosed to the recipient's bladder with running sutures using 5-0 absorbable suture via the Lich-Gregoir technique with a 3–4.7 Fr double J stent. All incisions were sutured subcutaneously using 3-0 absorbable sutures. The blood loss of all patients was collected using a negative pressure suction device during surgery. Blood loss and abdominal fluid drainage were precisely measured using a self-control precision metering drainage bag (**Figure 3F**). The short right renal vein was extended by reconstruction using the vena cava.

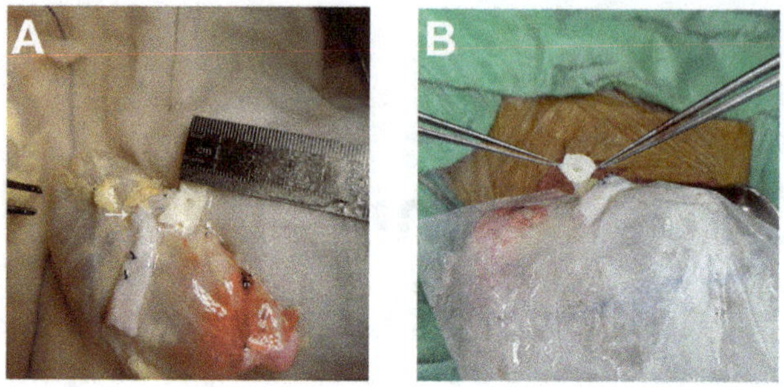

FIGURE 1 | A careful back-table preparation of the kidney. **(A)** The short right renal vein was extended by reconstruction using the vena cava (white arrow). **(B)** Tailored aortic patch.

CKT

Conventional pediatric Gibson's technique has been practiced for years (from 2008 to 2021, 60–100 pediatric kidney transplantations per year) in our transplantation center, with an incision ~8–14 cm in length in the lower right abdomen (**Figures 2D,E**). The inferior abdominal vessels and ovoid ligament were ligated, and the spermatic cord was dissociated. Through the skin and muscular layers, with wide extraperitoneal exposure of the internal/external iliac artery and external iliac vein, the lymphatic trunks alongside the vessels and the small branches of peripheral blood vessels were ligated. The remaining surgical steps were applied in a similar manner to the patients in the SMIPKT group.

Postoperative Management

All postoperative patients were admitted to the ICU of the kidney transplantation ward for 5 days. Central venous cannulation, with catheter placement by either the subclavian or internal jugular vein, has been well-established to monitor central venous pressure. Continuous non-invasive blood pressure monitoring is necessary during the 1st week after surgery, and the blood pressure is allowed to fluctuate between 100/60 and 120/80 mmHg. The drainage fluid and urine output were recorded per hour.

Immunosuppression Protocol

All recipients received a reduced dose of anti-human T lymphocyte rabbit immunoglobulin + methylprednisolone (cumulative 18–21 mg/kg) for preoperative induction and postoperative prevention of rejection. A triple immunosuppressive regimen of CNI combined with mycophenolate mofetil (MMF) and prednisone was administered postoperatively. The initial dose of tacrolimus was determined

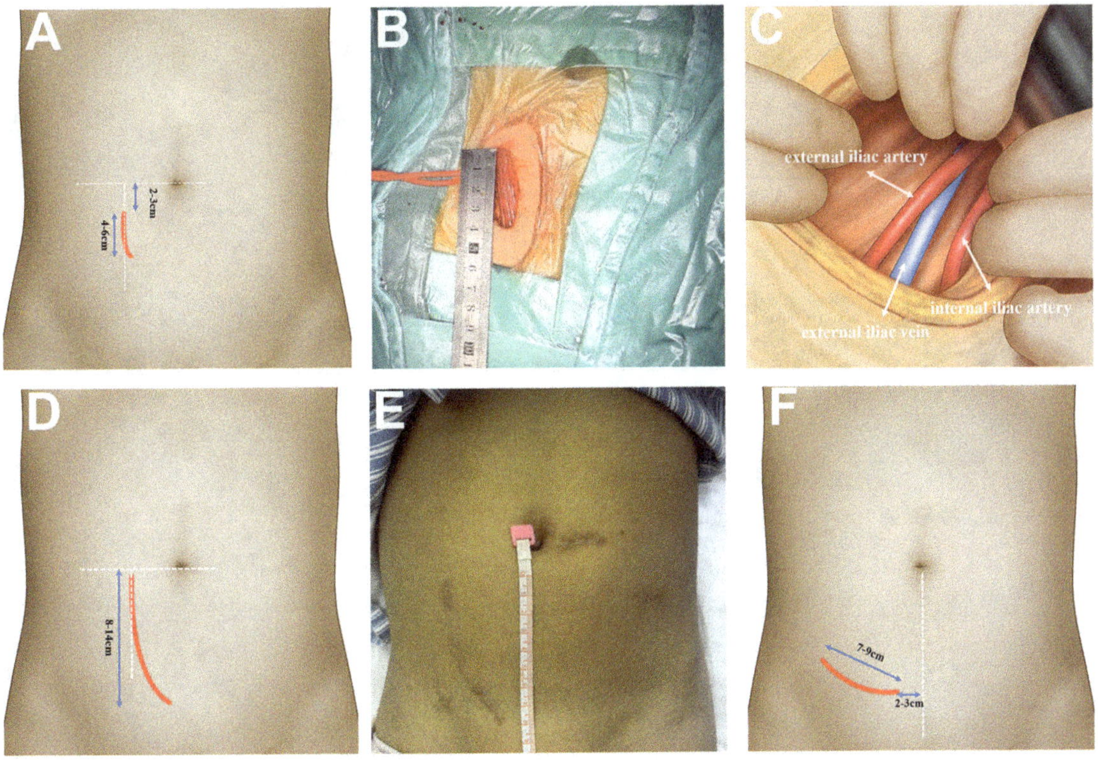

FIGURE 2 | The operative approach of SMIPKT and CKT. **(A)** The operative approach of SMIPKT. **(B)** A ~4 cm incision in SMIPKT in a 9-year-old patient. **(C)** The internal iliac artery and the external iliac vein were fully exposed and dissected free in a minimalistic fashion in SMIPKT. **(D)** The operative approach of CKT. **(E)** A ~8.5 cm incision in CKT (final result 2 years post-transplant in a 9-year-old patient). **(F)** The transverse incision of MIKT by Oyen and Kim.

according to the CYP3A5 genotype, and the target tacrolimus trough concentrations were monitored weekly during the first 3 months.

Statistical Analysis

The data were analyzed using SPSS for Windows (SPSS, version 19; IBM Corporation, Armonk, NY, USA). Parametric and non-parametric data are presented as mean ± standard deviation (SD) or median with range. Categorical variables are expressed as frequencies and percentages. We used the *t*-test to compare the parametric continuous variables. Meanwhile, the Mann-Whitney *U*-test was used for non-parametric continuous variables. Statistical significance was set at $p < 0.05$.

RESULTS

The median age was 13 years in the SMIPKT group and 14 in the CKT group, and 64.7% of the patients were male. Among the SMIPKT and CKT groups, other clinical characteristics, including DRWR, the choice of dialysis modality, pretransplant dialysis time, body mass index (BMI), renal artery number, cause of ESRD, DGF, length of the kidney, and cold ischemic time were statistically insignificant (all $P > 0.05$) (**Table 1**). More details are shown in **Table 2**.

Naturally, the SMIPKT skin incision was much shorter, and there were significant differences in terms of operative time, intraoperative bleeding, postoperative drainage volume within 24 h, and Vancouver scar scale at 1 month (all $P < 0.05$). Considering the effect of immunosuppressants on wound healing, tacrolimus trough concentration was monitored on postoperative days 3 and 7, and there was no significant difference between the SMIPKT and CKT groups ($P > 0.05$). Although the serum creatinine level at 1 month in the SMIPKT group was slightly lower than that in the CKT group, there was no statistically significant difference between the two groups ($P > 0.05$) (**Table 1**).

During the 30 days follow-up, there was no wound infection, wound dehiscence, incisional hernia, or lymphocele. However, one pediatric recipient with a diagnosis of urologic stenosis in the SMIPKT group and one with a diagnosis of urine leakage in the CKT group was confirmed by computerized tomography (CT) urography. A child with urologic stenosis underwent early ureteral reimplantation. Two pediatric recipients with stable graft renal function and no hypertension (1 in each group, $P = 1.000$) had a confirmed vascular complication of transplant renal artery stenosis on CT angiography.

The primary diseases of all patients are shown in **Table 1**. However, two patients showed non-surgical-related complications. One patient in each group relapsed with focal

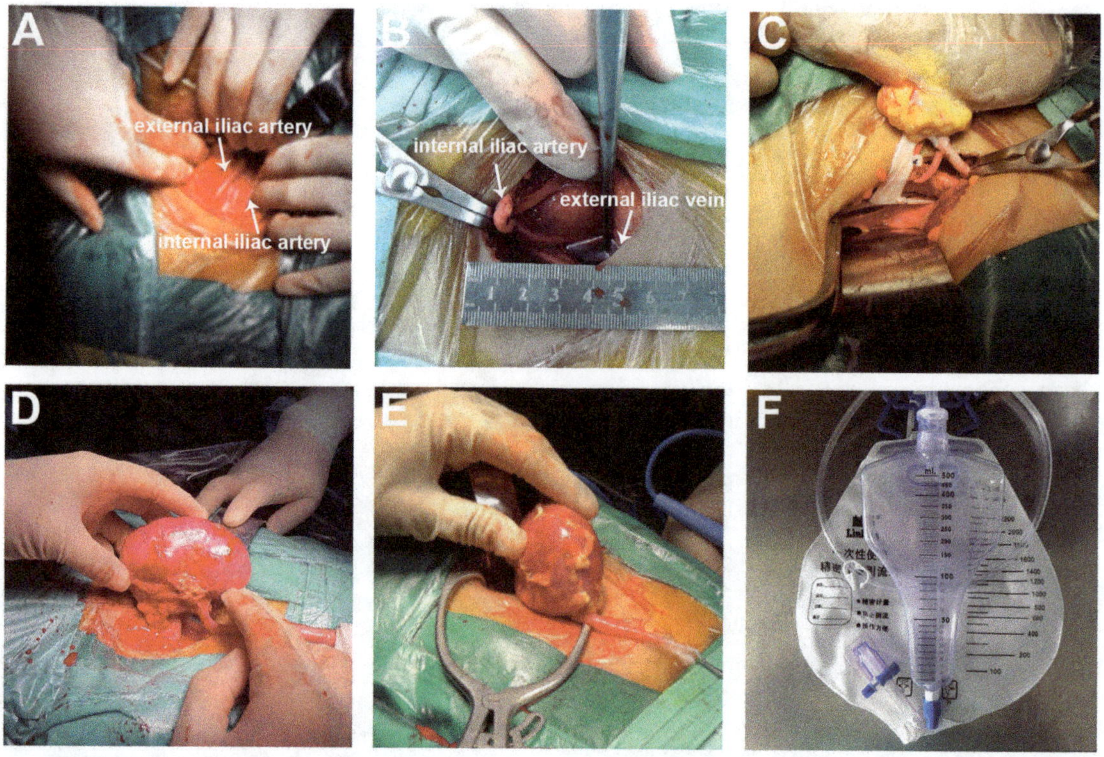

FIGURE 3 | The SMIPKT surgical technique. **(A,B)** Full exposure with minimal dissection of the external iliac artery (white arrow), iliac artery (white arrow), and the external iliac vein (white arrow). **(C)** The two vascular anastomoses were performed with renal graft in a custom-made ice bag wrapped in ice sludge. **(D)** Minimal incision can be smaller than the kidney. **(E)** The upper pole of renal graft was placed into the iliac fossa at first. **(F)** Blood loss and postoperative drainage volume are precisely measured through a self-control precision metering drainage bag.

segmental glomerular sclerosis (FSGS) in the early postoperative period after kidney transplantation.

DISCUSSION

A major point of the present MIS is the reduction of tissue trauma by using limited-sized incisions to obtain less pain and scarring, and a faster recovery period compared to traditional surgery (7, 8). Surprisingly, the original open technique of an oblique Gibson incision of ~20 cm in length remains the gold standard since kidney transplantation was first successfully performed in the 1950's.

MIKT, using a 7–9 cm transverse incision, 3–5 cm above the inguinal ligament, was first described in 21 kidney transplants by Oyen in 2006 (6). Kim (5), Kacar (9), and other similar series published later confirmed that MIKT is feasible and safe (10). Although there are few publications about MIKT in adults, we believe that SMIPKT is feasible and a more obvious choice for several reasons. First, pediatric recipients with end-stage renal disease often experience anemia, hypoalbuminemia, edema, chronic malnutrition, and growth retardation. Furthermore, immunosuppressive drugs must be taken daily or twice daily; in particular, steroids and mycophenolate acid significantly impair wound healing ability. Therefore, pediatric kidney transplant recipients may have a higher risk of wound infection, poor wound healing, and other wound complications than non-immunosuppressed patients after open surgery. Second, some children, especially younger ones, have poor compliance. The advantages of SMIPKT include reduced tissue trauma and pain, faster recovery, and better compliance. Third, the long-term mental health of children after kidney transplantation is important, and small incisions with cosmetic results can weaken the impact of kidney transplants. Fourth, the majority of pediatric candidates in our transplantation center were underweight, with a low BMI ($\leq$20 kg/m^2) due to chronic malnutrition. Moreover, the surgical field could be adequately exposed and clearly visible. Fifth, all renal grafts from pediatric donors after cardiac death were small for size, with an average diameter of 6.4 $\pm$ 1.0 cm in the SMIPKT group and 6.3 $\pm$ 1.1 cm in the CKT group, which did not require a large surgical space. Thus, a smaller incision approach could be easier to achieve.

In our study, among the baseline clinical characteristics, age, sex, DRWR, choice of dialysis modality, pretransplant dialysis time, BMI, renal artery number, cause of ESRD, DGF, length of the kidney and cold ischemic time, tacrolimus concentration at days 3 and 7, serum creatinine at 1 month were found to be statistically insignificant. However, the length of the incision, operation time, intraoperative bleeding, postoperative drainage volume within 24 h, and Vancouver

TABLE 1 | Characteristics of patients.

Variable	SMIPKT group ($n = 17$)	CKT group ($n = 17$)	*P*-value
Age (y), median (IQR)	13.0 (6.5–14.5)	14.0 (10.0–15.0)	0.198
Men, *n* (%)	11 (64.7)	11 (64.7)	1.000
DRWR	1.07 (0.54–1.43)	0.93 (0.45–1.14)	0.234
Dialysis, *n* (%)			0.814
HD	6 (35.3)	7 (41.2)	
PD	9 (52.9)	9 (52.9)	
Preemptive	2 (11.8)	1 (5.9)	
Pretransplant dialysis time (months), median (IQR)	9.0 (6.0–24.0)	12.5 (8.5–17.5)	0.342
BMI (kg/m^2), median (IQR)	15.8 (14.5–17.5)	16.7 (15.0–17.9)	0.428
Multiple renal arteries (≥2), *n* (%)			0.368
2	2 (11.8)	2 (11.8)	
3	0 (0.0)	1 (5.9)	
4	1 (5.9)	0 (0.0)	
Cause of ESRD, *n* (%)			0.765
Primary glomerular diseases	9 (52.9)	8 (47.1)	
Secondary glomerular disease	6 (35.3)	5 (29.4)	
Hereditary nephropathy	1 (5.9)	1 (5.9)	
No data	1 (5.9)	3 (17.6)	
DGF, *n* (%)	0 (0.0)	0 (0.0)	-
Cold ischemic time (h), mean ± SD	12.5 ± 3.0	12.7 ± 2.6	0.913
Length of the kidney (cm), mean ± SD	6.4 ± 1.0	6.3 ± 1.1	0.861
Wound infections	0 (0.0)	0 (0.0)	-
Wound dehiscence	0 (0.0)	0 (0.0)	-
Incisional hernia	0 (0.0)	0 (0.0)	-
Lymphocele	0 (0.0)	0 (0.0)	-
Urologic complications	1 (5.9)	1 (5.9)	1.000
Vascular complications	1 (0.0)	1 (0.0)	1.000
Length of the incision (cm), median (IQR)	4.5 (4.0–5.0)	12 (9.5–13.5)	<0.001
Operation time (min), mean (IQR)	130 (116–143)	162 (136–190)	0.014
Intraoperative bleeding (ml), median (IQR)	40 (30–50)	60 (35–175)	<0.001
Postoperative drainage volume within 24 h (ml), median (IQR)	60 (35–175)	160 (93–360)	0.007
Vancouver scar scale at 1M, median (IQR)	6 (5–6)	7 (6–8)	<0.001
Tacrolimus concentration (ng/ml)at 3d, mean ± SD	13.0 ± 5.0	10.8 ± 3.0	0.137
Tacrolimus concentration (ng/ml)at 1w, mean ± SD	11.1 ± 2.5	10.0 ± 1.7	0.122
Serum creatinine (μmol/L) at 1M, median (IQR)	82 (54–103)	94 (69–124)	0.215

SMIPKT, super-minimal incision technique in pediatric kidney transplantation; CKT, conventional kidney transplantation; DGF, delay graft function; DRWR, donor/ recipient weight ratio.
"-": the two groups were not compared.

scar scale at 1 month were statistically significant between the SMIPKT and CKT groups. We thought that SMIPKT may cause a higher complication rate in vascular and urinary complications, but there were no statistically significant differences in urologic complications (i.e., urologic stenosis or urine leakage), vascular complications (anastomotic stenosis), lymphocele, wound dehiscence, wound infections, and incisional hernia between SMIPKT and CKT groups, which is similar to other reports (6, 9).

Although there was no statistically significant difference in BMI between the SMIPKT and CKT groups, whether BMI really affects SMIPKT is unclear. Despite some limitations in space in obese patients using the small incision technique, there is no drawback in performing the anastomoses in overweight patients up to a BMI of 30 kg/m^2 in Claas Brockschmidt's and >30 kg/m^2 in Oyen's report (4, 6). However, in a subsequent study by Kim, a BMI <25 kg/m^2 was the inclusion criterion for MIKT recipients to ensure adequate exposure to the surgical field (5). Although SMIPKT has been proven successful in pediatric candidates with a BMI >25 kg/m^2 in our transplantation center, it should be noted that the majority of pediatric candidates in our group were lean, with a BMI of <20 kg/m^2, which was much lower than the previously described results. This may be a beneficial factor for SMIPKT. However, considering the limitations in surgical space in obese patients, candidates with a BMI ≥ 30 are still recommended for traditional kidney transplantation technique.

It has not been established whether DRWR mismatch truly affects the application of the super-minimal incision technique. According to our clinical experience with pediatric kidney transplantation, a DRWR mismatch ≤ 3.0 (maximum in this study) is not critical to preventing the use of the super-minimal incision technique. The width of the transplanted kidney (not kidney length) and the length of the recipient internal iliac artery that is sufficient to anastomose the graft artery (end to end) are the two key factors for the successful use of the super-minimal incision technique. However, considering the DRWR > 3, we prefer to recommend the CKT technique.

The operative approach is the key to SMIPKT. Oyen and Kim made a 7–9 cm transverse incision (**Figure 2F**). It is located 3–5 cm above the groin, with the medial endpoint of the incision 2–3 cm from the midline (5, 6). The difference was that the graft artery was anastomosed to the internal iliac artery at our transplant center. Hence, we used an incision starting 2–3 cm below the umbilicus and extending 4–6 cm along the outer edge of the rectus abdominis in SMIPKT. Only the "conjoined tendon" and hardly any muscular tissue were divided. The origin of the internal iliac artery and its terminal branch, the external iliac vein, and the bladder can be fully exposed and dissected in a minimalistic fashion. Currently, the minimum age and weight of the pediatric recipients using the super-minimal incision technique at our transplant center are 1 year old and 5 kg. However, in very young recipients with extremely low body weight ≤ 5 kg or <1 year old, the graft artery is often anastomosed with the common iliac artery or the distal aorta (end-to-side). The super-minimal

TABLE 2 | Detailed clinic characteristics of patients.

	Sex		Age (years)		Weight (kg)		BMI (kg/m^2)	
n	SMIPKT group	CKT group	SMIPKT group	CKT group	SMIPKT group	CKT group	SMIPKT group	CKT group
1	Male	Female	14	15	35.0	45.0	15.7	17.8
2	Male	Female	11	14	30.0	47.0	14.8	17.7
3	Male	Male	9	15	32.0	41.0	15.8	21.2
4	Male	Male	17	14	53.0	40.0	17.5	16.6
5	Female	Male	6	16	19.0	47.0	17.2	16.2
6	Male	Female	13	5	41.0	12.0	18.7	10.9
7	Male	Male	16	15	38.0	46.0	14.5	16.7
8	Male	Male	15	15	40.0	55.0	16.6	22.0
9	Female	Male	14	14	24.0	27.0	14.2	15.9
10	Female	Female	4	9	14.0	20.0	14.3	14.9
11	Female	Male	8	13	25.0	43.0	17.4	17.9
12	Male	Male	16	14	49.0	34.0	18.4	18.7
13	Female	Female	13	9	51.6	24.4	21.8	14.0
14	Female	Female	14	17	40.0	39.0	16.0	17.3
15	Male	Male	2	11	10.5	24.0	14.5	14.2
16	Male	Male	7	9	20.0	21.0	14.4	15.1
17	Male	Male	4	14	14.0	41.0	14.9	17.1

incision does not provide sufficient surgical space for easy dissection of the distal aorta and vascular anastomosis, as well as vesicoureteral replantation using the Lich-Gregoir technique. Therefore, the traditional pediatric kidney transplantation is recommended for very young recipients with extremely low body weight ≤ 5 kg or <1 year old. Moreover, venous anastomosis sites should be evaluated before transplant surgery. A suitable venous anastomosis site and well-tailored allograft vein can avoid kinking. Meanwhile, after reperfusion of the transplanted kidney, the final position of the transplanted kidney can also be adjusted (including adjusting the angle of the allograft or allograft was implanted higher in the retroperitoneal iliac fossa) to avoid kinking.

Another criticism of SMIPKT is that it does not sufficiently cool renal grafts before revascularization. To avoid this, the kidney space was pre-cooled with ice sludge for 5 min in advance. The kidney was then placed with the retroperitoneal pouch into the iliac fossa, and all three anastomoses were performed in the final position. It is not possible to move the kidney from a nearly fitted retroperitoneal pouch. Compared to CKT, the duration of MIKT may be prolonged for all three anastomoses. Studies have revealed that prolonged anastomosis time leads to significantly inferior long-term graft outcomes and patient survival (11, 12). Furthermore, if the renal hilum is bleeding after reperfusion, the kidney needs to be removed from the incision for hemostasis and must be reimplanted into the iliac fossa. When the original incision is insufficient, it must be extended. Therefore, we prefer to perform the two vascular anastomoses outside of the retroperitoneal cavity with renal graft in a custom-made ice bag wrapped in ice sludge, leaving more space, better vision, a simpler inspection of the kidney, and hemostasis after reperfusion.

Our results showed that SMIPKT has a shorter operating time and more favorable cosmetic effects. Moreover, its use seems particularly promising among the immunosuppressed population. Based on our positive experience with SMIPKT, we found it to be technically feasible, and it can be executed safely and quickly by any experienced kidney transplant surgeon after a very short learning curve. Considering that SMIPKT is not only suitable for pediatric recipients with the end-stage renal disease but can also weaken the impact of kidney transplants in children's growth (especially in younger children), we believe that SMIPKT is worth recommending.

The shortcomings of the experimental design are as follows. First, the research took place at a single center with a small number of cases, which needs to be further supplemented. Second, the patients were followed up for a short time; hence, long-term follow-up is still needed.

AUTHOR CONTRIBUTIONS

WS: conceived, designed, and supervised the study. WS, JW, and LZ: performed the experiments. JW: performed data analysis and wrote the paper. All authors revised and reviewed the paper. All authors contributed to the article and approved the submitted version.

ACKNOWLEDGMENTS

The incision pictures were taken by JW and are included with the written authorization of the patients' parents. I would like to thank them all for allowing us to publish the pictures.

REFERENCES

1. Iaria M, Capocasale E, Dalla VR, Mazzoni MP, Sianesi M. Laparoscopic versus open donor nephrectomy. An appraisal on surgical outcome and post-operative course. *Ann Ital Chir.* (2009) 80:449–51. doi: 10.1097/SLA.0b013e318153fd13
2. Klop KW, Dols LF, Kok NF, Weimar W, Ijzermans JN. Attitudes among surgeons towards live-donor nephrectomy: a European update. *Transplantation.* (2012) 94:263–8. doi: 10.1097/TP.0b013e3182577501
3. Pelizzo G, Bernardi L, Carlini V, Pasqua N, Mencherini S, Maggio G, et al. Laparoscopy in children and its impact on brain oxygenation during routine inguinal hernia repair. *J Minim Access Surg.* (2017) 13:51–6. doi: 10.4103/0972-9941.181800
4. Brockschmidt C, Huber N, Paschke S, Hartmann B, Henne-Bruns D, Wittau M. Minimal access kidney transplant: a novel technique to reduce surgical tissue trauma. *Exp Clin Transplant.* (2012) 10:319–24. doi: 10.6002/ect.2012.0045
5. Kim SD, Kim JI, Moon IS, Park SC. Comparison of minimal skin incision technique in living kidney transplantation and conventional kidney transplantation. *Chin Med J.* (2016) 129:917–21. doi: 10.4103/0366-6999.179800
6. Oyen O, Scholz T, Hartmann A, Pfeffer P. Minimally invasive kidney transplantation: the first experience. *Transplant Proc.* (2006) 38:2798–802. doi: 10.1016/j.transproceed.2006.08.102
7. Gandaglia G, Ghani KR, Sood A, Meyers JR, Sammon JD, Schmid M, et al. Effect of minimally invasive surgery on the risk for surgical site infections: results from the National Surgical Quality Improvement Program (NSQIP) Database. *J Am Med Assoc Surg.* (2014) 149:1039–44. doi: 10.1001/jamasurg.2014.292
8. Nicholson ML, Kaushik M, Lewis GR, Brook NR, Bagul A, Kay MD, et al. Randomized clinical trial of laparoscopic versus open donor nephrectomy. *Br J Surg.* (2010) 97:21–8. doi: 10.1002/bjs.6803
9. Kacar S, Eroglu A, Tilif S, Guven B. Minimally invasive kidney transplantation. *Transplant Proc.* (2013) 45:926–8. doi: 10.1016/j.transproceed.2013.02.079
10. Phillips SH, Hill SK, Lipscomb LD, Africa JB. Altering the approach: open minimally invasive renal transplant in obese patients through the anterior rectus sheath. *Urology.* (2017) 105:192–6. doi: 10.1016/j.urology.2017.03.011
11. Weissenbacher A, Oberhuber R, Cardini B, Weiss S, Ulmer H, Bosmuller C, et al. The faster the better: anastomosis time influences patient survival after deceased donor kidney transplantation. *Transpl Int.* (2015) 28:535–43. doi: 10.1111/tri.12516
12. Marzouk K, Lawen J, Alwayn I, Kiberd BA. The impact of vascular anastomosis time on early kidney transplant outcomes. *Transplant Res.* (2013) 2:8. doi: 10.1186/2047-1440-2-8

7

Oral Spermine Supplementation in Gestated Rabbit: A Study on Villi Height of Immature Intestines

Riana Pauline Tamba* and Yefta Moenadjat

Faculty of Medicine, Department of Surgery Cipto Mangunkusumo General Hospital, Universitas Indonesia, Jakarta, Indonesia

Correspondence:
Riana Pauline Tamba
rianatamba@gmail.com

Introduction: Immature intestines are the major problem in prematurity. Postnatal oral spermine has been shown in studies to improve intestinal maturation in rats and piglets. This study aimed to find out the efficacy of spermine in rabbits during gestation.

Method: An experimental study was done in an unblinded, randomized manner on those treated with and without spermine administration. A morphological examination of hematoxylin–eosin-stained villi was performed under a light microscope with a focus on villi height. Data were subjected to analysis.

Results: The median of the spermine-treated group was found to be higher at 24, 26, and 28 days than the non-spermine group, but was not significantly different.

Conclusion: Oral spermine supplementation during gestation might improve intestinal villi height in immature rabbit intestines.

Keywords: spermine, rabbit, gestation, immature intestines, villi height

INTRODUCTION

Premature birth was associated with a high risk of developing gut-derived infection and intestinal immaturity, as well as a 50% risk of death (1). According to one study, 90% of neonatal deaths were caused by gut-derived infections associated with intestinal immaturity (1). Thus, intestinal immaturity is a major problem in premature infants (2). In the term neonate, intestinal maturity is found in the first 3 weeks of life. However, premature babies' maturity takes longer, although there is no clear definition. The various anatomical and physiological structures of the cells/tissues constructing the digestive tract are not fully developed yet in immaturity. The epithelium of fetuses has not yet developed into the adults' type of epithelium, which is found in four types: enterocytes, entero(neuro)-endocrine, goblet cells, and Paneth cells, and no mucosal integrity assembling the epithelial lining. Likewise, microfold cells (M cells) and Peyer patches, lymphoid tissue in the lamina propria as gut-associated lymphoid tissue, play a role in inducing the defense system, in addition to the insufficient mucus layer (3, 4). Lamina muscularis, which plays a role in propulsion, is also found to be insufficient. Oral intake, including breastfeeding, is frequently delayed in this condition because it may be followed by severe effects associated with propulsion (3). On the other hand, the homeostasis of commensal bacteria, which is influenced by oral intake, has not been achieved. In contrast, commensal bacteria are known to induce maturity and gastrointestinal mucosa's natural defense system as well (4–7).

In addition, mucin insufficiency, and mucosal permeability that is not achieved due to unassembled integrity of epithelial lining, allow bacterial translocation. Thus, immaturity of the gastrointestinal leads to sepsis, which is fatal (3). Besides sepsis, the clinical entity associated with intestinal immaturity in preterm neonates is necrotizing enterocolitis (NEC), which is also fatal (8, 9). The immature intestine reacts to molecular patterns of colonizing bacteria and endogenous inflammatory stimuli by mounting excessive inflammation, a hallmark of NEC, due to developmental immaturity in the innate immune response gene (3).

Studies focused on gastrointestinal immaturity have shown a positive effect of oral spermine administration followed by intestinal maturation in mice (10–13) and piglets (14, 15). Polyamines (spermine, spermidine) are ubiquitous low-molecular-weight polycationic compounds that play an essential role in cell proliferation, growth, and differentiation in various cells/tissues (16, 17). In the digestive tract, spermine is known to interact with the constituent proteins of the intestinal barrier and play an essential role in wound healing and the immune system (13, 15, 18). The role of spermine was the interplay of molecules resembling epithelial junctions of the intestinal mucosa and associated cytoskeleton molecules responsible for providing an intestinal barrier. These studies showed achievement of intestinal maturity following postnatal spermine administration with different parameters. The morphological parameters investigated were villi height and crypt depth (19). Another study focused on biochemically showing the permeability and expression of junctional proteins, cytokines, etc (20, 21). However, spermine administration's efficacy during gestation is yet unknown. Therefore, this study focused on spermine administration during gestation to determine the efficacy of postnatal maturation in premature newborns, focused on the height of intestinal villi. It was hypothesized that the maturity level of newborns soon after delivery is achieved, but not a mature level in the first 3 weeks of a newborn's life.

MATERIALS AND METHODS

An experimental study was carried out on 3 kg weighted New Zealand White adult female rabbits (*Oryctolagus cuniculus*) prepared for a study by The Animal Lab, Ciawi, Bogor. Twenty-four rabbits were enrolled in the study. They were fed with standard DM20 pellets, bred, and handled with care during gestation. These rabbits were assigned in an unblinded, randomized manner to those treated with spermine administration and non-spermine administration. The subjects were randomly selected and set in the treatment and control groups, respectively. Spermine of 20 mg per kg body weight once daily was supplemented with food during the gestation period. The dose was set based on a previous study by Peulen et al., converted to a rabbit dose using a human equivalent dose conversion (22). In this study, the crew fed one rabbit and waited for it to finish its food before moving on to the next rabbit to ensure all rabbits ate the whole portion of their meal. Feeding was proceeded with close monitoring to assure these animals take the food completely, which was given once daily.

TABLE 1 | Ileal villi height in spermine and non-spermine treated groups.

	Villi height (μm)	Spermine (μm) Median (min-max)	Non-spermine (μm) Median (min-max)	*p*-value
Control	380	–	–	
24 days	–	143 (68–207)	117 (74–135)	0.344
26 days	–	108 (78–115)	95 (72–138)	1.000
28 days	–	138 (137–139)	92.5 (60–164)	0.355

The prematurity was established at various times, namely 24, 26, and 28 days of gestation, which represents the third trimester of pregnancy in humans, 28–38 weeks. These prematurely born fetuses were enrolled in a parallel assigned, non-masking randomized manner. The gestation was terminated by Cesarean section. The Cesarean section was carried out with ketamine of 10–40 mg per kg body weight and xylazine 3–5 mg per kg body weight, intramuscularly. Fifty fetuses of these rabbits were prematurely born. Furthermore, laparotomy was carried out on the newborn under ketamine per kg body weight and 1.5 mg of xylazine per kg body weight. A sample of terminal ileum measuring 5–6 cm was taken as the specimen for the study. Following laparotomy, the newborns were sacrificed according to the regulations in the animal lab. The control group referred to those normally delivered.

The specimens were stained with hematoxylin-eosin and examined under a light microscope (OptiLab Advance, Miconos) at 10 times objective magnification to determine villi height. The height of the villi of a fetus of a 14-days-old fetus was used as the control (23). Data was subjected to analysis using the ANOVA test. This study was approved by the Committee of Ethics, Faculty of Medicine, University of Indonesia with reference number 18-03-0249. The study was registered on ClinicalTrials.gov (No. NCT04004091).

RESULTS

Of the spermine-treated group, seven specimens were 24 days, four specimens were 26 days, and two specimens were 28 days. Of the non-spermine group, four specimens were 24 days, three specimens were 26 days, and four specimens were 28 days. The mean of villi height in 24–, 26–, and 28-days spermine groups was 100 μm + 23.5, 135 μm + 39.142, and 138 μm + 1.0, respectively. While the mean of villi height in non-spermine groups of 24–, 26–, and 28 days were 100.33 μm + 14.88, 102.25 μm + 36.75, and 106.28 μm + 1.0, respectively. The distribution was not the normal one, median (min–max) was used for statistical analysis purposes (**Table 1**, **Figures 1**, **2**). The difference was not significantly different with *p* values of 24–, 26–, and 28 days were 0.344, 1.000, and 0.355, respectively.

DISCUSSION

This study is the first investigation focused on the immature ileum of premature rabbits. Unlike the previous studies on mice

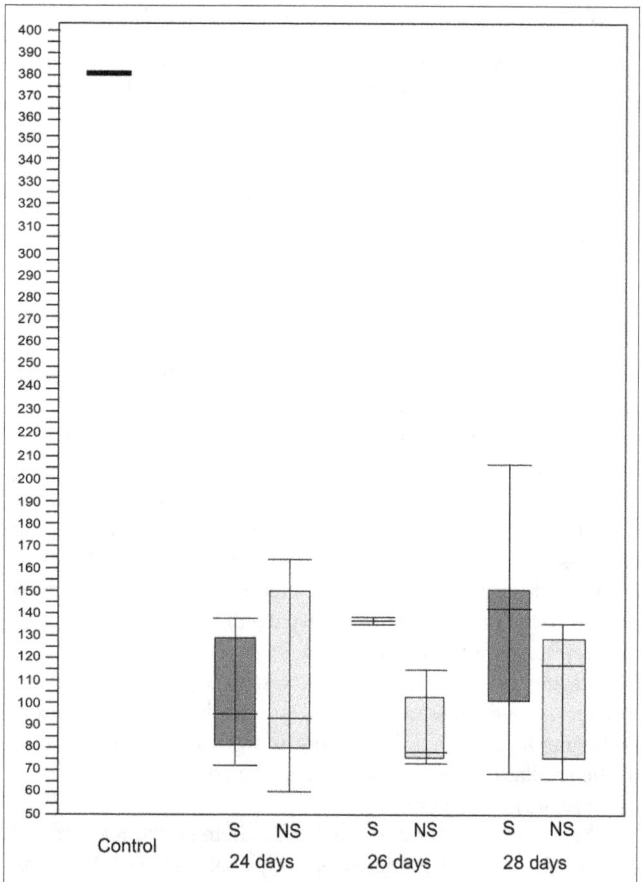

FIGURE 1 | Box–Whisker plot showing the difference in villi height between the spermine-treated and non-spermine groups in the immature intestines. The median of the spermine-treated group was higher than the non-spermine groups in three treated periods, namely 24, 26, and 28 days, though this difference was not statistically significant. For details, see the text.

and piglets, focusing on intestinal maturation after oral spermine administration in the postnatal period, the present study had a different approach. Firstly, this experiment was carried out on rabbits. There were references directly comparing rat and human intestinal epithelial cells, but to date, there are fewer studies carried out on rabbits, particularly those focused on spermine. Although rat intestines' morphology closely resembles humans' intestines, rabbit intestines resemble pH 7.5 as in humans, and the microflora in the intestines is similar to humans (24). For this reason, we use rabbits for study. Overall, rabbits are phylogenetically closer to primates and have a more diverse genetic background than inbred and outbred rodent strains (25). This makes the model a better overall approximation of humans, mimicking human genetic diversity more accurately (26).

Secondly, the treatment, i.e., spermine supplemented food, was given during the gestation period, and the outcome was observed in the intestine of the premature newborn rabbit. Previous studies have shown the efficacy of oral spermine supplementation in intestinal maturation. Maturation is a complex process that may be explained differently, namely, morphologically, and biochemically. Morphologically, the villi height of the crypt represents the parameters observed using a conventional hematoxylin-eosin-stained specimen. However, Goblet cells, Paneth cells, and M cells require a particular staining method. Another aspect is the absorptive parameter, representing the barrier integrity and intestinal permeability using fluorescence and other biochemical properties, such as the expression of some molecules that build the epithelial junctions.

To date, those studies have been carried out on mice and piglets. Because no other parameters exist for rabbits, this study concentrated on villi height and crypt depth as parameters; they are simple, feasible, and reliable for representing maturation. Maturation is the development of cells' individual characteristics through growth, while growth is a physical and quantifiable process in development, which is measurable. Studies have shown that DNA methylation, for instance, shows that maturation represents the development of fetal cells into well-developed (matured) cells (27). Somehow, development is closely related to morphogenesis.

The study by Sabater–Molina et al. showed that the mucosa's polyamine concentration is followed by deepening of the intestinal crypt but is not significantly associated with the mucosa's concentration (14). The study by Peulen et al. empowered the statement (28). Furthermore, Peulen's study showed that the maturation is associated with microflora that synthesized the mucosa's polyamine and uptake by the stem cells in the crypts (29). The regulation, as well as the utilization, is then associated with average growth and development. In rabbits, the crypts can be seen as an invagination of a villi base in the duodenum of a 1-day-old rabbit. Villi, goblet cells, and other glands develop later at the end of gestation. Primitive villi could be seen in the first 21 postnatal days, much higher in 22 days, resembling a cylindric shape in the first 28 days. The villi height increased within days in both the spermine-treated and non-spermine groups, according to the study (30). However, intestinal structure development starts earlier in humans in the first trimester of gestation, and maturation is achieved during delivery (30). The maturation remains, and the maturation remains in process. Thus, insignificancy in the analysis is not a big issue as maturation refers to a dynamic process.

Despite the controversy, most studies have shown the efficacy of oral supplementation, referring to close contact with the mucosa—particularly intestinal villi—associated with an increase in villi height (4, 31), as in this present study. The unanswered question was the influence of spermine supplementation during gestation as the aim of the study. The present study was not designed to determine the evidence regarding polyamines, both maternal and fetal or placental. The reason is that there was sufficient information regarding the ability to cross the placenta barrier (32–34).

In summary, we found that oral supplementation in gestated rabbits showed increased intestinal villi height in the premature rabbit's ileum, achieving a mature newborn's height. Still, the achievement was not mature intestines because, in a mature

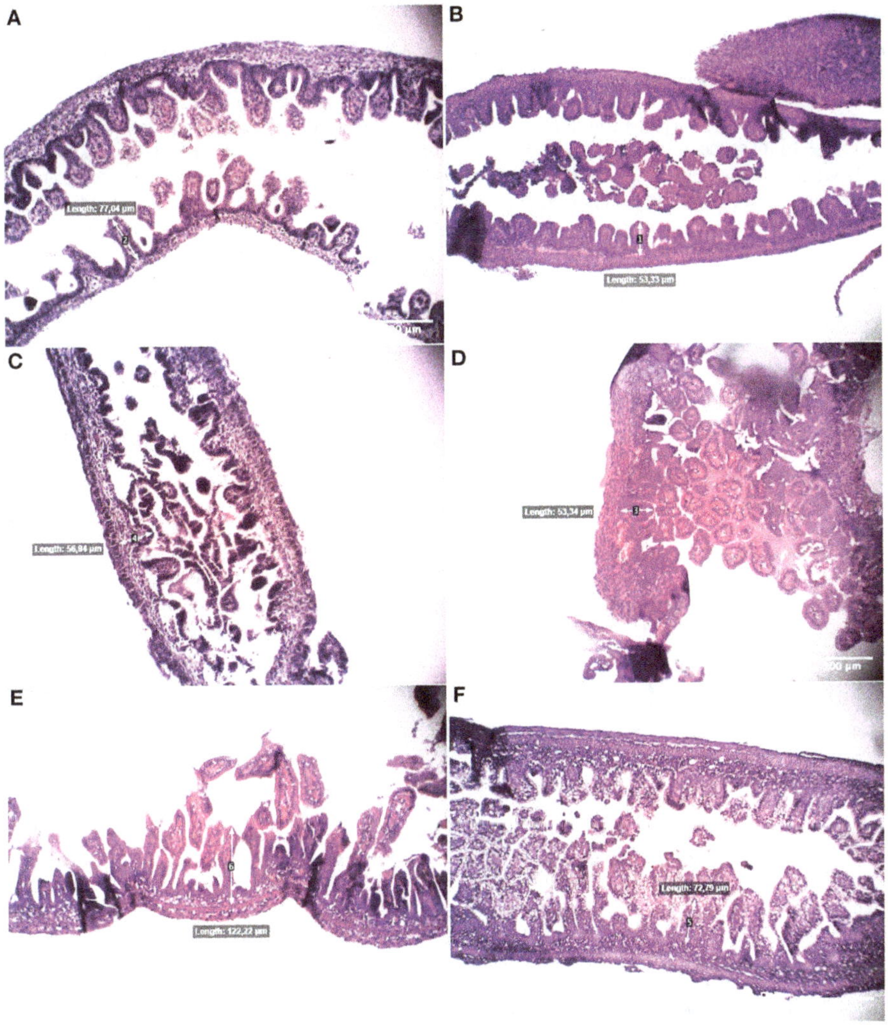

FIGURE 2 | Morphological presentation of villi height in hematoxylin-eosin (HE) stained specimens of immature rabbit's ileum at 24 days **(A,B)**, 26 days **(C,D)**, and 28 days postnatal **(E,F)** under objective magnification of 10 times. The left-sided figures show those of the spermine-treated group, and the right-sided figures represent the non-spermine group. It is shown that the spermine group's ileal villi are longer than the non-spermine group and more regularly. The spermine group's regular-shaped villi are configured by day 28 postnatal, whereas the non-spermine group remains discretely distributed.

newborn, intestinal maturation is achieved within the first 3 weeks of life. In other words, Spermine improves intestinal maturity intrauterine—although this finding is not significant.

However, there are limitations to the study. Firstly, the small sample size concerned the 3Rs regulations on using experimental animals. Secondly, the problem of broodstock led to finding samples with appropriate gestation periods and, consequently, different samples in each group. Thirdly, the unanswered question regarding the influence of spermine on intrauterine needs to be elaborated further through an investigation into epithelial molecular junctions.

CONCLUSION

During gestation, oral spermine supplementation might improve intestinal maturity of intestinal villi in immature rabbits, as indicated by an increase in height.

AUTHOR CONTRIBUTIONS

RT designed the study and performed the experiments. YM analyzed the data. RT and YM wrote the manuscript. Both authors contributed to the article and approved the submitted version.

REFERENCES

1. Collins A, Weitkamp JH, Wynn JL. Why are preterm newborns at increased risk of infection? *Arch Dis Child - Fetal Neonatal Ed.* (2018) 103:391–4. doi: 10.1136/archdischild-2017-313595
2. WHO. Born Too Soon. The global action report on preterm birth 2012. *World Heal Organ.* (2012) 29:283–7. doi: 10.1055/s-0031-1295659
3. Shi HN, Walker WA. Development and physiology of the intestinal mucosal defense. In: Mestecky J, Russell MW, Cheroutre H, Strober W, Kelsall BL, Lambrecht BN, editors. *Mucosal Immunology.* (2015) 4:9–29. doi: 10.1016/B978-0-12-415847-4.00002-1
4. Weström B, Arévalo Sureda E, Pierzynowska K, Pierzynowski SG, Pérez-Cano FJ. The immature gut barrier and its importance in establishing immunity in newborn mammals. *Front Immunol.* (2020) 11:1153. doi: 10.3389/fimmu.2020.01153
5. Gleeson M, Cripps AW. Development of mucosal immunity in the first year of life and relationship to sudden infant death syndrome. *FEMS Immunol Med Microbiol.* (2004) 42:21–33. doi: 10.1016/j.femsim.2004.06.012
6. Moore RE, Townsend SD. Temporal development of the infant gut microbiome. *Open Biol.* (2019) 9:2–7. doi: 10.1098/rsob190128
7. Hill DR, Huang S, Nagy MS, Yadagiri VK, Fields C, Mukherjee D, et al. Bacterial colonization stimulates a complex physiological response in the immature human intestinal epithelium. *Elife.* (2017) 4:e29132. doi: 10.7554/eLife.29132
8. Lee JH. An update on necrotizing enterocolitis: pathogenesis and preventive strategies. *Korean J Pediatr.* (2011) 54:368–72. doi: 10.3345/kjp.2011.54.9.368
9. Ma B, Mccomb E, Gajer P, Yang H, Humphrys M, Okogbule-Wonodi AC, et al. Microbial biomarkers of intestinal barrier maturation in preterm infants. *Front Microbiol.* (2018) 9:2755. doi: 10.3389/fmicb.2018.02755
10. Buts JP, De Keyser N, Kolanowski J, Sokal E, Van Hoof F. Maturation of villus and crypt cell functions in rat small intestine - Role of dietary polyamines. *Dig Dis Sci.* (1993) 38:1091–8. doi: 10.1007/BF01295726
11. Wild GE, Daly AS, Sauriol N, Bennett G. Effect of exogenously administered polyamine on the structural maturation and enzyme ontogeny of the postnatal rat intestine. *Biol Neonate.* (1993) 63:246–57. doi: 10.1159/000243938
12. Ter Steege JCA, Buurman WA, Forget PP. Spermine induces maturation of the immature intestinal immune system in neonatal mice. *J Pediatr Gastroenterol Nutr.* (1997) 25:332–40. doi: 10.1097/00005176-199709000-00017
13. Dufour C, Dandrifosse G, Forget P, Vermesse F, Romain N, Lepoint P. Spermine and spermidine induce intestinal maturation in the rat. *Gastroenterology.* (1988) 95:112–6. doi: 10.1016/0016-5085(88)90298-3
14. Sabater-Molina M, Larqué E, Torrella F, Plaza J, Lozano T, Muñoz A, et al. Effects of dietary polyamines at physiologic doses in early-weaned piglets. *Nutrition.* (2009) 25:940–6. doi: 10.1016/j.nut.2009.01.017
15. Van Wettere WHEJ, Willson NL, Pain SJ, Forder REA. Effect of oral polyamine supplementation pre-weaning on piglet growth and intestinal characteristics. *Animal.* (2016) 10:1655–9. doi: 10.1017/S1751731116000446
16. Jänne J, Pösö H, Raina A. Polyamines in rapid growth and cancer. *BBA - Rev Cancer.* (1978) 473:241–93. doi: 10.1016/0304-419X(78)90015-X
17. Porter CW, Ganis B, Dworaczyk D, Weiser MM. Polyamines and biosynthetic enzymes in the rat intestinal mucosa and the influence of methylglyoxal-bis(guanylhydrazone). *Cancer Res.* (1980) 40:2330–5.
18. Chen J, Li X, Bai Z, Fang F, Hua J, Li Y, et al. Association of fluid accumulation with clinical outcomes in critically ill children with severe sepsis. *PLoS ONE.* (2016) 5:e0160093. doi: 10.1371/journal.pone.0160093
19. Muñoz-Esparza NC, Latorre-Moratalla ML, Comas-Basté O, Toro-Funes N, Veciana-Nogués MT, Vidal-Carou MC. Polyamines in food. *Front Nutr.* (2019) 6:108. doi: 10.3389/fnut.2019.00108
20. Fang T, Jia G, Zhao H, Chen X, Tang J, Wang J, et al. Effects of spermine supplementation on the morphology, digestive enzyme activities, and antioxidant capacity of intestine in weaning rats. *Anim Nutr.* (2016) 2:370–5. doi: 10.1016/j.aninu.2016.09.002
21. Liu G, Mo W, Cao W, Wu X, Jia G, Zhao H, et al. Effects of spermine on ileal physical barrier, antioxidant capacity, metabolic profile and large intestinal bacteria in piglets. *RSC Adv.* (2020) 10:26709–16. doi: 10.1039/c9ra10406b
22. Peulen O, Dandrifosse G. Spermine-induced maturation in wistar rat intestine: a cytokine-dependent mechanism. *J Pediatr Gastroenterol Nutr.* (2004) 38:524–32. doi: 10.1097/00005176-200405000-00012
23. Yu B, Chiou PWS. The morphological changes of intestinal mucosa in growing rabbits. *Lab Anim.* (1997) 31:254–63. doi: 10.1258/002367797780596301
24. Hatton GB, Yadav V, Basit AW, Merchant HA. Animal farm: considerations in animal gastrointestinal physiology and relevance to drug delivery in humans. *J Pharm Sci.* (2015) 104:2747–76. doi: 10.1002/jps.24365
25. Graur D, Duret L, Gouyt M. Phylogenetic position of the order lagomorpha (rabbits, hares and allies). *Nature.* (1996) 379:333–5. doi: 10.1038/379333a0
26. Den Hondt M, Vanaudenaerde BM, Delaere P, Vranckx JJ. Twenty years of experience with the rabbit model, a versatile model for tracheal transplantation research. *Plast Aesthetic Res.* (2016) 3:223. doi: 10.20517/2347-9264.2015.117
27. Soda K. Spermine and gene methylation: a mechanism of lifespan extension induced by polyamine-rich diet. *Amino Acids.* (2020) 52:213–24. doi: 10.1007/s00726-019-02733-2
28. Peulen O, Gharbi M, Powroznik B, Dandrifosse G. Differential effect of dietary spermine on alkaline phosphatase activity in jejunum and ileum of unweaned rats. *Biochimie.* (2004) 86:487–93. doi: 10.1016/j.biochi.2004.06.002
29. Peulen O, Deloyer P, Grandfils C, Loret S, Dandrifosse G. Intestinal maturation induced by spermine in young animals. *Livest Prod Sci.* (2000) 66:109–20. doi: 10.1016/S0301-6226(00)00218-9
30. Dutta S, Sengupta P. Rabbits and men: relating their ages. *J Basic Clin Physiol Pharmacol.* (2018) 29:427–35. doi: 10.1515/jbcpp-2018-0002
31. Arévalo Sureda E, Weström B, Pierzynowski SG, Prykhodko O. Maturation of the intestinal epithelial barrier in neonatal rats coincides with decreased FcRn expression, replacement of vacuolated enterocytes and changed Blimp-1 expression. *PLoS ONE.* (2016) 11:e0164775. doi: 10.1371/journal.pone.0164775
32. Bell AW, Ehrhardt RA. Regulation of placental nutrient transport and implications for fetal growth. *Nutr Res Rev.* (2002) 15:211–30. doi: 10.1079/nrr200239
33. Lopez-Garcia C, Lopez-Contreras AJ, Cremades A, Castells MT, Peñafiel R. Transcriptomic analysis of polyamine-related genes and polyamine levels in placenta, yolk sac and fetus during the second half of mouse pregnancy. *Placenta.* (2009) 30:241–9. doi: 10.1016/j.placenta.2008.12.004
34. Vaughan OR, Fowden AL. Placental metabolism: substrate requirements and the response to stress. *Reprod Domest Anim.* (2016) 51:25–35. doi: 10.1111/rda.12797

8

Congenital Abdominal Aortic Aneurysm

Zhibin Zhou†, Yongqiang Yue†, Ke Ma, Zhaohui Hua and Zhen Li**

Department of Endovascular Surgery, The First Affiliated Hospital of Zhengzhou University, Zhengzhou, China

***Correspondence:**
Zhaohui Hua
huazhaohuisfy@163.com
Zhen Li
lizhen1029@hotmail.com

Congenital abdominal aortic aneurysm is a rare disease with unknown etiology, and the common symptoms are abdominal pulsatile mass and pain caused by aneurysm rupture. The disease has a high mortality rate and fewer reports of surgical treatment. Here, we present a case of an idiopathic congenital abdominal aortic aneurysm. A 4-year-old boy had an abdominal pulsatile mass, and computed tomography angiography revealed an isolated infrarenal abdominal aortic aneurysm. To prevent rupture of the aneurysm, we repaired the aneurysm with artificial graft transplantation. No genetic mutation of the known congenital aneurysmal diseases was found in the whole-exome sequencing of the patient and his parents. There was no graft obstruction, and the patient grew well 40 months after surgery. Open surgery is the best treatment for idiopathic congenital abdominal aortic aneurysms. Surgical details such as timing and graft selection need to be further explored.

Keywords: aortic aneurysm, aortic diseases, congenital, children, surgical treatment

INTRODUCTION

Abdominal aortic aneurysms in children are very rare. The common causes are congenital connective tissue disorders, vasculitis, traumatic umbilical artery intubation, and infection, while congenital abdominal aortic aneurysms (cAAAs) is rarely reported and has an unknown etiology and high mortality. This article reports the case of a 4-year-old child with isolated cAAA and the results of a 40-month follow-up of open surgery.

CASE DESCRIPTION

In June 2018, a 4-year-old boy was hospitalized because of the discovery of a left abdominal pulsatile mass for 2 months. Computed tomography angiography (CTA) revealed an isolated infrarenal AAA with a maximum diameter of 67 mm (**Figure 1**). The patient was 112 cm tall and weighs 23 kg and he had no family history of aneurysmal disease, connective tissue disorders, a history of trauma, umbilical cannulation, and infection. Laboratory tests revealed no abnormalities, and blood pressure was normal.

DIAGNOSTIC ASSESSMENT, THERAPEUTIC INTERVENTION, FOLLOW-UP, AND OUTCOME

In July 2018, we repaired the AAA using open surgery to prevent aneurysm rupture. When we blocked the blood flow at both ends of the aneurysm and opened the aneurysm through a midline

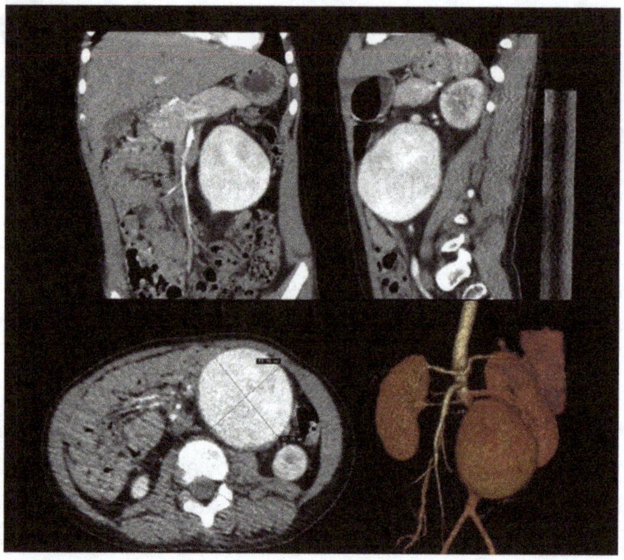

FIGURE 1 | Computerized tomography angiography demonstrated isolated infrarenal abdominal aortic aneurysm.

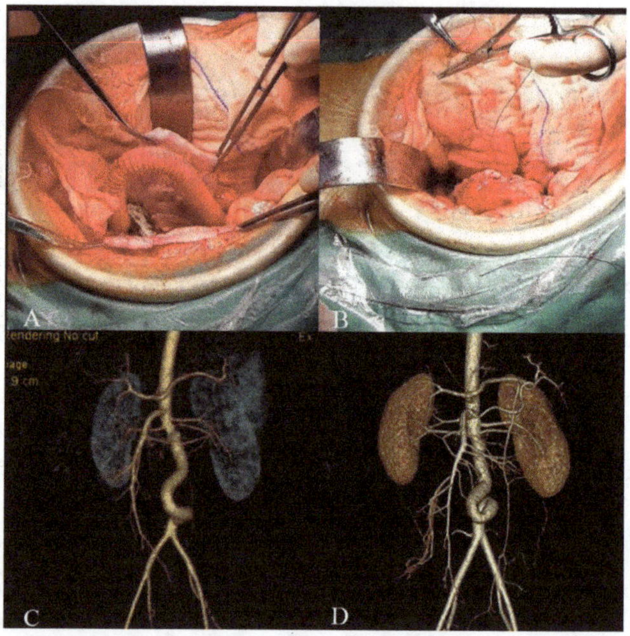

FIGURE 2 | Intraoperative and follow-up images. **(A)** A 10 mm Dacron aorto-aortic tube graft replace the AAA with a "C" shape. **(B)** The aneurysmal sac was wrapped around the graft. **(C)** CTA 7 days after surgery. **(D)** CTA 40 months after surgery showed twisted but unobstructed graft.

incision, we found that the intima of the aneurysm was smooth without thrombus. We then used a 10-mm Dacron aorto-aortic tube graft to replace the AAA; the graft was oversized by 6 cm and formed a "C" shape to allow aortic growth. The aneurysmal sac was wrapped around the graft to avoid aortoduodenal fistula. The patient recovered well after the operation. Whole-exome sequencing of the boy and his parents revealed no genetic mutations of the known congenital aneurysmal diseases. The patients had frequent follow-ups outside the hospital, and at 40 months post-operative follow up without any antiplatelet drugs, the patient was 140 cm tall and weighs 43 kg, and the CTA revealed that the graft blood flow was unobstructed (**Figure 2**).

DISCUSSION

AAA is more common in the elderly with arteriosclerosis, and is rare in children and infants, and is commonly caused by congenital connective tissue disorders, vasculitis, umbilical cannulation, and infection, while cAAA is extremely rare and has an unknown etiology. One relevant hypothesis is that cAAA results from a developmental defect during embryogenesis that creates a focal narrowing of the abdominal aorta, which leads to poststenotic turbulent blood flow and subsequent aneurysm formation (1). There are no epidemiological data related to cAAA, and as of December 2021, only 31 cases have been reported (**Table 1**) (2–8). There are fifteen patients diagnosed before 1 year of age, eight patients were diagnosed after 1 year of age, and the remaining eight patients were diagnosed at 19–30 weeks of gestation. The male-to-female ratio was 18:10, 20 of 31 patients had infrarenal AAA, and 19 of 30 patients had other aneurysms. The reason for admission of patients is usually abdominal pulsatile mass or rupture of aneurysm; suspected diseases should receive vital imaging examination, such as ultrasound, which can provide a clear diagnosis.

The histopathological changes in the intima of cAAA include calcifications, thromboses, and ulcerations and ruptures of the layers (2, 9). Molecular genetic defects considered to be associated with AAA, Marfan's syndrome, and Loeys-Dietz syndrome are caused by mutations in the genes encoding TGF-β2 or TGF-β receptor (TGFBR) I or II. Mutations in the fibrillin-1(FBN1) gene have also been found to be associated with the occurrence of coronary aneurysms (10–13). Unfortunately, no similar genetic or molecular changes have been found in cAAA, including this case.

The mortality caused by cAAA rupture and renal failure was 30.76% (2). There is no universal approach to the management of cAAA. Although steroids, cyclophosphamide, antihypertensive drugs, non-steroidal anti-inflammatory drugs, and statins have certain curative effects, the reported mortality of conservative treatment is still as high as 57.14% (4/7). It is still unclear how to judge the diameter of aneurysms in the intervention, and the uncertainty of children's activity cannot refer to the surgical standards of adults. Surgical repair after diagnosis should be considered. Endovascular aneurysm repair (EVAR) is not feasible in infants or children because of the lack of an appropriate endograft and the impact on patients' growth and development. Artificial grafts and allografts were most frequently selected for revascularization, and in the past, 13 cases were reported using Dacron graft or polytetrafluoroethylene (PTFE) graft, 4 cases of allografts, and 1 case of native vessels. Although allografts have the advantages of high long-term patency and low risk of

TABLE 1 | Previously reported cases of idiopathic congenital abdominal aortic aneurysms.

Author	Gender	Age at discovery	Location	Other aneurysms	Other aneurysms	Surgical treatment	Outcome
Howorth Jr. MB	Female	1 day	Infrarenal	None	Large abdominal mass, vomiting, anorexia	Exploratory laparotomy	Ruputure and death during operation
Darden WA	Male	2.5 years	Infrarenal	None	None	Dacron aortic graft	Died of pneumonitis at 5 months after surgery
Sterpetti AV	Male	19 years	Infrarenal	None	Middle epigastric pain, abdominal fullness, dysuria, abdominal pulsatile mass	Dacron aortic graft 18 mm	Died of pneumonitis at 5 months after surgery
Odagiri S	Male	1 year	Infrarenal	Multiple left renal artery aneurysrre, bilateral corrmon iliac artery aneurysms	None	Dacron aortic graft 12 mm	Healthy at 10 months after surgery
Latter D	Male	1 month	Infrarenal	None	Pulsatile abdominal mass	Polytetrafluoroethylene tube graft 8 mm	Healthy at 10 months after surgery
Saad SA	Male	6 weeks	Infrarenal	Left common iliac artery aneurysm mass	Pulsatile abdominal mass	Aneurysmorrhaphy	Healthy at 3 months after surgery
Myrmel T	Male	30 years	Infrarenal	None	Pulsatile abdominal mass, acute abdominal pain	Albumin coated USCI graft sized 16 × 8 mm	Healthy at 1 year after surgery
Malee MP	Female	32 weeks' gestation	Juxtarenal	Aneurysmal dilation of the bilateral iliac artery (details unknown)	Palpable abdominal mass, ileus compression from an aneursysm	None	Died of acute pulmonary hypertension and cardiac dysfuncticn at age 9 days
Kim ES	Female	9 days	Juxtarenal	None	None	Nono	Died of heart failure secondary to renovascular hypertension at age 20 days
Mehall JR	Male	6 weeks	Juxtarenal	Right common iliac artery aneurysm	None	Bifurcated GoreTex graft 7–4 mm	Healthy at 1 month after surgery
Laing AJ	Male	12 months	Infrarenal	None	Pale, shocked, in an urresponsive state, vomiting, abdominal distention	Exploratory laparotomy	Rupture and death during operation
Dittrick K	Male	12 years	Infrarenal	None	None	Collagen impregnated Dacron aortic graft 14 mm	Healthy at 2 years after surgery
Bell P	Female	1 day	Infrarenal	None	Billous vomiting, large abdominal mass	Cryopreserved allograft 5 mm	Healthy at 14 months after surgery
Cheung SCW	Male	6 months	Juxtarenal	Bilateral common and external iliac artery aneurysms, right internal iliac artery aneurysm	None	None	Progression of thrombosis of the aneurysm and renal dysfunction at age 3 years
Buddingh KT	Male	1 day	Juxtarenal	Descending thoracic aortic aneurysm, left common iliac artery aneurysm	Bilous vomiting, anorexia, pulsatile abdominal mass	None	Alive at 7 months, aneurysm has grown to a maximum diameter of 93 mm
Kim JI	None reported	21 weeks' gestation	Infrarenal	Bilateral common iliac artery aneurysms, left internal iliac artery aneurysm	None	Dacron aortic graft 12 mm	Uneventful postoperative recovery
Malikov S	Male	28 weeks' gestation	Juxtarenal	None	Pulsatile abdominal mass	Repair with native iliac vessels	Healthy at 39 months after surgery

(Continued)

TABLE 1 | Continued

Author	Gender	Age at discovery	Location	Other aneurysms	Other aneurysms	Surgical treatment	Outcome
Cantinotti M	None reported	22 weeks' gestation	Unspecified	None reported	None reported	None reported	None reported
Tsunematsu R	Male	25 weeks' gestation	Unspecified	None	Pulsatile abdominal mass	None	Stable after 6 months follow up
McAteer J	Female	32 weeks' gestation	Thoracoab dominal	None	None	None	Died of rupture at age 4 weeks
Cho YP	Male	23 months	Infrarenal	None	Irritability, vomiting, poor oral intake, diffuse tenderness, palpable pulsatile abdominal mass	Cryopreserved cadaveric artery 7 mm	Healthy at 10 months after surgery
Meyers RL	None reported	Neonate	Infrarenal	None	None	Decellularised, antigen reduced cryopreserved allograft	Healthy at 29 months after surgery
Ko Y	Male	2 months	Supraceliac	Two descending thoracic aortic aneurysms	None reported	Dacron aortic graft 10 mm	Uneventful postoperative recovery
Fettah ND	Female	1 day	Infrarenal	None	Vomiting, abdominal distention, palpable pulsatile abdominal mass	Repair with polytetrafluorethylene patch	Died of sepsis and cardiopulmonary insufficiency at 4 weeks after surgery
Bivins HS	Male	19 weeks' gestation	Infrarenal	Iliac artery aneurysms (details unknown)	Large abdominal mass	None	Died of renal failure at age 12 days
Bansal A	Male	1 year	Infrarenal	None	Abdominal distension	Dacron aortic graft 10 mm	Uneventful postoperative recovery
Sirisabya A	Female	1 day	Infrarenal	Left common iliac artery aneurysm, two small right renal artery aneurysms	Marked abdominal distension with a large pulsatile mass	Gore-Tex vascular graft	Thrombosis of the aortic graft and bilateral common iliac, internal iliac, and external iliac arteries at 13 months after surgery. Living a fairly normal life at 26 months after surgery
Kuboi T	Female	Neonate	Infrarenal	None	Lower back mass (subcutaneous vascular malformation)	None reported	None reported
Higuchi K	Female	4 years	Infrarenal	Multiple intracranial aneurysms, bilateral hypogastric artery aneurysms, left renal artery aneurysm	Palpable pulsatile abdominal mass	Dacron aortic graft 10 mm	Healthy at 21 months after surgery
Tanga C F	Male	11 years	Infrarenal	Bilateral common iliac artery aneurysms, bilateral internal iliac artery aneurysm	Abdominal pain, shock	Dacron aortic graft 12 mm	Healthy at 10 months after surgery
LeNguyen A	Female	36 weeks' gestation	Infrarenal	Bilateral common iliac artery aneurysms, bilateral internal iliac artery aneurysm	None	Cryopreserved cadaveric artery 5 mm	Healthy at 12 months after surgery

Modified from Wang and Tao (2).

postoperative graft infection, there are difficulties with the long-term use of immune-suppressants and allograft sources. Malikov reported a successful case of revascularization with native iliac vessels (14).

The common complications of artificial vascular grafts are graft stenosis and obstruction. The diameter of the artificial graft should be considered to match with the artery and ensure blood supply to the lower limbs. At present, the reported diameter is mostly between 8 and 12 mm, which is easier for older children to choose. There is a high risk of synthetic vascular graft occlusion with a diameter of <6 mm for a neonatal patient; it may, therefore, be more appropriate to delay surgery for smaller aneurysms to produce better results and prevent the need for follow-up surgery (15). It is necessary to reserve appropriate length for artificial grafts to adapt to the patient's growth; however, most reports do not indicate the specific appropriate length. Dueppers et al. (16) reserved 4-cm graft to meet the growth needs of children. We considered the patient's age, preoperative aortic diameter and adult physique estimated from his parents' physique, and decided to use 10-mm Dacron graft to reconstruct the diseased artery with a 6-cm long graft reserved to form a "C" shape; our length selection principle is to keep a certain length on the premise of avoiding angulation.

The average follow-up time of the 16 patients who underwent surgical repair with follow-up records was 19 months. The longest follow-up time with artificial grafts under the age of 18 years was 26 months. Of these 16 patients, two died of infection during follow-up, an anastomotic stenosis of allografts occurred 7 days after surgery, and one PTFE graft was completely occluded 13 months after the operation. The graft patency rate was 93.3% (14/15). There is no literature recommending the routine use of anticoagulant or antiplatelet drugs for AAA patients with reconstructed branches. LeNguyen et al. (8) continued to use low-molecular-weight heparin for patients with anastomotic stenosis, resulting in graft patency at 1-year follow-up.

During the 40-month follow-up in our case, the artificial graft was twisted, but there was no obvious angulation and it remained unobstructed. The patient's physical development was not affected. We will continue to follow up the patient to observe graft patency.

CAAA is rare and has unknown etiology, and for patients with confirmed aneurysms, it is suggested to improve the systemic examination and long-term follow-up to exclude other lesions. Due to the high mortality rate, the long-term results of open repair in children are still unclear. The patency of grafts also requires long-term follow-up observations and necessary drug adjuvant treatment. In cases of complications, timely and effective interventions are necessary.

ETHICS STATEMENT

The studies involving human participants were reviewed and approved by Medical Ethical Committee of the First Affiliated Hospital of Zhengzhou University. Written informed consent to participate in this study was provided by the participants' legal guardian/next of kin. Written informed consent was obtained from the minor(s)' legal guardian/next of kin for the publication of any potentially identifiable images or data included in this article.

AUTHOR CONTRIBUTIONS

ZZ was wrote the manuscript and was assistant in surgery. KM and YY were assistant in surgery and participate in editing the articles. ZH and ZL designed the operation and revising the manuscript. All authors contributed to the article and approved the submitted version.

REFERENCES

1. Lee BB, Laredo J, Lee TS, Huh S, Neville R. Terminology and classification of congenital vascular malformations. *Phlebology.* (2007) 22:249–52. doi: 10.1177/026835550702200605
2. Wang Y, Tao Y. Diagnosis and treatment of congenital abdominal aortic aneurysm: a systematic review of reported cases. *Orphanet J Rare Dis.* (2015) 10:4. doi: 10.1186/s13023-015-0225-x
3. Bansal A, Mitra A, Bisoi AK, Agarwala S. Surgical repair of congenital abdominal aortic aneurysm in a 1-year-old child with literature review. *J Indian Assoc Pediatr Surg.* (2017) 22:176–8. doi: 10.4103/jiaps.JIAPS_258_16
4. Sirisabya A, Trinavarat P, Namchaisiri J, Punnahitanonda S, Thaithumyanon P. Congenital abdominal aortic aneurysm in a term neonate: a case report. *Nephron Clin Pract.* (2017) 11:163–7. doi: 10.5372/1905-7415.1102.548
5. Kuboi T, Miyagi M, Kondo S, Arioka M, Yamato S, Sadamura T, et al. Congenital abdominal aortic aneurysm discovered incidental to a lower back mass. *Pediatr Int.* (2018) 60:98–9. doi: 10.1111/ped.13458
6. Higuchi K, Furukawa K, Nakamura E, Imamura H, Gi T, Nakamura K. Congenital abdominal aortic aneurysm in a four year old girl. *EJVES Vasc Forum.* (2020) 48:12–8. doi: 10.1016/j.ejvsvf.2020.05.004
7. Tanga CF, Fakhoury E, Ham PB III, Dosluoglu HH, Harris LM. Ruptured abdominal aortic aneurysm in an 11-year-old with multiple peripheral artery aneurysms. *J Vasc Surg Cases Innov Tech.* (2020) 6:539–42. doi: 10.1016/j.jvscit.2020.07.015
8. Le-Nguyen A, Joharifard S, Cote G, Borsuk D, Ghali R, Lallier M. Neonatal microsurgical repair of a congenital abdominal aortic aneurysm with a cadaveric graft. *Eur J Pediatr Surg Rep.* (2021) 9:e23–7. doi: 10.1055/s-0041-1723019
9. Ye C, Yin H, Lin Y, Zhou L, Ye R, Li X, et al. Abdominal aorta aneurysms in children: single center experience of six patients. *Ann Thorac Surg.* (2012) 93:201–5. doi: 10.1016/j.athoracsur.2011.08.038
10. Gentilini D, Oliveri A, Fazia T, Pini A, Marelli S, Bernardinelli L, et al. NGS analysis in Marfan syndrome spectrum: Combination of rare and common genetic variants to improve genotype-phenotype correlation analysis. *PLoS ONE.* (2019) 14:e0222506. doi: 10.1371/journal.pone.0222506
11. Mariucci E, Bonori L, Lovato L, Graziano C, Ciuca C, Pacini D, et al. Coronary artery aneurysms in patients with marfan syndrome: frequent, progressive, and relevant. *Can J Cardiol.* (2021) 37:1225–31. doi: 10.1016/j.cjca.2021.03.002
12. Forte A, Galderisi U, Cipollaro M, De Feo M, Della Corte A. Epigenetic regulation of TGF-β1 signalling in dilative aortopathy of the thoracic ascending aorta. *Clin Sci.* (2016) 130:1389–405. doi: 10.1042/CS20160222
13. Verstraeten A, Perik M, Baranowska AA, Meester JAN, Van Den Heuvel L, Bastianen J, et al. Enrichment of rare variants in Loeys-Dietz Syndrome Genes in spontaneous coronary artery dissection but not in severe fibromuscular dysplasia. *Circulation.* (2020) 142:1021–4. doi: 10.1161/CIRCULATIONAHA.120.045946
14. Malikov S, Delarue A, Fais PO, Keshelava G. Anatomical repair of a congenital aneurysm of the distal abdominal aorta in a newborn. *J Vasc Surg.* (2009) 50:1181–4. doi: 10.1016/j.jvs.2009.05.022
15. Barral X, de Latour B, Vola M, Lavocat MP, Fichtner C, Favre JP. Surgery of the abdominal aorta and its branches in children: late follow-up. *J Vasc Surg.* (2006) 43:1138–44. doi: 10.1016/j.jvs.2006.01.033

9

Uniportal Thoracoscopic Debridement for Children with Refractory Pleural Empyema: Case Series of 21 Patients

Jin-Xi Huang [1,2,3,4], *Qiang Chen* [1,2,3,4], *Song-Ming Hong* [1,2,3,4], *Jun-Jie Hong* [1,2,3,4] and *Hua Cao* [1,2,3,4*]

[1] *Department of Cardiothoracic Surgery, Fujian Branch of Shanghai Children's Medical Center, Fuzhou, China,* [2] *Fujian Children's Hospital, Fuzhou, China,* [3] *Fujian Maternity and Child Health Hospital, Affiliated Hospital of Fujian Medical University, Fuzhou, China,* [4] *Fujian Key Laboratory of Women and Children's Critical Diseases Research, Fujian Maternity and Child Health Hospital, Fuzhou, China*

Correspondence:
Hua Cao
caohua0791@163.com

Purpose: The effectiveness of video-assisted thoracic surgery (VATS), even uniportal VATS (U-VATS), in the treatment of pleural empyema has recently been demonstrated. However, few works have evaluated its safety and feasibility for children. We review our experience with U-VATS in the treatment of pleural empyema for children under 11 years old.

Methods: From January 2019 to December 2020, we consecutively enrolled 21 children with stage II and stage III pleural empyema in our institution. A 1.0 cm utility port was created in the 5th intercostal space at the anterior axillary line. A rigid 30°5 mm optic thoracoscope was used for vision, and two or three instruments were used through the port. Surgery was based on three therapeutic columns: removal of pleural fluid, debridement, and decortication. A chest tube was inserted through the same skin incision. Perioperative data and outcomes were summarized.

Results: The procedures were successful, and satisfactory debridement of the pleural cavity was achieved in all cases. The mean age was 4.1 years (range: 6 months to 11 years old). The mean operating time was 65.7 ± 23.2 min. No intraoperative conversion or major complications were identified among the patients. The mean hospital stay was 5.0 ± 0.6 days. At a follow-up of more than 4 months after operating, all patients had recovered well without recurrence.

Conclusion: According to our experience, U-VATS debridement is feasible for the surgical management of stage II and III empyema in the pediatric population. Indeed, U-VATS permits easier performance and complete debridement and decortication, with a very low risk for conversion.

Keywords: video-assisted thoracoscopic surgery, uniportal, children, pleural empyema, pyothorax

INTRODUCTION

Pleural empyema is defined as the presence of purulent fluid in the pleural cavity. It is due to pleural space infection resulting from post-bacterial pneumonia in the majority of cases (1). According to its radiological (X-ray, computed tomography scan, and ultrasonography) features, empyema is classified into three stages (2): Stage I: Parapneumonic effusion, with an increase in pleural effusion; Stage II: Fibrinopurulent stage with loculations of pleural fluid and fibrinous septa formation; Stage III: Chronic organizing stage with scar adhesions and progressive constriction resulting in incarcerated lung. For patients with advanced disease (Stages II and III), early surgical intervention is beneficial to avoid more complex surgical procedures, higher morbidity, mortality, and longer disease duration (3). For pleural empyema in children: A systematic review of 44 retrospective studies comparing different treatment strategies (4). They were chest tube therapy (16 studies, 611 cases), chest tube with fibrinolytic drug (10 studies, 83 cases), video-assisted thoracic surgery (VATS) (22 studies, 449 cases) and thoracotomy (13 studies, 226 cases). This study found that patients who received VATS or thoracotomy had shorter hospital stays than those who were non-operatively treated. The American Association for Thoracic Surgery (AATS) recommends VATS debridement rather than open thoracotomy for the surgical management of empyema in the pediatric population (5).

Articles on surgical vs. non-surgical treatment have been widely reported in recent years. A 2017 meta-analysis (6) included eight randomized controlled trials with a total of 391 participants. The authors concluded that there was insufficient evidence to assess the impact of fibrinolytic therapy and that VATS may reduce the length of hospital stay compared to thoracostomy drainage. To date, very few works have evaluated the role of the uniportal VATS (U-VATS) approach in the treatment of pleural empyema in children, even though it currently represents the most innovative and less invasive thoracoscopic approach (7). We report our experience with U-VATS in the treatment of pleural empyema in children.

PATIENTS AND METHODS

The present study was approved by the ethics committee of our hospital and adhered to the tenets of the Declaration of Helsinki. Additionally, written informed consent was obtained from the parents of the patients.

Patients

From January 2019 to December 2020, 39 children with empyema were treated in our department. Our inclusion criteria were as follows: (1) patients with primary pleural empyema; (2) no surgical treatment received before admission to our hospital; and (3) Stage II and Stage III empyema with no improvement after conservative treatment. The exclusion criteria were patients with other pre-operative complications, such as congenital heart disease, immunocompromised state, restrictive or obstructive chest wall disease, and patients with additional foci of infection. The diagnosis and the stages of empyema were confirmed by chest X-ray plus ultrasound and then further verified by computed tomography (CT) scan (**Figure 1**). Thirteen of them had Stage I empyema, which improved after chest drainage and anti-infection treatment. One child was referred to our hospital after surgery in another hospital. Four children had other pre-operative complications. Once the diagnosis of pleural empyema was determined, a further ultrasound scan was performed to identify the presence of fibrinous septa and loculated fluid. Patients underwent closed placement of chest drainage and antibiotic therapy as the first procedure. If the following clinical and radiological examinations showed the failure of medical therapy with persistence of septic status, trapped lung or several loculations of pleural fluid and the presence of fibrinous septa, U-VATS treatments were performed. Finally, after eliminating contraindications such as the inability to tolerate one lung ventilation and severe coagulopathy (5), 21 patients received U-VATS during the study period (**Figure 2**). Their clinical information is summarized in **Table 1**.

Surgical Technique

All patients were consecutively operated on by the same team of thoracic surgeons. We used a uniportal approach as described and defined by Migliore et al. (8). All patients were operated on under general anesthesia with selective one-lung ventilation using a single-lumen endotracheal tube with a bronchial blocker (Tappa, Hangzhou, China). The patients were positioned in the full lateral decubitus position, and the surgeon always stood at the ventral side of the patient. A 1.0 cm utility port was created in the 5th intercostal space (ICS) at the anterior axillary line. A wound protector (disposable wound protectors, Changzhou Anker Medical Co., LTD, Changzhou, China) was applied at the utility port. A rigid 30° 5 mm optic thoracoscope was used for vision, and two or three instruments, such as suction/irrigator devices, electrocantery, endoscopic graspers or scissors, endoscopic ultrasonic scalpels or open surgical instruments, were used through the utility port. The operation proceeded with septal rupture, debridement, and removal of all adhesions and inflammatory effusions from the diaphragmatic and parietal pleura to the apex of the chest cavity with the aim of creating a unique pleural cavity (without septa and loculations) and restoring the physiological movement of the lung. Multiple washings with warm physiological solution were carried out to eliminate all the residual effusion and organized pus from the visceral pleura. Under thoracoscopic control, lung inflation was performed to evaluate the efficacy of decortication. One chest tube was placed for pleural drainage after surgery. The chest tube was removed when there was no air leak, and when the amount of daily drainage was <1 mL/kg (9). Patients were discharged 1 day after removal of the chest tube if the follow-up chest X-ray showed no signs of pneumothorax and no signs of complications.

Statistical Analysis

Continuous data are presented as the mean ± standard deviation and range, while categorical variables are presented as frequencies (%). SPSS Statistics (Windows version 19.0 IBM Corp., Armonk, NY) was used for analysis.

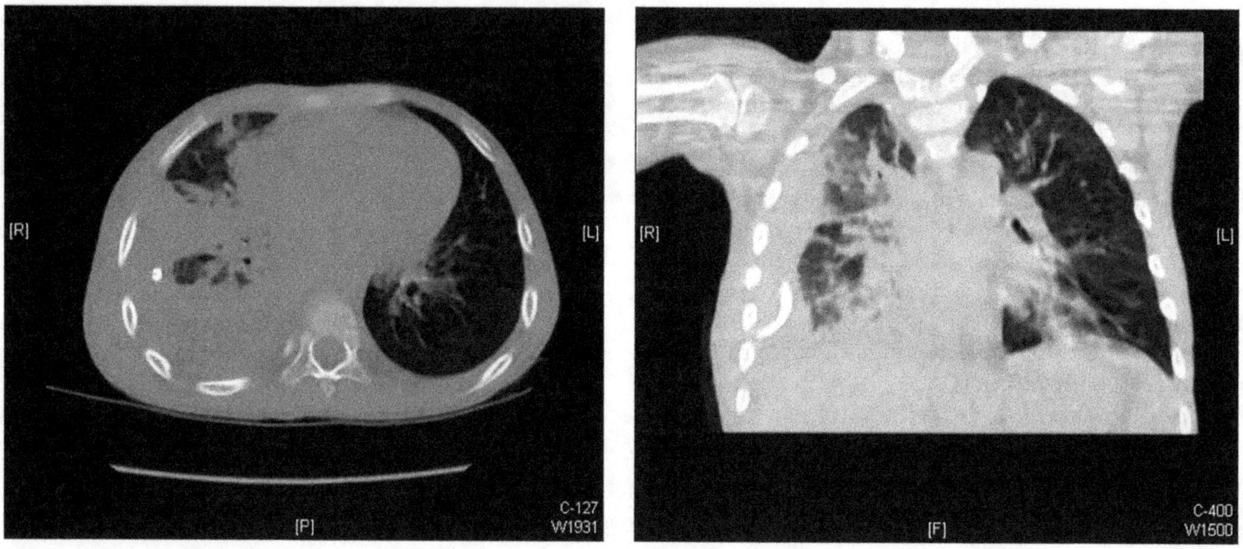

FIGURE 1 | CT image of pleural empyema.

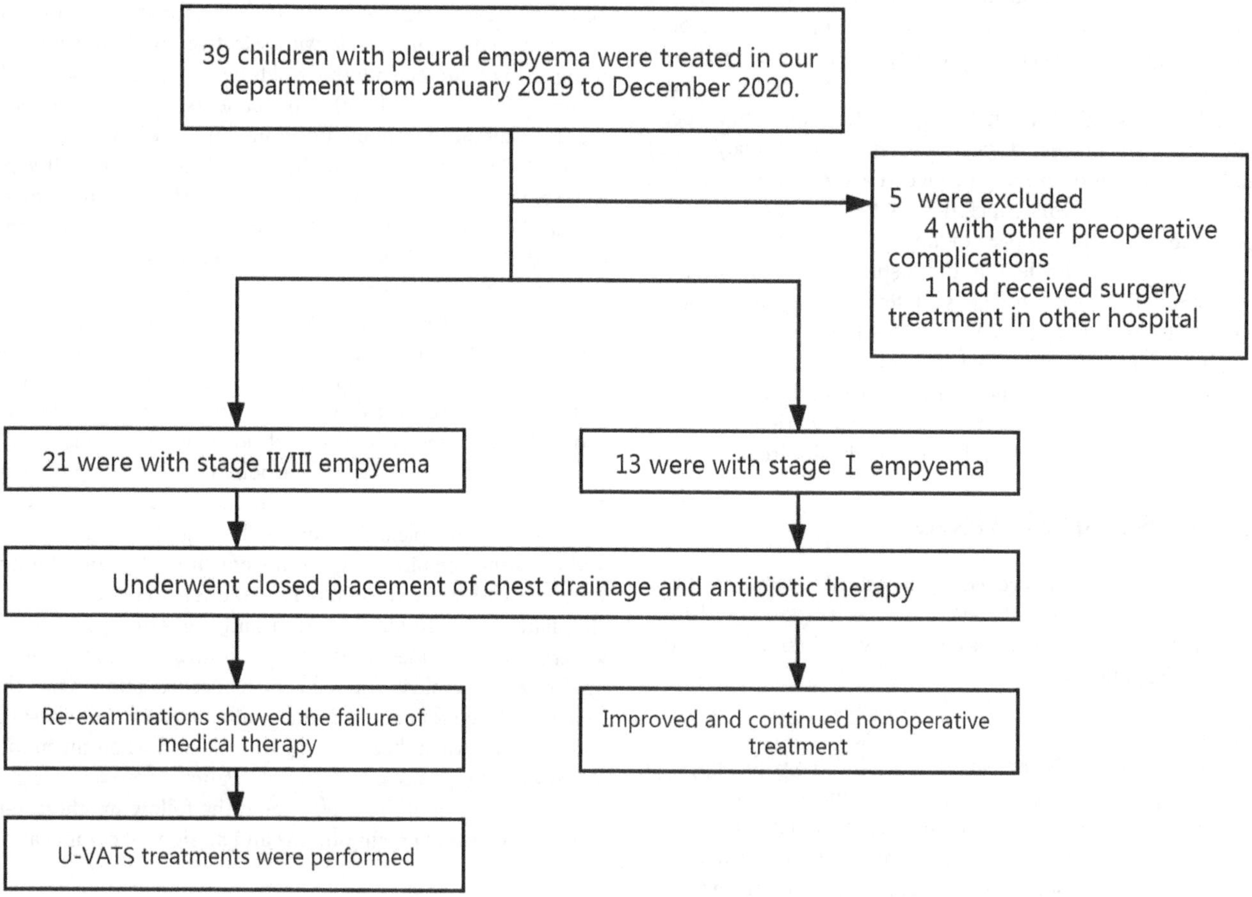

FIGURE 2 | CONSORT flow diagram of participants.

TABLE 1 | Demographical and clinical characteristics of the patients.

Patient number	Age (years)	Gender	Weight (kg)	Location	Empyema stage	Duration of post-operative fever (days)	Operative time (min)	Drainage duration (days)	Hospital stay (days)	Post-operative complications
1	3	F	15	R	Stage II	13	60	3	4	No
2	4	M	16.5	L	Stage II	15	60	4	5	No
3	11	F	24	L	Stages III	12	110	3	4	No
4	3	F	13.9	R	Stage II	13	120	4	5	No
5	10	M	22	R	Stages III	14	100	4	5	No
6	2	M	12.5	L	Stage II	15	50	3	4	No
7	2	M	13	R	Stages III	12	55	3	4	No
8	6	M	21	L	Stage II	13	60	5	6	Subcutaneous emphysema
9	3	M	15.5	L	Stages III	10	65	5	6	Pneumothorax
10	5	M	19	L	Stage II	14	70	4	5	No
11	1	M	9	R	Stages III	10	95	4	5	No
12	1	F	11	R	Stage II	14	75	5	5	No
13	0.6	M	7	R	Stages III	10	120	5	6	No
14	0.5	F	6.5	L	Stages III	12	100	4	5	No
15	3	M	14.5	L	Stages III	10	50	4	5	No
16	2	F	13	R	Stage II	12	55	5	5	No
17	5	F	20.5	R	Stages III	8	60	4	5	No
18	7	M	25	L	Stage II	12	65	5	6	Subcutaneous emphysema
19	6	M	22	L	Stages III	8	70	4	5	No
20	9	F	23	R	Stages III	13	100	3	5	No
21	3	F	11	R	Stages III	12	50	3	5	No
	4.1 ± 3.0	M: 57.1%	15.9 ± 5.5	R: 42.9%	Stage II: 42.9%	12 ± 2.0	65.7 ± 23.2	4 ± 0.76	5 ± 0.62	3 (14.3%)

RESULTS

The mean age of the patients was 4.1 years (range 6 months to 11 years old), and 57.1% (12 patients) were males. Twelve patients (57.1%) presented Stage III empyema, and 9 patients (42.9%) presented Stage II empyema. All cases were related to complicated parapneumonic effusion. Pleural culture was positive in 6 (28.6%) patients. The main aetiologic agents were Staphylococcus aureus (2 patients), Streptococcus pneumoniae (3 patients), and Streptococcus viridans (1 patient). Of the 2 patients with Staphylococcus aureus, 1 had methicillin-resistant strain. All patients were treated with broad-spectrum antibiotic therapy. A chest tube was placed to evacuate pleural effusion, provided microbiologic insights. No fibrinolytic therapy had been administered. Among patients treated with chest tube insertion, 19 patients (90.5%) showed a trapped lung. All patients were treated with antibiotics plus thoracic drainage for at least 2 weeks (range 14–21 days), and with the failure of these medical treatments, the operation was carried out. The mean operation time for the U-VATS approach was 65.7 ± 23.3 min. Complete debridement and decortication were obtained in all patients, and no conversion or further access was needed for any reason. Post-operative complications occurred in 3 patients, including pneumothorax (air leakage >2 days) in 1 patient and subcutaneous emphysema in 2 patients. The drainage tube was removed after 4.0 ± 0.8 days, and patients were discharged after 4.9 ± 0.7 days. The long-term outcome was excellent in all cases, and all patients were alive with no recurrence.

DISCUSSION

To our knowledge, this is the first report of children with pleural empyema undergoing U-VATS for treatment. In 2001, Waller and his colleagues (10) concluded that VATS was proven to be as effective as open surgery in the treatment of Stage III empyema and had the advantages of being minimally invasive, plus reduced pain and hospitalization. Some authors (11–14) reported that the clinical effect of VATS decortications was better than that of thoracotomy. A recent meta-analysis (15) reviewed 14 published articles in 2010, and the results showed that VATS was superior to open surgery in terms of post-operative pain, complications, morbidity, 30-day mortality, and length of stay, with no significant difference in recurrence rates. U-VATS was first reported by Rocco in 2004 and has often been performed (16). Mahmoud Ismail and his colleagues (7) concluded that U-VATS allows for an easier performance, complete debridement

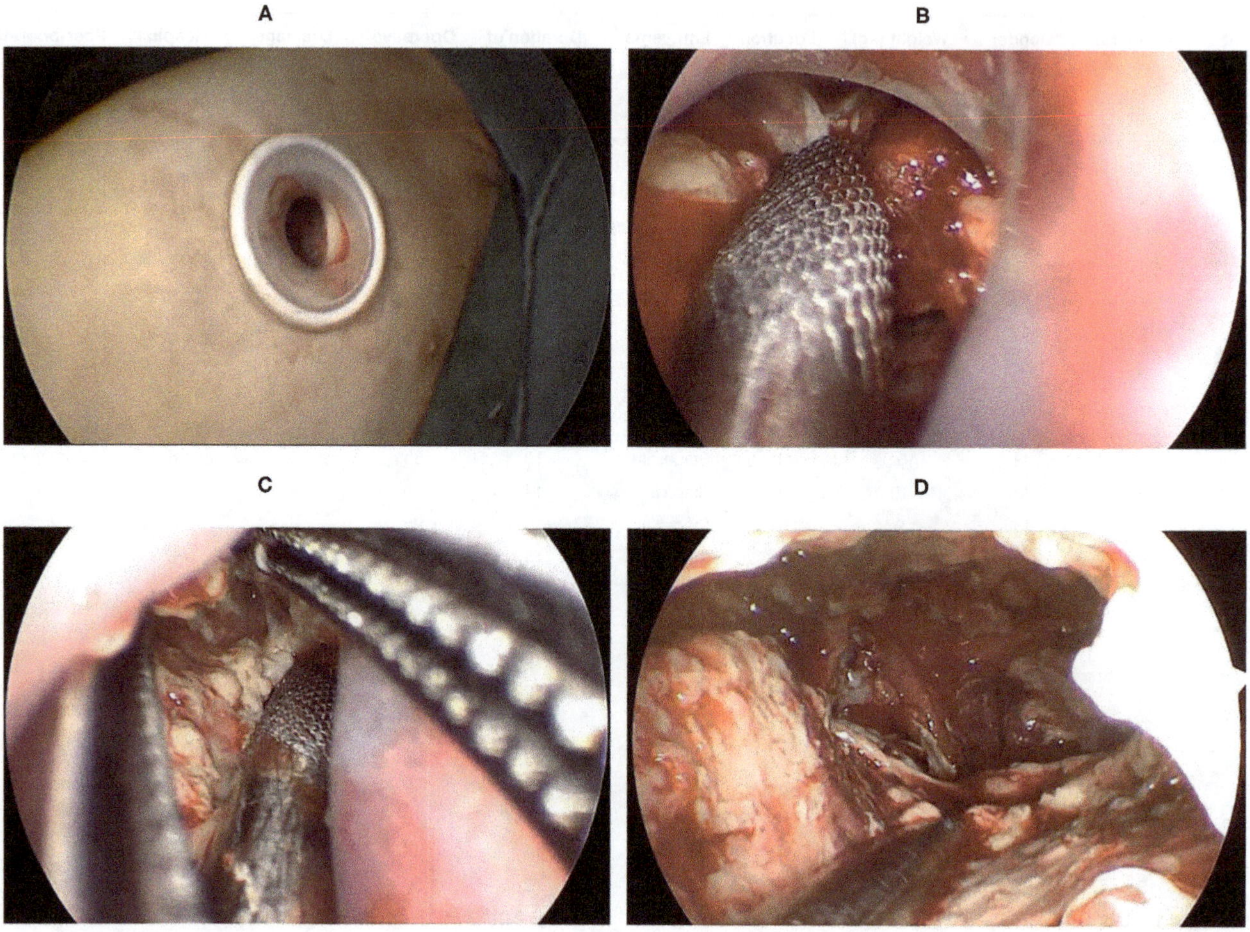

FIGURE 3 | (A) A 1.0 cm port created in the 5th ICS at the anterior axillary line. **(B)** The aspirator was used to suck and remove the tissue around the incision. **(C)** Debride the area around the incision with aspirator and curved forceps. **(D)** Create a suitable surgical space.

and decortication, with a very low risk for conversion and excellent post-operative outcomes in terms of less pain, faster recovery, and cosmetic results. However, beyond that, few studies have evaluated the usefulness of the U-VATS method in the treatment of pleural empyema in children, and all the above reports are adult cases. Hung Do Manh and his colleagues (17) described a single trocar thoracoscopic surgery for pediatric pleural empyema, in which a 10 mm trocar was inserted with a scope and a single instrument for pleural dissection. Although different from the U-VATS as defined (8), some good results have been achieved. We tried to use a similar method and found that the main difficulty was that just one instrument could not perform debridement while aspirating the blood and pus at the same time.

Martin-Ucar and Socci (18) reported the advantages of U-VATS in many factors, including post-operative pain, post-operative recovery, view of the thoracic cavity, angle of vision, no rotational effect, and the ergonomic position of the operating surgeon. When performing U-VATS for children with pleural empyema, we noticed the above advantages and found some others from our single-center experience. How to expose the surgical field was the first question we faced. All the cases had severe pleural adhesions, and the surgeon needed to create a surgical space at the beginning of the operation. Tander et al. (19) reported a balloon-aided single-port thoracoscopic technique to achieve a wider field of vision, and a satisfactory conclusion was obtained. We found that the separation of adhesions from the edge of the incision using double-joint instruments of different curvatures could also gradually create a satisfactory surgical area (**Figure 3**).

There are some characteristics of the children's chest, including small cavum space and narrow intercostal space. The distance between the surgical area and the chest surface was short, which resulted in a limited angle of instrument activity. Angulated and narrow-shaft double-hinged instruments have become essential instruments for U-VATS, while articulating instruments help bring the operative fulcrum inside the chest. It is worth mentioning that, after early exploration, we found that a small incision is unique in its instrumentation requirement. Customized double-hinged surgical instruments with a 4-mm rod diameter were used in our U-VATS, and electrocantery was able to change the angle at will with a rod diameter of 2 mm. All the instruments made it advantageous to operate from multiple angles and to multiple regions.

Although pulmonary collapse would not be good due to pleural adhesion, we still recommend bronchial occlusion in our experience. Because the degree of lung collapse is gradually restored with debridement, without tracheal occlusion, the surgical space would be limited. There is a propensity for bleeding during empyema debridement and decortication, which can result in limited vision of the surgical field, making the procedure dangerous, especially near the hilum. We considered it safe and effective to perform debridement and aspirate the blood at the same time. When multiportal VATS or single-port VATS is performed, the chest is a closed environment. Although the surgical procedure is exercisable under artificial pneumothorax, the use of an aspirator would significantly reduce the surgical space, which is not a concern for U-VATS with tracheal occlusion. In addition, two or three instruments can simultaneously perform operative procedures such as suction, exposure, separation and hemostasis. Due to the limitation of retrospective studies, its superiority needs to be confirmed by further prospective research.

The application of the U-VATS technique marked a milestone innovation in thoracic surgery. However, there is often a long learning curve for the conversion from conventional multiportal VATS to U-VATS. Our surgeons have had many years of experience in U-VATS, so we conducted this study and aimed to evaluate the safety and feasibility of U-VATS for children with pleural empyema. As a result of the 21 successful cases mentioned, our experience was limited. We are also moving forward with more cases and more complex U-VATS procedures to further confirm our findings with prospective, comparative studies.

CONCLUSIONS

The U-VATS approach is safe and feasible for children with pleura empyema. We presented U-VATS for the surgical management of Stage II and III empyema with satisfactory perioperative results.

AUTHOR CONTRIBUTIONS

J-XH and HC made a significant contribution to the conception and design of the work. J-JH and S-MH drafted the work and revised it critically for important intellectual content. QC and J-XH are responsible for all aspects of the work and ensure that questions related to the accuracy or integrity of any part of the work are appropriately investigated and resolved. All authors read and approved the final manuscript.

ACKNOWLEDGMENTS

We thank all doctors in our center for their helpful advice and discussions.

REFERENCES

1. Ferguson AD, Prescott RJ, Selkon JB, Watson D, Swinburn CR. The clinical course and management of thoracic empyema. *QJM.* (1996) 89:285–9. doi: 10.1093/qjmed/89.4.285
2. Scarci M, Abah U, Solli P, Page A, Waller D, van Schil P, et al. EACTS expert consensus statement for surgical management of pleural empyema. *Eur J Cardiothorac Surg.* (2015) 48:642–53. doi: 10.1093/ejcts/ezv272
3. Reichert M, Hecker M, Witte B, Bodner J, Padberg W, Weigand MA, et al. Stage-directed therapy of pleural empyema. *Langenbecks Arch Surg.* (2017) 402:15–26. doi: 10.1007/s00423-016-1498-9
4. Gates RL, Caniano DA, Hayes JR, Arca MJ. Does VATS provide optimal treatment of empyema in children? A systematic review. *J Pediatr Surg.* (2004) 39:381–6 doi: 10.1016/j.jpedsurg.2003.11.045
5. Shen KR, Bribriesco A, Crabtree T, Denlinger C, Eby J, Eiken P, et al. The American Association for Thoracic Surgery consensus guidelines for the management of empyema. *J Thorac Cardiovasc Surg.* (2017) 153:e129–46. doi: 10.1016/j.jtcvs.2017.01.030
6. Redden MD, Chin TY, van Driel ML. Surgical versus non-surgical management for pleural empyema. *Cochrane Database Syst Rev.* (2017) 3:CD010651. doi: 10.1002/14651858.CD010651.pub2
7. Ismail M, Nachira D, Meacci E, Ferretti GM, Swierzy M, Englisch JP, et al. Uniportal video-assisted thoracic surgery in the treatment of pleural empyema. *J Thorac Dis.* (2018) 10(Suppl. 31):S3696–703. doi: 10.21037/jtd.2018.05.10
8. Migliore M, Halezeroglu S, Molins L, Van Raemdonck D, Mueller MR, Rea F, et al. Uniportal video-assisted thoracic surgery or single-incision video-assisted thoracic surgery for lung resection: clarifying definitions. *Future Oncol.* (2016) 12:5–7. doi: 10.2217/fon-2016-0370
9. St PS, Tsao K, Spilde TL, Keckler SJ, Harrison C, Jackson MA, et al. Thoracoscopic decortication vs tube thoracostomy with fibrinolysis for empyema in children: a prospective, randomized trial. *J Pediatr Surg.* (2009) 44:106–11. doi: 10.1016/j.jpedsurg.2008.10.018
10. Waller DA, Rengarajan A. Thoracoscopic decortication: a role for video-assisted surgery in chronic postpneumonic pleural empyema. *Ann Thorac Surg.* (2001) 71:1813–6. doi: 10.1016/S0003-4975(01)02471-7
11. Tong BC, Hanna J, Toloza EM, Onaitis MW, D'Amico TA, Harpole DH, et al. Outcomes of videoassisted thoracoscopic decortication. *Ann Thorac Surg.* (2010) 89:220–5. doi: 10.1016/j.athoracsur.2009.09.021
12. Marks DJ, Fisk MD, Koo CY, Pavlou M, Peck L, Lee SF, et al. Thoracic empyema: a 12-year study from a UK tertiary cardiothoracic referral centre. *PLoS ONE.* (2012) 7:e30074. doi: 10.1371/journal.pone.0030074
13. Swanson SJ, Meyers BF, Gunnarsson CL, Moore M, Howington JA, Maddaus MA, et al. Video-assisted thoracoscopic lobectomy is less costly and morbid than open lobectomy: a retrospective multIInstitutional database analysis. *Ann Thorac Surg.* (2012)93:1027–32. doi: 10.1016/j.athoracsur.2011.06.007
14. Schneider CR, Gauderer MW, Blackhurst D, Chandler JC, Abrams RS. Video-assisted thoracoscopic surgery as a primary intervention in pediatric parapneumonic effusion and empyema. *Am Surg.* (2010) 76:957–61. doi: 10.1177/000313481007600928
15. Chambers A, Routledge T, Dunning J, Scarci M. Is videoassisted thoracoscopic surgical decortication superior to open surgery in the management of adults with primary empyema? *Interact Cardiovasc Thorac Surg.* (2010) 11:171–7. doi: 10.1510/icvts.2010.240408

16. Mineo TC, Ambrogi V. A glance at the history of uniportal video-assisted thoracic surgery. *J Visual Surg.* (2017) 3:157. doi: 10.21037/jovs.2017.10.11
17. Do H, Nguyen Q, Nguyen L, Nguyen L. Single trocar thoracoscopic surgery for pleural empyema in children. *J Laparoendosc Adv Surg Tech A.* (2020). doi: 10.1089/lap.2019.0637. [Epub ahead of print].
18. Martin-Ucar AE, Socci L. Why perform uniportal video-assisted thoracic surgery?-multiple considerations. *J Vis Surg.* (2016) 2:108. doi: 10.21037/jovs.2016.06.01
19. Tander B, Ustun L, Ariturk E, Rizalar R, Ayyildiz SH, Bernay F, et al. Balloon-assisted single-port thoracoscopic debridement in children with thoracic empyema. *J Laparoendosc Adv Surg Tech A.* (2007) 17:504–8. doi: 10.1089/lap.2006.0180

10

Incision and Drainage with Primary Fistulotomy of Perianal Abscess is Safe and Effective in Neonates: A Long-Term Follow-Up Study

Wanbin Yin [1], Laian Li [1], Lin Su [2] and Shuai Wang [1]*

[1] Department of Anorectal Surgery, Affiliated Hospital of Jining Medical University, Jining, China, [2] Department of Pediatric Surgery, Affiliated Hospital of Jining Medical University, Jining, China

Correspondence:
Shuai Wang
jyfyws@126.com

Objective: Perianal abscess (PA) in neonates is poorly understood, and its management remains controversial. The aim of this study was to compare incision and drainage (ID) with or without primary fistulotomy in the management of neonatal first-time PA.

Methods: A retrospective comparative study was conducted for neonates with first-time PA treated with incision and drainage with primary fistulotomy (IDF) vs. ID between 2008 and 2017.

Results: In total, 138 patients (137 boys and 1 girl) were identified; 65 in the IDF group and 73 in the ID group. The median follow-up was 6.5 years (range 4–13 years). Baseline characteristics were similar between the 2 groups. The cure rate in the IDF group (98.5%, 64/65) was significantly higher than that in the ID group (80.8%, 59/73; $p = 0.001$). The rate of fistula formation in the IDF group (1.5%, 1/65) was significantly lower than that in the ID group (13.7%, 10/73; $p = 0.01$). The rate of abscess recurrence was not statistically different ($p = 0.12$), even though the IDF group (0%, 0/65) seemed to have a better outcome than the ID group (5.5%, 4/73). No fecal incontinence was observed in any of our patients.

Conclusions: First-time PA in neonates can be treated safely and effectively by the IDF or by ID alone. The former may be advantageous over the latter in terms of the rate of cure and fistula formation.

Keywords: neonates, perianal abscess, incision and drainage, fistulotomy, fistula formation, abscess recurrence, long-term, follow-up

INTRODUCTION

A perianal abscess (PA) in neonates is a relatively common disease, but it is poorly understood. It is usually considered a trivial disease by physicians. Nevertheless, the discovery of perianal swelling in a neonate can be a source of anxiety for parents. Parents' excessive worry and physicians' insufficient experience make the management of neonatal PA very challenging. However, only rare literature is devoted to it. Therefore, the treatment is usually based on the studies of PA in infants and children.

The management of PA in infants and children is controversial. It has traditionally been treated surgically by incision and drainage (ID) (1–11). However, in the past two decades, some studies have shown that the conservative management appears to be effective in selected cases (12–23). On the other hand, the other studies have recommended that the surgical procedure should involve a careful identification for the fistula and treatment of that by fistulotomy (24–32). Thus, at present, the optimal management has not yet been established.

At our center, PA in infants can be treated either in the department of anorectal surgery or in the department of pediatric surgery. Some infants experienced fistula formation after ID, and were transferred to the department of anorectal surgery. Is ID enough? Is incision and drainage with primary fistulotomy (IDF) better than ID? These ideas prompted us to complete this long-term comparative study.

To the best of our knowledge, no published study in PubMed has directly compared the outcomes of IDF vs. ID for neonatal PA. This study aimed to compare the efficacy and safety of IDF and ID for PA in neonates.

MATERIALS AND METHODS

A retrospective case note review was carried out for all consecutive neonates with PA at a single tertiary center between January 2008 and December 2017. At our center, all neonates admitted to the department of anorectal surgery underwent IDF, while all neonates admitted to the department of pediatric surgery underwent ID. Patients with PA undergoing IDF were assigned to the IDF group, and those undergoing ID were assigned to the ID group. Although group allocation was not randomized, it was naturally formed according to the department in which the patients were hospitalized. Neonates with PA received intravenous antibiotics routinely (Ceftazidime in the IDF group and Cefathiamidine in the ID group) for 3–5 days.

The present study was approved by the Affiliated Hospital of Jining Medical University Institutional Review Board. Written informed consent was obtained from all parents.

Diagnostic Criteria

Perianal abscess was diagnosed by the presence of a firm or fluctuant tender mass close to the anus. Fistula-in-ano (FIA) was diagnosed by the presence of a hole with or without pus drainage at the site of the anus, persisting more than 3 weeks postoperatively. A recurrence of PA was defined as an abscess developed at the original location again after wound healing. New-onset PA was defined as a new abscess that developed at other locations.

Inclusion and Exclusion Criteria

Inclusion criteria were neonatal patients with first-time PA who presented to our center during the first 28 days after birth and underwent IDF or ID. Exclusion criteria were patients whose age at symptom onset is younger than 28 days but the age at admission was older than 28 days, inpatients discharged without surgery due to parental refusal, patients who had undergone prior surgical treatment at other centers, or patients lost to follow-up.

Incision and Drainage

A small incision was made through the dome of the abscess and pockets within the cavity were delicately broken by gentle exploration with a hemostatic forceps under local anesthesia.

Incision and Drainage With Primary Fistulotomy

Subsequent fistulotomy was performed right after ID with the patient in the left lateral decubitus position under conscious sedation and local anesthesia. The most important step was to identify the internal opening. A fine probe was gently introduced through the abscess cavity to the affected anal crypt, then the fistula tract was unroofed and laid open with diathermy. If the internal opening could not be probed, then the corresponding internal opening, which was in the same location as the center of the abscess was laid open. All of the fistulas were low-type.

Follow-Up

Short-term follow-up was conducted by outpatient reviews within 3 weeks of discharge. Given the coronavirus disease 2019 (COVID-19) pandemic, long-term follow-up data were mainly obtained *via* telephone interview, supplemented by outpatient review and a home visit. As we all know, a high percentage of completed follow-up is essential for long-term outcomes and is necessary to minimize any bias that might result from failure to contact patients. Therefore, we made every effort to make contact with each parent.

Data Collection

Collected data included baseline characteristics, length of follow-up, fistula formation, recurrence of abscess, new-onset abscess, and fecal incontinence.

Statistical Analysis

Quantitative variables were summarized as mean ± standard deviation (SD) or median with interquartile range (IQR). Categorical variables were summarized as percentages. Comparisons between 2 groups were made by using the 2-tailed *t*-test or Mann–Whitney *U*-test for continuous variables. The chi-square test and Fisher's exact test were used for comparing categorical variables. Differences were considered statistically significant at $p < 0.05$. Data were analyzed using the SPSS software, version 18.0.

RESULTS

A total of 147 hospitalized neonates with PA were identified from January 2008 to December 2017 (**Figure 1**). Of the 9 excluded patients, 5 were excluded because parents refused surgery. Of the 138 included patients, 65 (47.1%) underwent IDF and 73 (52.9%) underwent ID. Follow-up data were available for all but one who had been excluded according to exclusion criteria. The median follow-up was 6.5 years (range 4–13 years).

Patient and abscess characteristics are summarized in **Table 1**. The 2 groups were similar in respect of gender, age of onset, duration of symptoms, age at admission, number of the abscess, location of the abscess, and length of stay. Of note, inpatient costs were higher in the IDF group vs. the ID group (3,774.0 vs. 2,416.0 Yuan, $p = 0.000$). Healing time (the time needed for the complete epithelialization of the wound bed) was about 3 and 2 weeks for the IDF group and ID group, respectively.

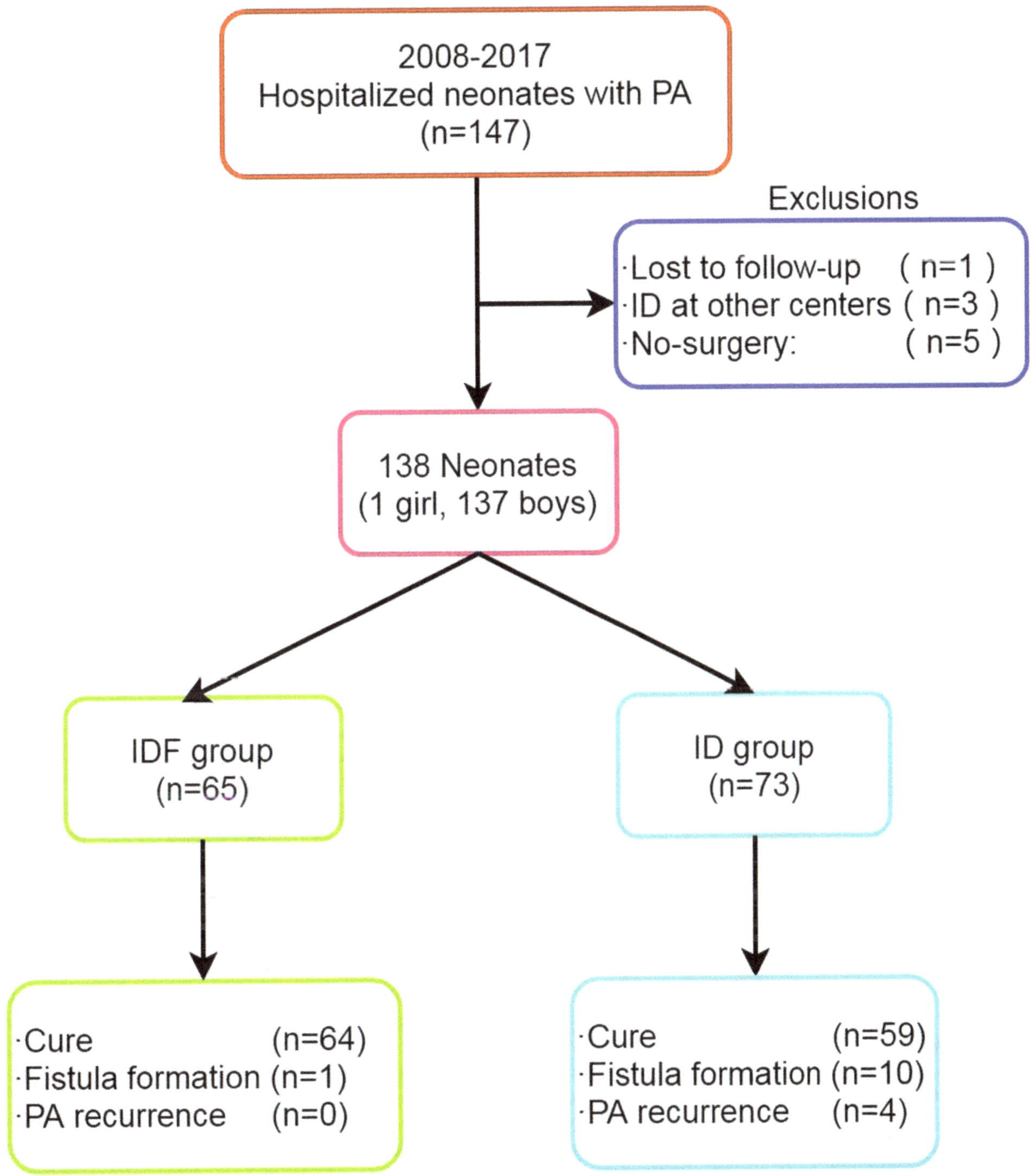

FIGURE 1 | Enrollment, treatment, and long-term outcomes of patients with PA. PA, perianal abscess; ID, incision and drainage; IDF, incision and drainage with primary fistulotomy.

A comparison of long-term outcomes between the 2 groups is shown in **Table 2**. The median follow-up for patients undergoing IDF and ID was 5.00 years (IQR, 4.00–7.50) and 7.00 years (IQR, 5.50–9.00), respectively ($p = 0.000$). Patients in the IDF group had a higher cure rate (98.46 vs. 80.82%, $p = 0.001$) and a lower fistula formation rate (1.54 vs. 13.70%, $p = 0.01$) than the ID group. After surgery, 11 patients developed FIA (**Figure 2**). Of the 3 patients developing FIA after ID, 2 patients were cured after more than 2 years of plaster and Chinese herbal preparations ointment (ingredients unknown), respectively. The

TABLE 1 | Clinical characteristics of neonates with PA.

Characteristics	IDF (*n* = 65)	ID (*n* = 73)	*P*
Male sex, *n* (%)	65 (100)	72 (98.63)	1.00
Age of onset, mean ± SD, d	18.62 ± 4.28	18.73 ± 4.00	0.87
Duration of symptoms, median (IQR), d	4.00 (2.00–5.50)	3.00 (2.00–5.00)	0.77
Age at admission, mean ± SD, d	22.71 ± 3.49	22.36 ± 4.51	0.61
Number of the abscess, *n* (%)			0.13
1	58 (89.23)	70 (95.89)	
2	6 (9.22)	3 (4.11)	
3	1 (1.54)	0 (0)	
Locations of the abscesses			0.76
3-o'clock, *n* (%)	21 (28.77)	25 (32.89)	
9-o'clock, *n* (%)	35 (47.95)	32 (42.11)	
Other locations	17 (23.29)	19 (25.00)	
Length of stay, median (IQR), d	6.00 (5.00–7.75)	6.00 (5.00–8.00)	0.37
Inpatient costs, median (IQR), *yuan RMB*	3,774 (3,497–4,007)	2,416 (1,884–3,245)	0.000

PA, perianal abscess; ID, incision and drainage; IDF, incision and drainage with primary fistulotomy; SD, standard deviation; IQR, interquartile range; RMB, renminbi, the currency of China.

TABLE 2 | Long-term outcomes of IDF vs. ID.

Long-term outcomes	IDF (*n* = 65)	ID (*n* = 73)	*P*
Follow-up time, median (IQR), y	5.00 (4.00–7.50)	7.00 (5.50–9.00)	0.000
Cure, *n* (%)	64 (98.46)	59 (80.82)	0.001
Fistula formation, *n* (%)	1 (1.54)	10 (13.70)	0.01
PA recurrence, *n* (%)	0 (0)	4 (5.48)	0.12

ID, incision and drainage; IDF, incision and drainage with primary fistulotomy; IQR, interquartile range; PA, perianal abscess.

third patient was cured with an ointment (ingredients and duration unknown).

None of the patients in the IDF group had a recurrence, while 4 patients in the ID group experienced recurrence (**Table 3**). Patients undergoing IDF seemed to have a lower abscess recurrence rate (0 vs. 5.48%; $p = 0.12$), albeit statistical significance was not achieved.

It is noteworthy that 2 (3.08%) patients developed new abscesses at the contralateral side of the anus in the IDF group, compared with 7 (9.59%) patients in the ID group (**Table 4**). However, the difference between the 2 groups is not statistically significant ($p = 0.17$).

No fecal incontinence was confirmed in any patients in our study. A 10-year-old boy (undergoing IDF in 2010) with mental illness was found to have stools in his underwear sometimes. It is not sure whether it was caused by surgery or mental illness.

DISCUSSION

Our long-term study showed that IDF was associated with a higher rate of cure and a lower rate of fistula formation compared with ID. In addition, patients in the IDF group seemed to have a lower rate of abscess recurrence and new-onset abscess, albeit statistical significance was not achieved.

In our study, the cure rate in the IDF group and ID group was 98.46 and 80.82%, respectively. That was similar to a previous report (29) that cure occurred in 61/66 (92%) in whom a fistula was identified and treated by fistulotomy at the initial operation, compared with 19/25 (76%) in whom a fistula was not identified (ID alone). The high cure rate is attributable to careful identification and laying opening of the coexisting fistula. The rate of fistula (between the PA and the anal crypt) identified at the time of primary drainage varies widely in different studies. The percentage of communication between the PA and the internal (anal) opening was <20% (1, 4, 6, 7, 11) or more than 60% (25, 27, 29–32). Our results (approximately 80%) support the latter.

In the IDF group, the fistula formation rate was 1.54% (1/65) and there were no recurrences after surgery. Our findings are supported by several studies. There were no recurrences (26, 27, 31) or the recurrence rate was <15% (29, 30, 32) in patients who underwent fistulotomy at the time of ID. These findings are in excellent agreement with ours. Given this, we recommend that ID and laying open of the coexisting fistulous tract be performed for PA in neonates.

Surprisingly, in the ID group, the rate of fistula formation and recurrence was 13.7 (10/73) and 5.48% (4/73), respectively. These results are better than we expected. Our study with a large sample size confirms that neonates may have a lower rate of fistula formation after ID than infants and children. We believe that our results are valuable to the clinician. In the literature, the rate of fistula formation and recurrence was 10.5 (4/38) and 7.9% (3/38) (5), 6 (2/33) and 12% (4/33) (7), 20 (20/100) and 27 (27/100) (8), 30 (15/50) and 4% (2/50) (9), 3.8 (1/26) and 3.8% (1/26) (23), and 28 (8/29) and 7% (2/29) (24), respectively. It is well-known that fistula formation and abscess recurrence are the two major challenges for PA therapy. Unfortunately, some studies did not distinguish between them (1–3, 11, 14, 18, 29–34). Of those studies, the rate of fistula formation or recurrence after ID varies widely, which was <20% in 2 studies (2, 3), between 20 and 50% in 7 studies (1, 18, 29–32, 34), and more than 50% in 2 studies (14, 33). Altogether, previous studies differed substantially regarding the rate of fistula formation or recurrence after ID. There are several potential reasons for this difference. First, some reports did not distinguish between fistula formation and abscess recurrence. Since fistula formation and abscess recurrence are different, we call for distinguishing them in future studies. Second, the indications for ID varied in the literature. Some surgeons argue that the abscess should be incised as soon as possible, while other surgeons recommend ID should be reserved for patients with failed conservative management, large abscess, or systemic signs of infection. Third, surgical techniques may differ in detail. Fourth, the sample size in some studies was small. Thus, these results should be viewed with caution.

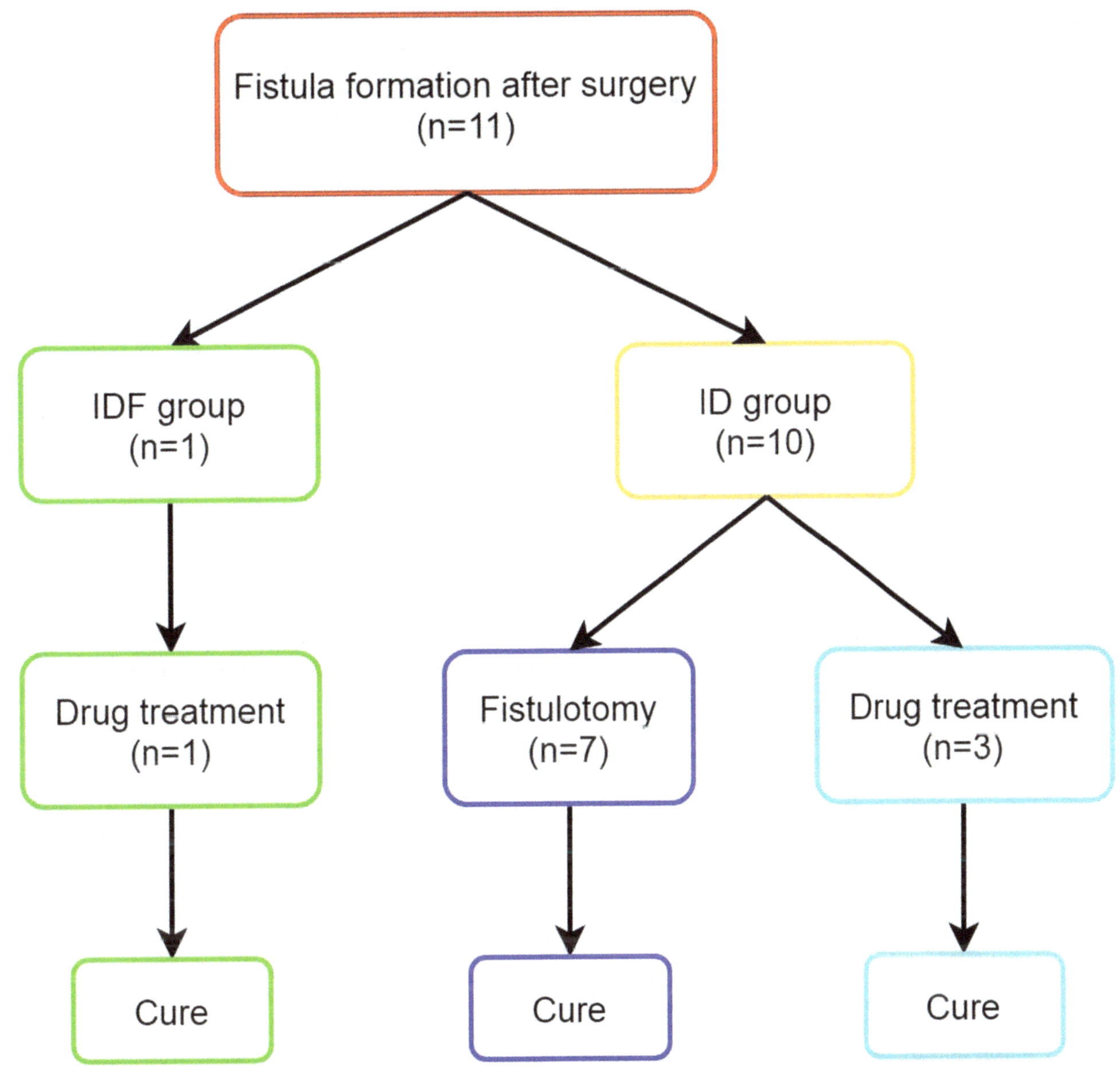

FIGURE 2 | Outcomes of patients with fistula formation after surgery. ID, incision and drainage; IDF, incision and drainage with primary fistulotomy.

Remarkably, in the present study, 6.5% (9/138) of patients developed new abscesses on the contralateral side of the anus. Several studies have previously reported a similar phenomenon (16, 21, 25, 35, 36), but the reason was unknown.

Some studies show that PA is a self-limited entity. In our study, 4 patients who were excluded, experienced spontaneous drainage, and their parents refused surgery. Notably, 3 patients among them were cured without surgery. Similar results have been reported in other studies (18, 22). However, two other studies have shown different results (10, 12). We believe that there is a possibility of a self-resolution of abscesses. In future studies, we will further investigate the safety and effectiveness of non-operative therapy for PA in neonates who spontaneously drained.

There are several strengths to our study. First, the subjects in this study were neonates with PA, excluding infants and children. It is well-known that different stages of life have different pathophysiological features. PA in neonates, infants, and children may have different clinical characteristics. Limiting the age to newborns helped reduce the potential confounding effects of age and made the conclusions more reliable. Second, to the best of our knowledge, this is the first study directly comparing the outcomes of IDF vs. ID for neonatal PA. Third, our sample size (138 neonates) was very large, which improved

TABLE 3 | Characteristics and course of recurrent patients after initial surgery[a].

Case	Time to recurrence	Location	Treatment	Outcome
1	15 d	Right front	Re-ID	Cure
2	18 d	Right	IDF	Cure
3	78 d	Right front	Re-ID	Fistula formation[b]
4	20 m	Right front	IDF	Cure

ID, incision and drainage; IDF, incision and drainage with primary fistulotomy; d, day; m, month.
[a] There was no recurrence among patients undergoing IDF.
[b] The patient was cured after subsequent IDF.

TABLE 4 | Characteristics and course of patients with new-onset abscess after initial surgery.

Case	Initial surgery	Time to new-onset	Location	Treatment	Outcome
1	IDF	36 d	Left	Re-IDF	Cure
2	IDF	1 y	Left	Re-IDF	Cure
3	ID	2 d	Left	Re-ID	Recurrence[a]
4	ID	3 d	Right	Re-ID	Cure
5	ID	4 d	Left	IDF	Cure
6	ID	15 d	Right	CHM	Cure
7	ID	17 d	Right	IDF	Cure
8	ID	Not clear	Right	Plaster	Fistula formation[b]
9	ID	Not clear	Left	Re-ID	Cure

ID, incision and drainage; IDF, incision and drainage with primary fistulotomy; CHM, Chinese herbal medicine; d, day; y, year.
[a] The patient was cured by conservative treatment.
[b] The patient was cured after 2 years of plaster.

the power of the analysis and reduced the bias to a certain extent. Fourth, follow-up data were available for all but one who had been excluded according to exclusion criteria. This is a long-term study with a median follow-up time of 6.5 years. Although various difficulties were encountered, with the aid of the public security bureau, all but one patient were successfully contacted due to the ingenuity, perseverance, and intense effort of our team. Finally, our study included detailed characteristics and course of patients with fistula formation, abscess recurrence, and new-onset abscess after initial surgery, which have not been reported previously.

Of course, some limitations in our study need to be recognized. First, it is a single-center retrospective study, potentially limiting the generalizability of our results. Second, long-term follow-up data were mainly obtained by telephone interviews instead of outpatient reviews. Considering the COVID-19 pandemic, this may be a reasonable alternative method. Third, patients' assignment was not randomized. However, we could be rather certain that it was not assigned by disease severity. At our center, PA in neonates can be treated at the department of anorectal surgery or the department of pediatric surgery. Why patients are admitted to a ward or to another depends on the cognition of the parents, not the severity of the disease. In addition, because of changes in the electronic medical records system, much data were not recorded consecutively, such as body temperature, abscess size, body mass index, white blood cell count, C-reactive protein, procalcitonin, and pus cultures. However, our results showed that important clinical characteristics that might influence the outcome were considerable between the 2 groups (**Table 1**). Thus, there was no inclusion bias. Fourth, not all the surgeries were performed by the same surgeon. Nevertheless, all of those were performed by experienced surgeons using the standardized technique in each group. Finally, the children are too young to cooperate, so anorectal manometry was not performed, which should be performed in the near future.

Unfortunately, PA in neonates and infants is generally considered a trivial condition. However, there are considerable unresolved questions surrounding it. Long-term prospective studies will be necessary to determine the optimal treatment.

CONCLUSION

Our long-term follow-up study demonstrated that IDF and ID are both safe and effective treatments for PA in neonates. IDF is associated with a higher rate of cure and a lower rate of fistula formation compared with ID. Our findings support the value of careful identification and laying opening of the coexisting fistula when ID is performed.

AUTHOR CONTRIBUTIONS

WY: study design, data collection, and drafting of the manuscript. LL: data collection and analysis, article revision, and quality control. LS: data collection, statistical analysis, and article revision. SW: study design, data collection, article revision, and overall responsibility for the article. All authors read and approved the final manuscript.

REFERENCES

1. Enberg RN, Cox RH, Burry VF. Perirectal abscess in children. *Am J Dis Child.* (1974) 128:360–1. doi: 10.1001/archpedi.1974.02110280090011
2. Charalampopoulos A, Zavras N, Kapetanakis EI, Kopanakis K, Misiakos E, Patapis P, et al. Surgical treatment of perianal abscess and fistula-in-ano in childhood, with emphasis in children older than 2 years. *J Pediatr Surg.* (2012) 47:2096–100. doi: 10.1016/j.jpedsurg.2012.06.032
3. Zhu YM, X FY. The pathogens and curative effects analysis of perianal abscess of infants under 3 months. *Turkish J Pediatr.* (2019) 61:40–3. doi: 10.24953/turkjped.2019.01.007
4. al-Salem AH, Qaisaruddin S, Qureshi SS. Perianal abscess and fistula in ano in infancy and childhood: a clinicopathological study. *Pediatr Pathol Lab Med.* (1996) 16:755–64. doi: 10.1080/15513819609169302

5. Nix P, Stringer MD. Perianal sepsis in children. *Br J Surg.* (1997) 84:819–21. doi: 10.1046/j.1365-2168.1997.02699.x
6. Macdonald A, Wilson-Storey D, Munro F. Treatment of perianal abscess and fistula-in-ano in children. *Br J Surg.* (2003) 90:220–1. doi: 10.1002/bjs.4017
7. Niyogi A, Agarwal T, Broadhurst J, Abel RM. Management of perianal abscess and fistula-in-ano in children. *Eur J Pediatr Surg.* (2010) 20:35–9. doi: 10.1055/s-0029-1241878
8. Afşarlar CE, Karaman A, Tanir G, Karaman I, Yilmaz E, Erdogan D, et al. Perianal abscess and fistula-in-ano in children: clinical characteristic, management and outcome. *Pediatr Surg Int.* (2011) 27:1063–8. doi: 10.1007/s00383-011-2956-7
9. Arditi M, Yogev R. Perirectal abscess in infants and children: report of 52 cases and review of literature. *Pediatr Infect Dis J.* (1990) 9:411–5. doi: 10.1097/00006454-199006000-00009
10. Abercrombie JF, George BD. Perianal abscess in children. *Ann R Coll Surg Engl.* (1992) 74:385–6.
11. Boenicke L, Doerner J, Wirth S, Zirngibl H, Langenbach MR. Efficacy of conservative treatment of perianal abscesses in children and predictors for therapeutic failure. *Clin Exp Pediatr.* (2020) 63:272–7. doi: 10.3345/cep.2019.00969
12. Rosen NG, Gibbs DL, Soffer SZ, Hong A, Sher M, Peña A. The nonoperative management of fistula-in-ano. *J Pediatr Surg.* (2000) 35:938–. doi: 10.1053/jpsu.2000.6931
13. Watanabe Y, Todani T, Yamamoto S. Conservative management of fistula in ano in infants. *Pediatr Surg Int.* (1998) 13:274–6. doi: 10.1007/s003830050315
14. Christison-Lagay ER, Hall JF, Wales PW, Bailey K, Terluk A, Goldstein AM, et al. Nonoperative management of perianal abscess in infants is associated with decreased risk for fistula formation. *Pediatrics.* (2007) 120:e548–52. doi: 10.1542/peds.2006-3092
15. Abbott MB. Surgeons say no to surgery for perianal abscesses in infants. *Pediatrics.* (2007) 120:646. doi: 10.1542/peds.2007-1295
16. Kubota M, Hirayama Y, Okuyama N. Usefulness of bFGF spray in the treatment of perianal abscess and fistula-in-ano. *Pediatr Surg Int.* (2010) 26:1037–40. doi: 10.1007/s00383-010-2664-8
17. Kawahara H, Nakai H, Yoneda A, Kubota A. Management of perianal abscess with hainosankyuto in neonates and young infants. *Pediatr Int.* (2011) 53:892–6. doi: 10.1111/j.1442-200X.2011.03395.x
18. Gong Z, Han M, Wu Y, Huang X, Xu WJ, Lv Z. Treatment of first-time perianal abscess in childhood, balance recurrence and fistula formation rate with medical intervention. *Eur J Pediatr Surg.* (2018) 28:373–7. doi: 10.1055/s-0037-1603092
19. Gosemann JH, Lacher M. Perianal abscesses and fistulas in infants and children. *Eur J Pediatr Surg.* (2020) 30:386–90. doi: 10.1055/s-0040-1716726
20. Ding W, Sun YR, Wu ZJ. Treatment of perianal abscess and fistula in infants and young children: from basic etiology to clinical features. *Am Surg.* (2021) 87:927–32. doi: 10.1177/0003134820954829
21. Sueyoshi R, Lane GJ, Kusafuka J, Yamataka A, Doi T. Combination therapy with traditional medicines for perianal abscess in children. *Pediatr Int.* (2019) 61:1025–9. doi: 10.1111/ped.13988
22. Samuk I, Avinadav E, Barak U, Seguier E, Steiner Z, Freud E. Perianal abscess in infants: amenable to conservative treatment in selected cases. *Pediatr Int.* (2019) 61:1146–50. doi: 10.1111/ped.13996
23. Hanada M, Furuya T, Sugito K, Ohashi K, Ikeda T, Koshinaga T, et al. Evaluation of the efficacy of incision and drainage versus hainosankyuto treatment for perianal abscess in infants: a multicenter study. *Surg Today.* (2015) 45:1385–9. doi: 10.1007/s00595-014-1058-2
24. Krieger RW, Chusid MJ. Perirectal abscess in childhood. A review of 29 cases. *Am J Dis Child.* (1979) 133:411–2. doi: 10.1001/archpedi.1979.02130040065014
25. Piazza DJ, Radhakrishnan J. Perianal abscess and fistula-in-ano in children. *Dis Colon Rectum.* (1990) 33:1014–6. doi: 10.1007/BF02139215
26. Festen C, van Harten H. Perianal abscess and fistula-in-ano in infants. *J Pediatr Surg.* (1998) 33:711–3. doi: 10.1016/S0022-3468(98)90193-2
27. Bałaz K, Trypens A, Polnik D, Pankowska-Wozniak K, Kaliciński P. Perianal abscess and fistula-in-ano in children - evaluation of treatment efficacy. Is it possible to avoid recurrence?. *Pol Przegl Chir.* (2020) 92:29–33. doi: 10.5604/01.3001.0013.8158
28. King SK. Should we seek a fistula-in-ano when draining a perianal abscess? *J Paediatr Child Health.* (2010) 46:273–4. doi: 10.1111/j.1440-1754.2009.01694.x
29. Buddicom E, Jamieson A, Beasley S, King S. Perianal abscess in children: aiming for optimal management. *ANZ J Surg.* (2012) 82:60–2. doi: 10.1111/j.1445-2197.2011.05941.x
30. Juth Karlsson A, Salö M, Stenström P. Outcomes of various interventions for first-time perianal abscesses in children. *Biomed Res Int.* (2016) 2016:9712854. doi: 10.1155/2016/9712854
31. Murthi GV, Okoye BO, Spicer RD, Cusick EL, Noblett HR. Perianal abscess in childhood. *Pediatr Surg Int.* (2002) 18:689–91. doi: 10.1007/s00383-002-0761-z
32. Tan Tanny SP, Wijekoon N, Nataraja RM, Lynch A, Pacilli M. Surgical management of perianal abscess in neonates and infants. *ANZ J Surg.* (2020) 90:1034–6. doi: 10.1111/ans.15801
33. Ezer SS, Oguzkurt P, Ince E, Hiçsönmez A. Perianal abscess and fistula-in-ano in children: aetiology, management and outcome. *J Paediatr Child Health.* (2010) 46:92–5. doi: 10.1111/j.1440-1754.2009.01644.x
34. al-Salem AH, Laing W, Talwalker V. Fistula-in-ano in infancy and childhood. *J Pediatr Surg.* (1994) 29:436–8. doi: 10.1016/0022-3468(94)90587-8
35. Laberge JM. Perianal abscess and fistula-in-ano in infants. *J Pediatr Surg.* (1998) 33:1848. doi: 10.1016/s0022-3468(98)90305-0
36. Serour F, Somekh E, Gorenstein A. Perianal abscess and fistula-in-ano in infants: a different entity?. *Dis Colon Rectum.* (2005) 48:359–64. doi: 10.1007/s10350-004-0844-0

11

Uniportal Video-Assisted Thoracoscopic Resection and Lobectomy for Infants with Pulmonary Sequestration: Case Series and Initial Experience

Jin-Xi Huang [1,2,3,4], Qiang Chen [1,2,3,4], Song-Ming Hong [1,2,3,4], Jun-Jie Hong [1,2,3,4] and Hua Cao [1,2,3,4]*

[1] Department of Cardiothoracic Surgery, Fujian Branch of Shanghai Children's Medical Center, Fuzhou, China, [2] Fujian Children's Hospital, Fuzhou, China, [3] Fujian Maternity and Child Health Hospital, Affiliated Hospital of Fujian Medical University, Fuzhou, China, [4] Fujian Key Laboratory of Women and Children's Critical Diseases Research, Fujian Maternity and Child Health Hospital, Fuzhou, China

***Correspondence:**
Hua Cao
caohua0791@163.com

Background: The present study aimed to evaluate the safety and feasibility of uniportal video-assisted thoracoscopic surgery (U-VATS) for infants with pulmonary sequestration (PS).

Methods: From January 2019 to July 2020, 19 infants with PS were admitted to a provincial hospital in the Fujian Province of China. A 1.5-cm utility port was created in the fifth intercostal space at the anterior axillary line. A rigid 30° 5-mm optic thoracoscope was used for vision, and two or three instruments were utilized through the port. Surgical options include standard lobectomy, wedge resection, and resection of the extralobar sequestration. Only one intercostal space was entered, and a chest tube was inserted through the same skin incision if necessary.

Results: The procedure was successful in all patients with an average operation duration of 58.3 ± 31.5 min. The length of post-operative hospital stay was 5.4 ± 1.5 days, and no post-operative deaths or serious complications were observed. The mean post-operative drainage volume was 164.6 ± 45.9 mL, and the mean post-operative thoracic tube indwelling duration was 5.5 ± 1.0 days. No intraoperative conversion, surgical mortality, or major complications were identified among the patients.

Conclusion: Our preliminary experience presented a series of U-VATS lobectomy, wedge resection, and resection of the PS for infants with satisfactory perioperative results.

Keywords: video-assisted thoracoscopic surgery, infant, lobectomy, pulmonary sequestration, uniportal

INTRODUCTION

Pulmonary sequestration (PS) is the second most common type of congenital dysplasia of the lungs and a non-functioning lung mass with an abnormal connection to tracheobronchial trees and an anomalous systemic artery supply (1, 2). The two subtypes of PS are intralobar sequestration (ILS) and extralobar sequestration (ELS). Patients with PS usually manifest upper airway syndrome, hemoptysis, or repeated lung infections (2). The infection rate in children with ILS was 71.17%, and that in children with ELS was 31.37% (3). The currently available data suggested that early (<6-months-old) surgery allows for ease of operative intervention, adequate recovery, and a reasonable time for compensatory lung growth while avoiding the potential infectious complications (4). Video-assisted thoracoscopic surgery (VATS) is a common and effective surgical method for PS, and lobectomy and lung-sparing resection are the two major operative approaches (3, 4).

Nearly a decade after the initial reports from Rocco et al. on the use of video-assisted thoracoscopic surgery (U-VATS) for intermediate therapeutic procedures in the form of non-anatomical wedge resection of nodules (5), the first lobectomy was performed by Gonzalez et al. (6), and Successive reports of anatomical segmentectomies (7), pneumonectomies (8), complex bronchial (9), and en bloc chest wall resections (10) followed. Shaqqura et al. (11) reported on U-VATS lobectomy in a 9-week-old patient, Chang SL reported three cases of one-lung ventilation using uniblocker bronchial blockers for infants in U-VATS (12), but no other study has yet described the U-VATS for infants with PS. The children's chest includes small cavum space and narrow intercostal space, making it challenging to perform U-VATS compared to other surgical procedures, such as multiportal VATS (13). Among clinical advantages, pain control after U-VATS has been reported to be superior to conventional, three-port access VATS (14). The survival and impact of the potentially limited immune response to trauma are areas that lack extensive studies, U-VATS lobectomy has been shown to reduce the humoral immune response to trauma (13). However, there was another answer to the question "why do a U-VATS lobectomy": embrace the challenge is the only way to grow (15). The aim of this study is to evaluate the safety and feasibility of U-VATS for infants. The results are encouraging.

PATIENTS AND METHODS

The present study adhered to the tenets of the Declaration of Helsinki and was approved by the Ethics Committee of our hospital. Additionally, the written informed consent was obtained from the parents of the patients.

Patients

The selection criteria were as follows: (1) Patients with PS, including ILS or ELS; (2) the ILS lesion was localized to only one pulmonary lobe; (3) all the patients were newly treated by surgery. The exclusion criteria were patients with other preoperative complications, such as congenital heart disease, immunocompromised state, restrictive or obstructive chest wall disease, and multiple lesions. From January 2019 to July 2020, two infants with complications (one with foregut cyst and another had coexistent left lower lobe ELS and left upper lung congenital cystic adenomatoid malformation) were excluded, and 19 infants with PS received U-VATS in our institution. Preoperative enhanced computed tomography (CT) was used to confirm the diagnosis, identify the lesions, and locate the systemic feeding artery. Routine examinations included a standard electrocardiogram, echocardiography, and blood tests. Subsequently, seven patients were found to be symptomatic, which included frequent respiratory infections and shortness of breath. Demographics, characteristics of PS (location, subtype, and origin of systemic artery), and perioperative data (operation time, blood loss, complications, duration of pleural drainage, and duration of post-operative hospital stay) were recorded for all patients.

Surgical Technique

All patients were consecutively operated on by the same experienced thoracic surgical team. Herein, we used a uniportal approach as described and defined by Migliore et al. (16). All patients were operated under general anesthesia with selective one-lung ventilation using a single-lumen endotracheal tube with a bronchial blocker. The patients were positioned in the full lateral decubitus position, and the surgeon always stood at the ventral side of the patient. A 1.5-cm utility port was created in the fifth intercostal space (ICS) at the anterior axillary line. A wound protector (Disposable wound protectors, Changzhou Anker Medical Co., Ltd., Changzhou, China) was applied at the utility port. A rigid 30° 5-mm optic thoracoscope was used for vision, and two or three instruments, such as suction/irrigator device, electrocautery, endoscopic grasper or scissors, and endoscopic ultrasonic scalpel or open surgical instruments, were used through the utility port.

The majority of the dissections were performed using endoscopic hook electrocautery and a 5-mm endoscopic ultrasonic scalpel (Harmonic Scalpel; Ethicon Endo-Surgery Inc., Cincinnati, OH, USA). The systemic feeding artery was the first structure dissected out. It was divided using Hem-o-Lok clips (Sinolinks clips; Sinolinks Medical Innovation Inc., Jiangsu, China) at the beginning of the operation. The extent of parenchymal resection depended on the extent of PS. The surgical options include standard lobectomy, wedge resection, and resection of the ELS. Endo-GIA (Covidien, Mansfield, MA, USA) and Hem-o-Lok were used to carry out lobectomy. Because of the small incision, we use a 3-mm thoracoscope and a 1.2-mm forceps for operation when Endo-GIA was used. When the lesion is large, we cut the specimen into small pieces before extracting out. One chest tube was placed for pleural drainage after lobectomy or wedge resection, and no chest tube was placed after resection of the ELS. The chest tube was removed when there was no air leak, and the amount of daily drainage was <20 mL. Patients were discharged 1 day after removal of the chest tube if the follow-up chest X-ray did not show any signs of complications, such as pneumothorax and hydrothorax.

TABLE 1 | Clinical data of infants undergoing U-VATS.

Patient number	Age (months)	Gender	Weight (kg)	Type (ILS/ELS)	Location	Origin of systemic artery	Symptomatic	Operation ways	Operative time (min)	Blood loss (mL)	Drainage duration (days)	Drainage volume (mL)	Hospital stay (days)
1	4	M	7.8	ILS	LLL	Thoracic aorta	Frequent respiratory infection	Wedge-shaped	60	20	6	220	7
2	4	F	10.1	ELS	RLL	Thoracic aorta	No		15	1			4
3	4	M	7.5	ILS	LLL	Thoracic aorta	No	Wedge-shaped	60	15	6	210	7
4	3	M	5.65	ELS	LLL	Thoracic aorta	Frequent respiratory infection		38	5			3
5	5	M	9.65	ILS	LLL	Thoracic aorta	Shortness of breath	Lobectomy	110	85	5	170	6
6	5	M	7.5	ILS	RLL	Thoracic aorta	Frequent respiratory infection	Lobectomy	120	80	4	120	5
7	6	F	6.9	ILS	LLL	Celiac trunk	No	Lobectomy	100	75	5	160	6
8	3	F	5.1	ELS	LLL	Superior mesenteric artery	No		40	10			4
9	4	M	6.9	ILS	RLL	Thoracic aorta	Frequent respiratory infection	Wedge-shaped	50	10	5	120	6
10	5	F	6.5	ILS	LLL	Thoracic aorta	No	Wedge-shaped	55	20	6	155	7
11	4	F	6.75	ELS	LLL	Abdominal aorta	No		20	1			4
12	6	M	9	ILS	LLL	Abdominal aorta	No	Wedge-shaped	60	20	6	200	7
13	3	M	5.5	ELS	RLL	Thoracic aorta	No		35	5			3
14	5	F	8	ILS	RLL	Thoracic aorta	Frequent respiratory infection	Wedge-shaped	65	25	7	220	8
15	5	M	7.5	ELS	LLL	Intercostal aorta	No		10	1			4
16	4	F	6.5	ILS	RLL	Thoracic aorta	Shortness of breath	Wedge-shaped	70	50	7	200	7
17	5	M	8.5	ILS	LLL	Thoracic aorta	No	Lobectomy	95	50	5	100	6
18	6	M	9.1	ILS	LLL	Abdominal aorta	No	Lobectomy	75	30	4	100	5
19	5	M	7.6	ELS	RLL	Abdominal aorta	No		30	2			4

RLL, right lower lobe; LLL, left lower lobe.

Statistical Analysis

Continuous data are presented as mean ± standard deviation and range, and the categorical variables are presented as frequencies (%). Clinical parameters are shown in **Table 1**. SPSS (Windows version 19.0 IBM Co., Armonk, NY, USA) was used for all statistical analyses.

RESULTS

Medical History and Diagnosis

A total of 19 infants (12 males and 7 females), aged 34.5 ± 0.9 (range: 3–6) months and weight 7.5 ± 1.4 (5.1–10.1) kg were recruited in this study. Most patients with PS had manifestations of lung infection, while some patients also presented dry cough and shortness of breath. PS was detected by prenatal ultrasonography in all patients. A total of 12 patients had ILS, and 7 had ELS. ILS was observed in the left lower lobe in 8 patients and the right lower lobe in 4 patients. Extralobar PS was detected near the left lower lobe in 4 patients and near the lower right lobe in 3 patients. The anomalous arterial blood supplies was via the thoracic aorta in 12 patients, abdominal aorta in 4, the celiac trunk in 1, intercostal aorta in 1, and superior mesenteric artery in 1 patient.

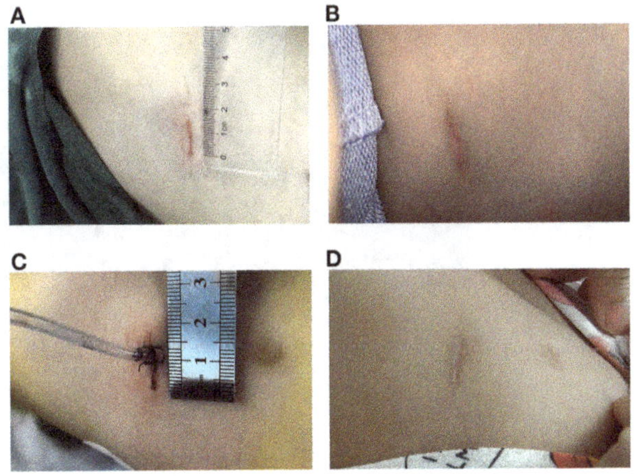

FIGURE 1 | Incisions were minor and cosmetic **(A)** Incision without tube. **(B)** Incision without tube 3 months after surgery. **(C)** Incision with a chest tube. **(D)** Incision with a chest tube 3 months after surgery.

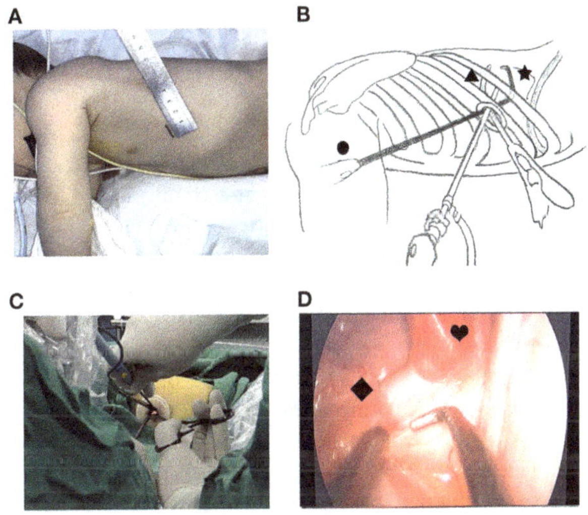

FIGURE 2 | Uniportal thoracoscopic resection of pulmonary sequestration. **(A)** Location and length of the U-VATS incision. **(B)** •, thoracoscope; ▲, angulated forceps; ★, plasticity electrocoagulation hook. **(C)** Operation photos. **(D)** Thoracoscopic image. ♥, PS; ♦, systemic feeding artery.

Intraoperative Conditions and Post-operative Management

The surgery was smooth in all 19 patients. The operative time was 58.3 ± 31.5 (10 120) min, and the intraoperative blood loss volume was 26.6 ± 27.9 (1–85) mL. All 7 patients with ELS underwent resection of the diseased lung tissues. Among 12 patients with ILS, lobectomy was performed in five patients and wedge-shaped lung resection in seven patients. Systemic artery identification and ligation were completed in all cases. The mean post-operative drainage volume was 164.6 ± 45.9 mL, and the mean post-operative thoracic tube duration was 5.5 ± 1.0 days. No intraoperative conversion, surgical mortality, or major complications were observed among these patients. However, in some patients, respiratory symptoms, such as shortness of breath and repeated pneumonia, were noted before surgery, but none displayed any symptoms after surgery. The operative findings and post-operative outcomes are summarized in **Table 1**.

Follow-Up

Follow-up and chest radiographs were performed 1-month post-surgery, and chest CT assessment was performed 1 year after surgery. All 19 patients were followed up for 1 year without loss. The symptoms had been either resolved totally or improved significantly in all symptomatic patients, and no complications were detected during the follow-up period. During a 2-year follow-up period after surgery, none of the patients developed symptoms. The incision in the chest was minor and cosmetic (**Figure 1**).

DISCUSSION

PS is an uncommon congenital anomaly due to the continuous advances in VATS. The approach has become the main surgical technique in treating PS (17). The surgical resection of the diseased lung is recommended for symptomatic patients and should also be performed for some asymptomatic patients to control and prevent recurrent pulmonary infection by blocking the inflammatory process and lowering the incidence of airway complications (1). The feasibility and safety of VATS lobectomy for PS have been investigated (18, 19).

For PS, U-VATS lobectomy has been applied to both ELS (20, 21) and ILS (22–24). However, these reported cases were all in adults and children after 1 year of age. Komori et al. examined long-term pulmonary function in 93 patients who underwent lobectomy between 2 days and 15 years of life (25).

A B

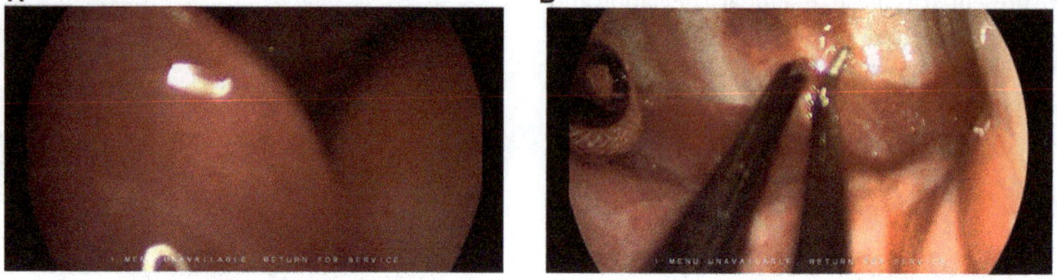

FIGURE 3 | (A,B) Expose the surgical area.

Alveolar growth (as opposed to emphysematous change) as measured by radionucleotide imaging was lower in patients who had undergone lobectomy after 1 year of age, suggesting an improvement in long-term pulmonary function in those who had undergone lobectomy before 1 year of age. Other than the case report from Shaqqura et al. (11), no studies have yet been reported about U-VATS in infants.

There is no consensus on the location and length of the U-VATS incision in infants. For adults, a 3 to 5-cm utility port was created in the fourth or fifth ICS at the anterior axillary line. In our opinion, a 4-cm incision is extremely traumatic for an infant. Hence, we recommend a 1.5-cm incision in the fifth ICS at the anterior axillary line for U-VATS. The pulmonary ligament and the aberrant systemic artery could be approached easily. Some characteristics of the infant's chest were small cavum space and narrow intercostal space. The distance between the surgical area and the chest surface was short, which resulted in a limited angle of instrument activities. Angulated and narrow-shaft double-hinged instruments have become a part of the essential armamentarium for the U-VATS, while articulating instruments bring the operative fulcrum inside the chest. The customized biarticular surgical instruments with a rod diameter of 4 mm were used in the current U-VATS, and the electrocoagulation hook was able to change the angle at will with a rod diameter of 2 mm. All the instruments made it advantageous to operate from multiple angles and in various regions (**Figure 2**).

The U-VATS for infants require close cooperation with the anesthesiologist and the camera-holding assistant. Maintaining the collapse of the lung on the operated side is also crucial. However, due to the small volume of the infant's chest cavity, the space with the collapsed lung was not sufficient to expose the surgical area. We also observed that the occlusion of the main bronchus, combined with the use of surgical instruments to remove the lobes blocking the view, produces satisfactory results. Notably, the lung tissue of the infants is vulnerable to being clipped by surgical instruments, and hence an angulated forceps holding a small piece of gauze was used to brush away the lobe from the surgical area (**Figure 3**).

The application of the U-VATS technique in thoracic surgery is a milestone innovation. However, there is often a long learning curve for the conversion from the conventional multiportal VATS to U-VATS. Our surgeons have had several years of experience in adult U-VATS; thus, we aimed to evaluate the safety and feasibility of U-VATS for infants in this study. Despite the success of 19 cases described above, the present study has many limitations; it was a single-center, small sample study, a retrospective analysis, and lacked a control group. Therefore, in the future, additional cases and complex U-VATS procedures, such as segmentectomy, are required to confirm the current findings using prospective, comparative studies.

CONCLUSION

Although U-VATS is challenging, the surgical approach is safe and feasible for infants with PS. Herein, we presented a series of U-VATS lobectomy, wedge resection, and resection of the PS for infants with satisfactory perioperative results.

AUTHOR CONTRIBUTIONS

J-XH participated in clinical practice, contributed to the collection and analysis of data, and drafting and revising the manuscript. J-JH carried out data collection. QC participated in clinical practice. S-MH helped in the study design and drafting of the manuscript. HC carried out patient recruitment and clinical practice, contributed to the conception and design of the study, and drafting and revising the manuscript. All authors read and approved the final manuscript.

REFERENCES

1. Corbett HJ, Humphrey GM. Pulmonary sequestration. *Paediatr Respir Rev.* (2004) 5:59–68. doi: 10.1016/j.prrv.2003.09.009
2. Van Raemdonck D, De Boeck K, Devlieger H, Demedts M, Moerman P, Coosemans W, et al. Pulmonary sequestration: a comparison between pediatric and adult patients. *Eur J Cardio Thorac Surg.* (2001) 19:388–95. doi: 10.1016/s1010-7940(01)00603-0
3. Zhang N, Zeng Q, Chen C, Yu J, Zhang X. Distribution, diagnosis, and

treatment of pulmonary sequestration: report of 208 cases. *J Pediatr Surg.* (2019) 54:1286–92. doi: 10.1016/j.jpedsurg.2018.08.054

4. Downard CD, Calkins CM, Williams RF, Renaud EJ, Jancelewicz T, Grabowski J, et al. Treatment of congenital pulmonary airway malformations: a systematic review from the APSA outcomes and evidence based practice committee. *Pediatr Surg Int.* (2017) 33:939–53. doi: 10.1007/s00383-017-4098-z
5. Rocco G, Khalil M, Jutley R. Uniportal video-assisted thoracoscopic surgery wedge lung biopsy in the diagnosis of interstitial lung diseases. *J Thorac Cardiovasc Surg.* (2005) 129:947–8. doi: 10.1016/j.jtcvs.2004.08.027
6. Gonzalez D, Paradela M, Garcia J, Dela Torre M. Single-port video-assisted thoracoscopic lobectomy. *Interact Cardiovasc Thorac Surg.* (2011) 12:514–5. doi: 10.1510/icvts.2010.256222
7. Gonzalez-Rivas D, Fieira E, Mendez L, Garcia J. Single-port video-assisted thoracoscopic anatomic segmentectomy and right upper lobectomy. *Eur J Cardio Thorac Surg.* (2012) 42:e169–71. doi: 10.1093/ejcts/ezs482
8. Gonzalez-Rivas D, Delgado M, Fieira E, Mendez L, Fernandez R, de la Torre M. Uniportal video-assisted thoracoscopic pneumonectomy. *J Thorac Dis.* (2013) 5(Suppl. 3):S246–52. doi: 10.3978/j.issn.2072-1439.2013.07.44
9. Gonzalez-Rivas D, Fernandez R, Fieira E, Rellan L. Uniportal video-assisted thoracoscopic bronchial sleeve lobectomy: first report. *J Thorac Cardiovasc Surg.* (2013) 145:1676–7. doi: 10.1016/j.jtcvs.2013.02.052
10. Huang CL, Cheng CY, Lin CH, Wang BY. Single-port thoracoscopic rib resection: a case report. *J Cardiothorac Surg.* (2014) 9:49. doi: 10.1186/1749-8090-9-49
11. Shaqqura B, Rumman N, Gonzalez Rivas D, Abu Akar F. Uniportal video-assisted thoracoscopic lobectomy in a 9-week-old patient. *Interact Cardiovasc Thorac Surg.* (2020) 30:327. doi: 10.1093/icvts/ivz263
12. Chang SL, Lai CH, Chen GY, Chou CM, Huang SY, Chen YM, et al. Case reports of one-lung ventilation using Fuji Uniblocker bronchial blockers for infants under one-year-old in uniportal video-assisted thoracoscopic surgery. *Medicine.* (2021) 100:e26325. doi: 10.1097/MD.0000000000026325
13. Martin-Ucar AE, Socci L. Why perform uniportal video-assisted thoracic surgery?—multiple considerations. *J Visual Surg.* (2016) 2:108. doi: 10.21037/jovs.2016.06.01
14. Tamura M, Shimizu Y, Hashizume Y. Pain following thoracoscopic surgery: retrospective analysis between single-incision and three-port video-assisted thoracoscopic surgery. *J Cardiothor Surg.* (2013) 8:153. doi: 10.1186/1749-8090-8-153
15. Andrade R. Commentary: why do uniportal video-assisted thoracoscopic lobectomy? *J Thorac Cardiovasc Surg.* (2020) 159:2496–7. doi: 10.1016/j.jtcvs.2019.11.081
16. Migliore M, Halezeroglu S, Molins L, Van Raemdonck D, Mueller MR, Rea F, et al. Uniportal video-assisted thoracic surgery or single-incision video-assisted thoracic surgery for lung resection: clarifying definitions. *Future Oncol.* (2016) 12:5–7. doi: 10.2217/fon-2016-0370
17. Ferland N, Couture C, Provencher S. Near-fatal haemoptysis as presentation of a giant intralobar pulmonary sequestration. *Eur Respir Rev.* (2015) 24:155–6. doi: 10.1183/09059180.00005914
18. Shen JF, Zhang XX, Li SB, Guo ZH, Xu ZQ, Shi XS, et al. Complete video-assisted thoracoscopic surgery for pulmonary sequestration. *J Thorac Dis.* (2013) 5:31–5. doi: 10.3978/j.issn.2072-1439.2013.01.01
19. Kestenholz PB, Schneiter D, Hillinger S, Lardinois D, Weder W. Thoracoscopic treatment of pulmonary sequestration. *Eur J Cardio Thorac Surg.* (2006) 29:815–8. doi: 10.1016/j.ejcts.2006.02.018
20. Tamura M, Shimizu Y, Hashizume Y. Single-incision video-assisted thoracic resection for extrapulmonary sequestration: a case report. *J Cardiothorac Surg.* (2014) 9:22. doi: 10.1186/1749-8090-9-22
21. Halezeroglu S, Okur E, Ergene G. Single-incision video-assisted thoracic surgery for an extralobar sequestration in a child. *Innovations.* (2016) 11:64–6. doi: 10.1097/imi.0000000000000239
22. Lin ZW, Xu ST, Wang Q. Uniportal video-assisted thoracic lobectomy in a semiprone position for the treatment of a large intralobar pulmonary sequestration. *Interact Cardiovasc Thorac Surg.* (2015) 21:542–4. doi: 10.1093/icvts/ivv158
23. Sihoe ADL, Luo Q, Shao G, Li Y, Li J, Pang D. Uniportal thoracoscopic lobectomy for intralobar pulmonary sequestration. *J Cardiothor Surg.* (2016) 11:27. doi: 10.1186/s13019-016-0425-z
24. Kim CW, Kim DH. Single-incision video-assisted thoracic surgery lobectomy in the treatment of adult communicating bronchopulmonary foregut malformation with large aberrant artery. *J Thorac Dis.* (2016) 8:E148–51. doi: 10.3978/j.issn.2072-1439.2016.01.36
25. Komori K, Kamagata S, Hirobe S, Toma M, Okumura K, Muto M, et al. Radionuclide imaging study of long-term pulmonary function after lobectomy in children with congenital cystic lung disease. *J Pediatr Surg.* (2009) 44:2096–100. doi: 10.1016/j.jpedsurg.2009.04.033

12

The Value of Hepatic Scintigraphy in the Diagnosis of Biliary Atresia

Wing Ki Chan [1], Patrick Ho Yu Chung [2] and Kenneth Kak Yuen Wong [2]*

[1] Li Ka Shing Faculty of Medicine, The University of Hong Kong, Hong Kong, China, [2] Department of Surgery, The University of Hong Kong, Hong Kong, China

Correspondence:
Patrick Ho Yu Chung
chungphy@hku.hk

Introduction: Biliary Atresia (BA) requires prompt diagnosis and surgical intervention to optimize its outcome. The aim of this study was to evaluate the accuracy of EHIDA in distinguishing between BA and other causes of cholestatic jaundice.

Methods: This was a retrospective study of all patients who underwent EHIDA in a tertiary center from 1997 to 2019. The sensitivity, specificity, Negative Predictive Value (NPV) and Positive Predictive Value (PPV) of EHIDA were evaluated. Factors that can potentially affect its accuracy were also analyzed.

Results: During the study period, 93 patients aged 10 to 110 days with cholestasis and suspected BA underwent EHIDA. The sensitivity and NPV were 91.2 and 85.3% while specificity and PPV were 80.6 and 88.1%. These results suggested that EHIDA is suboptimal in both diagnosing or excluding BA. Out of 59 patients who showed no tracer activities in the intestines after 24 h, 56 were subjected to surgical exploration and 52 (92.9%) were eventually diagnosed BA. The accuracy of EHIDA scan were different by the maturity of the patient, age at testing and severity of cholestasis.

Conclusions: EHIDA has a limited accuracy and surgical exploration remains the gold standard to establish the diagnosis of BA. Potential confounding factors that may affect the accuracy of EHIDA were identified but require further studies with larger sample sizes to validate.

Keywords: Biliary Atresia (BA), laparoscopy, neonatal cholestasis, Kasai portoenterostomy, hepatic scintigraphy

INTRODUCTION

Biliary Atresia (BA) is a congenital disorder characterized by destructive inflammatory obliterative cholangiopathy of the entire biliary system resulting in life-threatening cholestasis (1). BA is one of the most challenging liver diseases in infants and a prompt diagnosis is required for the best outcome. There have been controversies regarding the diagnostic pathway for BA. The current gold standard for the diagnosis of BA is surgical exploration with or without liver biopsy to demonstrate the presence of an atretic bile duct as well as peribiliary fibrosis and ductular proliferation. A high sensitivity of 100%, specificity of 94.3% and an accuracy rate of 96.9% have been reported for this diagnostic approach (2, 3). Over the years, there is still no single non-invasive test that can effectively diagnosis BA. Hepatic scintigraphy (EHIDA) is a functional radioisotope study that has commonly been performed as one of the investigations for the evaluation of neonatal cholestasis. Some centers depend on the result of EHIDA scan for the decision to initiate surgical referral for suspected BA. The study required intravenous administration of radioisotopes such as

Tc-99m Mebrofenin and Disofenin. The hepatic uptake, excretion of tracer via the liver, bile ducts and intestines are subsequently evaluated. The absence of tracer activity in the intestines after 24 hours is a feature suggestive of extrahepatic occlusive disorders including BA (4). A previous study reported that the sensitivity and specificity of EHIDA was 98.7% and 37–74% respectively, revealing a doubtful reliability (5). Furthermore, misinterpretation of EHIDA scan has also been reported (6). The potential inaccuracy of EHIDA may lead to a delayed Kasai portoenterostomy. It was estimated that about 70% of the BA patients can establish bile flow if KPE is performed within the first 60 days of life; while only 25% of them can restore biliary drainage if KPE is performed after 90 days of life (3). Furthermore, treatment is different for other non-BA causes of neonatal cholestasis and therefore it is important to differentiate between the causes of cholestatic jaundice (7). The aim of this study was to evaluate the diagnostic accuracy of EHIDA in patients with suspected BA due to persistent cholestasis, as well as highlighting the limitations associated with EHIDA scan to reinforce the fact that it should not delay or replace surgical exploration for a diagnosis of BA. Furthermore, we attempted to examine factors that can potentially affect the accuracy of EHIDA scan.

METHODS

This was a retrospective study conducted in a tertiary referral center for BA. All infants aged 10 to 110 days who underwent EHIDA for conjugated hyperbilirubinemia in our institute from September 1997 to October 2019 were included. During the study, each patient was given an intravenous injection of 99m Tc-Mebrofenin. Imaging was then carried out on a Gamma Camera with the patient lying supine. Serial images were acquired at 15 min, 30 min, 45 min and 60 min for 3 h. If there is non-excretion of the radiotracer in the intestines, a delayed image would be acquired at 24 h for confirmation. Non-excretion of 99m Tc-mebrofenin in the intestines in the 24-h delayed image was considered a feature suggestive of BA. This was also the definition of positive EHIDA result in this study. For patients with drainage of radiotracer in the intestines or having inconclusive findings, they were defined as having a negative EHIDA result. In all patients, the diagnosis of BA was confirmed by laparoscopic exploration to reveal the presence of an atretic bile duct. If necessary, an intra-operative cholangiogram was also performed to examine the biliary patency. For the analysis, we determined the sensitivity, specificity, NPV and PPV of EHIDA in diagnosing BA. Factors that can potentially affect the diagnostic accuracy of EHIDA were also analyzed (prematurity, age of life to conduct EHIDA, conjugated bilirubin level latest to performing EHIDA, concomitant heart disease). Continuous and categorical variables were expressed as medians with range and frequency with percentage respectively. All descriptive analysis and statistical calculations were performed with SPSS Statistics Version 24 (SPSS Inc., Chicago, IL., USA). This study was performed in accordance with the Declaration of Helsinki.

TABLE 1 | Correlation between EHIDA results and the diagnosis.

	BA positive	BA negative
EHIDA positive	52	7
EHIDA negative	5	29

A positive EHIDA result means "BA cannot be excluded" due to the absence of Mebrofenin in the intestines in the 24-h delayed image; whereas a negative EHIDA result means either the presence of tracer activities in the intestines after 24 h or inconclusive findings, suggesting BA was unlikely.

RESULTS

EHIDA Results in All Patients

There was a total of 93 patients who underwent EHIDA during the study period, of which 32 (34.4%) were male and 61 (65.6%) were female. The median age at performing the scan was 45 days of life. We first analyzed the based on the diagnosis. Fifty-seven (61.3%) patients were confirmed to have BA and 36 (38.7%) had other causes of cholestasis including neonatal hepatitis and choledochal cysts. Among the 57 BA patients, 52 (91.2%) and 5 (8.8%) had positive and negative EHIDA results respectively. For the 5 EHIDA negative cases, two of them had an early EHIDA examination (<the median time of 45 days of life) while the other 3 had EHIDA after 45 days of life (on day 56, 57 and 109 respectively).

We then performed the analysis based on the EHIDA findings. EHIDA was considered positive in 59 patients, of which 56 (94.9%) subsequently proceeded to surgical exploration at a median age of 65 days of life, while the median age for all patients was 59 days of life. Fifty-two (92.9%) patients were eventually diagnosed with BA. For the 3 EHIDA positive patients who did not undergo surgical exploration, cholestasis resolved in two patients prior to surgery while the other one defaulted our subsequent follow up. Out of the 34 EHIDA negative patients, 9 (26.5%) of them required surgical exploration and 5 (14.7%) of them were subsequently confirmed to suffer from BA.

The sensitivity, specificity, NPV and PPV of EHIDA scan in BA diagnosis were therefore 91.2, 80.6, 85.3, and 88.1% respectively (**Table 1**).

Analysis of Factors That May Affect the Accuracy of EHIDA

Prematurity

Prematurity was defined as delivery before 37 weeks of gestation. In our study, 18 (19.4%) were premature babies while 75 (80.6%) were born at term. Among the premature patients, there were 1 false negative (5.6%) and 4 false positives results (22.2%). As for the term babies, there were 4 false negative (5.3%) and 3 false positive (4%) results (**Table 2**).

Age of Life to Conduct EHIDA

The age to conduct EHIDA of our subjects ranged from 10 to 110 days of life. We have classified them into examination before or after 45 days of life according to the median value for all ages of examination. For the 48 patients (51.6%) who had EHIDA before 45 days of life, there were 2 false negative (4.2%) and 1

TABLE 2 | Diagnostic accuracy of EHIDA in the context of different variables (Prematurity, age of life to conduct EHIDA, conjugated bilirubin level and concomitant heart disease).

	N (%)	True positive rate (%)	False positive rate (%)	True negative rate (%)	False negative rate (%)
Prematurity					
Premature	18 (19.4%)	22.2	22.2	*50*	5.6
Term	75 (80.6%)	64	*4*	*26.7*	5.3
Timing of EHIDA (days of life)					
≤45	48 (51.6%)	64.6	2.1	29.2	4.2
> 45	45 (48.4%)	46.7	13.3	33.3	6.7
Level of conjugated bilirubin (μmol/L)					
≤66	48 (51.6%)	31.3	14.6	54.2	0
>66	45 (48.4%)	82.2	0	6.7	*11.1*
Concomitant heart disease					
Present	14 (15.1%)	*21.4*	14.3	*64.3*	0
Absent	79 (84.9%)	*62.2*	6.3	*25.3*	*6.3*

N, Number of corresponding subjects.

false positive result (2.1%). For the 45 patients (48.4%) who had EHIDA after 45 days of life, there were 3 false negative (6.7%) and 6 false positive (13.3%) results respectively.

Conjugated Bilirubin Level

The conjugated bilirubin level prior to EHIDA scan of our subjects ranged from 10 to 238 μmol/L. We have divided our patients into 2 groups according to the median value of conjugated bilirubin level latest to performing EHIDA. For the 48 patients (51.6%) who had conjugated bilirubin level of <66 μmol/L, there were no false negative but 7 (14.6%) false positive results. For the remaining 45 patients (48.4%) who had conjugated bilirubin of more than 66 μmol/L, there were 5 (11.1%) false negative but no false positive results respectively.

Concomitant Heart Disease

There were 79 patients (84.9%) without concomitant heart disease. For the 14 patients (15.1%) who suffered from concomitant heart diseases, their cardiac diagnoses were valvular heart disease such as patent ductus arteriosus and atrial/ventricular septal defects and cardiac arrhythmias. Among those with concomitant heart disease, there were 2 false positives (14.3%) but no false negative results. As for those without heart disease, there were 5 false positive (6.3%) and negative results.

DISCUSSION

EHIDA scan is a common investigation ordered for suspected BA. Many clinicians still depend on its result before the activation of BA management protocol. However, our data have revealed that this investigation is inaccurate for the diagnosis of BA, which reinforces the findings from previous studies (8). Among all parameters, the specificity is the lowest, suggesting the absence of radiotracer in the intestines should not be regarded as the pathognomonic of BA. More importantly, patients with EHIDA positive result should still be surgically explored for the definitive diagnosis (3, 9). On the other hand, false negative result can potentially delay the diagnosis of BA and the narrow treatment window by KPE is missed. Misinterpretation of EHIDA should also be considered. It has been reported that tracer activities in the urinary bladder and kidneys were mistaken as bowel activities in previous studies (6, 10).

In some centers, the availability of radionuclide scan is limited and takes time to be scheduled. KPE could have been delayed should BA be the underlying diagnosis and this is unfavorable as the prognosis is influenced by the timing of surgery. A better alternative is to proceed to surgical exploration with high clinical suspicion of BA after initial non-invasive and readily available investigations such as liver function test and abdominal ultrasound. Although there are additional surgical and anesthetic risks associated with surgical exploration in comparison to the use of EHIDA, the highest diagnostic accuracy has outweighed the disadvantages as BA is a lethal condition. With the advances of minimally invasive surgery in infants, surgical trauma is minimized. KPE can also be readily performed once the diagnosis is confirmed. If BA is excluded, intra-operative liver biopsy, which is often required to look for alternative diagnosis for the liver dysfunction, can be performed during the same operation. In our opinion, laparoscopic exploration can be considered a tool to achieve an earlier diagnosis of BA.

Despite a diminishing role of EHIDA scan in the diagnosis of BA, we attempted to identify the factors that may influence the accuracy of this investigation. Prematurity was evaluated because it may affect the hepatic uptake of radiotracer. Both the true and false positive rate were low in premature patients that suggested a higher diagnostic inaccuracy among premature patients. A postulation is that premature patients have underdeveloped liver function that reduces the hepatic uptake of the radiotracer during EHIDA study, leading to potential inaccuracy in evaluating the tracer activities in the bile ducts and intestines. On the other hand, as BA is a disease that evolve during peri-natal period, the biliary obstruction could have happened after the EHIDA scan is performed. However, there was an unequal distribution of patients across the two groups and further analysis with more evenly distributed sample is required. We also evaluated the impact of conjugated bilirubin level because of a postulation that Mebrofenin only allows biliary visualization on EHIDA images with bilirubin level up to 30 to 40 mg/dL, which suggested that a grossly elevated bilirubin level decreases the diagnostic accuracy of EHIDA (11). Milder jaundice seems to have a higher chance of false positive result. We next analyzed if the age of examination affects the accuracy of the scan. We found out that a delayed scan may result in higher false positive result. In advanced liver disease, the hepatic uptake an excretory function could be impaired that give rise to a false positive result. Last but not least, we evaluated if concomitant heart disease may affect liver function due to cardiac cirrhosis. Although there were differences in comparisons for this factor, as in the comparison for maturity, we could not draw a definitive conclusion due to the unequal distribution of samples.

As the passage of white stool is the first noticeable features of BA, stool color screening has been introduced in some regions as a non-invasive modality to screen for BA. It has been adopted as a screening programme in Taiwan and a high accuracy has been reported (12). This policy has also led to earlier diagnosis, treatment by Kasai operation and subsequently improved the 3-year jaundice-free survival in their population. Subsequently, the programme has been extended to other places that show similar efficacy. However, its applicability in regions with low prevalence of BA is limited due to a doubtful cost-effectiveness. Another issue concerns the compliance of using stool color cards and attending follow-ups for further management as it involves parents' incentive to use them. Nevertheless, we feel that for jaundiced-baby passing white color stool, direct proceed to surgical exploration without waiting for EHIDA scan should be considered.

The utilization of multiple non-invasive tests has been proposed to achieve an early diagnosis of BA (13). An example of this suggestion is the combination of B-US (high likelihood ratio+) and MRCP/hepatobiliary scintigraphy (low likelihood ratio-). The advantages of dual tests are the non-invasiveness in nature as well as improved diagnostic performances (14). However, there are also potential problems including the limited availability of MRCP in public institutions which may also lead to the delayed diagnosis of BA.

This study has several limitations. First, the study was only conducted in a single center and the analysis was performed in a retrospective manner. Second, the decision to refer a patient for EHIDA scan is subjective and there might be some patients who suffered from cholestasis but were not scanned and hence not evaluated in this study. The interpretations of the scan were done by a few radiologists and the interpretation of tracer activities in the intestines can be inconsistent throughout the study period.

CONCLUSION

In conclusion, the accuracy of EHIDA scan in the diagnosis of BA is limited and maybe affected by prematurity, age at testing and the severity of cholestasis during examination. Future study with larger and more evenly distributed samples is required to identify factors that would improve its accuracy. For the best outcome of the patients, the decision of surgical exploration should not be delayed by EHIDA scan.

AUTHOR CONTRIBUTIONS

WC manuscript writing, data acquisition, and data analysis. PC contributed to study design and critical revision. KW supervised the study. All authors contributed to the article and approved the submitted version.

REFERENCES

1. Hartley JL, Davenport M, Kelly DA. Biliary atresia. *Lancet.* (2009) 374:1704–13. doi: 10.1016/S0140-6736(09)60946-6
2. Russo P, Magee JC, Boitnott J, Bove KE, Raghunathan T, Finegold M, et al. Design and validation of the biliary atresia research consortium histologic assessment system for cholestasis in infancy. *Clin Gastroenterol Hepatol.* (2011) 9:357–62 e2. doi: 10.1016/j.cgh.2011.01.003
3. Fawaz R, Baumann U, Ekong U, Fischler B, Hadzic N, Mack CL, et al. Guideline for the evaluation of cholestatic jaundice in infants: joint recommendations of the north american society for pediatric gastroenterology, hepatology, and nutrition and the european society for pediatric gastroenterology, hepatology, and nutrition. *J Pediatr Gastroenterol Nutr.* (2017) 64:154–68. doi: 10.1097/MPG.0000000000001334
4. Snyder E, Kashyap S, Lopez PP. *Hepatobiliary Iminodiacetic Acid Scan.* Treasure Island, FL: StatPearls. (2021).
5. Mandelia A, Lal R, Mutt N. Role of hepatobiliary scintigraphy and preoperative liver biopsy for exclusion of biliary atresia in neonatal cholestasis syndrome. *Indian J Pediatr.* (2017) 84:685–90. doi: 10.1007/s12098-017-2408-z
6. Kim H, Park S, Ha S, Kim JS, Kim DY, Oh M. False-negative hepatobiliary scintigraphy for biliary atresia. *Nucl Med Mol Imaging.* (2019) 53:356–60. doi: 10.1007/s13139-019-00606-w
7. Venigalla S, Gourley GR. Neonatal cholestasis. *Semin Perinatol.* (2004) 28:348–55. doi: 10.1053/j.semperi.2004.09.008
8. He JP, Hao Y, Wang XL, Yang XJ, Shao JF, Feng JX. Comparison of different noninvasive diagnostic methods for biliary atresia: a meta-analysis. *World J Pediatr.* (2016) 12:35–43. doi: 10.1007/s12519-015-0071-x
9. Wildhaber BE. Biliary atresia: 50 years after the first kasai. *ISRN Surg.* (2012) 2012:132089. doi: 10.5402/2012/132089
10. Bridoux V, Schwarz L, Kianifard B, Moutel G, Herve C, Tuech JJ. Systematic review and meta-analysis of randomized clinical trials of self-expanding metallic stents as a bridge to surgery versus emergency surgery for malignant left-sided large bowel obstruction (Br J Surg 2012; 99: 469-476). *Br J Surg.* (2012) 99:1464; author reply–5. doi: 10.1002/bjs.8929
11. MettlerJr F, Guiberteau M. *Essentials of Nuclear Medicine and Molecular Imaging* (Seventh Edition). New Mexico, TX: Elsevier (2019).
12. Lien TH, Chang MH, Wu JF, Chen HL, Lee HC, Chen AC, et al. Effects of the infant stool color card screening program on 5-year outcome of

biliary atresia in Taiwan. *Hepatology.* (2011) 53:202–8. doi: 10.1002/hep.24023

13. Wang L, Yang Y, Chen Y, Zhan J. Early differential diagnosis methods of biliary atresia: a meta-analysis. *Pediatr Surg Int.* (2018) 34:363–80. doi: 10.1007/s00383-018-4229-1
14. Sung S, Jeon TY, Yoo SY, Hwang SM, Choi YH, Kim WS, et al. Incremental value of MR cholangiopancreatography in diagnosis of biliary atresia. *PLoS ONE.* (2016) 11:e0158132. doi: 10.1371/journal.pone.0158132

13

High Anal Canal Pressure and Rectal Washouts Contribute to the Decrease of Anal Basal Pressure After Botulinum Toxin Injections in Paediatric Patients with Chronic Constipation

Ge Sun[1], *Monika Trzpis*[1*] *and Paul M. A. Broens*[1,2]

[1] Department of Surgery, Anorectal Physiology Laboratory, University of Groningen, University Medical Center Groningen, Groningen, Netherlands, [2] Department of Surgery, Division of Pediatric Surgery, University of Groningen, University Medical Center Groningen, Groningen, Netherlands

***Correspondence:**
Monika Trzpis
m.trzpis-bremer@umcg.nl

Introduction: Chronic constipation can be treated by injecting botulinum toxin into the anal sphincter to decrease anal basal pressure. To assess the effect of botulinum toxin, we investigated the factors that contribute to changes in anal basal pressure after injection.

Methods: This was a retrospective study conducted in a tertiary hospital in the Netherlands. We included children with chronic constipation treated with botulinum toxin injections and measured anal basal pressure before and after each injection. Multivariable linear regression analyses were used.

Results: We investigated 30 cases with idiopathic constipation. Their median age was 20.5 (7.75–53.25) months. Anal basal pressure decreased after injection in 20 cases. The mean decrease of anal basal pressure after injection was 18.17 ± 35.22 mmHg. The anal basal pressure change was linearly correlated with preinjection pressure ($R^2 = 0.593$, $P < 0.001$). A significant decrease of pressure was observed in patients with preinjection pressure > 70 mmHg. Preinjection anal basal pressure ($\beta = -0.913$, $P < 0.001$) and rectal washouts ($\beta = -21.015$, $P = 0.007$) contributed significantly to pressure changes. Changes in anal basal pressure were also significantly associated with patients' weights ($\beta = 0.512$, 95% CI, 0.011–1.013) and sex ($\beta = 22.971$, 95% CI, 9.205–36.736).

Conclusions: Botulinum toxin significantly decreases anal basal pressure when preinjection pressure is higher than 70 mmHg. In patients with severely elevated anal basal pressure, we recommend rectal washouts to promote the decrease of anal basal pressure.

Keywords: pediatric constipation, manometry, physiology, rectal washout, anal basal pressure, botulinum toxin

INTRODUCTION

Chronic constipation is often encountered in children and can be present as idiopathic constipation or as a result of an organic problem, such as anorectal malformation or Hirschsprung's disease (1–4). Dietary fibers, laxatives and enemas are often prescribed to treat idiopathic chronic constipation (5). If necessary, these remedies are also used to support defecation in children with organic constipation who have already been treated for the organic cause. Alternatively, if a child does not respond to conservative treatment, botulinum toxin injections in the anal sphincter can be administered (2, 3, 5–9). The idea underlying botulinum toxin therapy for treating chronic constipation stems from the assumption that elevated anal basal pressure indicates chronic contraction of the anal sphincter, disabling its relaxation when emptying the rectum is appropriate and thus hampering defecation (10, 11). Indeed, there are studies that confirm the association between elevated anal basal pressure and chronic constipation (12, 13). Botulinum toxin was introduced to force the anal sphincter to relax, thereby decreasing pressure in the anal canal and thus relieving intractable constipation (14, 15). This type of treatment, however, is not effective in all constipated patients (3). In the case of children, the efficacy regarding symptom improvement varies between 17 to 91% (16). This wide range may be the result of the different methodological designs of studies and of the fact that efficacy is based primarily on symptom improvement which, in case of children and toddlers in particular, relies mostly on their parents' opinions and might therefore be subjective. Nevertheless, it is undeniable that some patients do not respond to botulinum toxin therapy. To date, no factor has been identified that significantly determines the efficacy of botulinum toxin to reduce anal basal pressure. Seeing that constipation itself is associated with demographic factors such as age and sex (17), it could be that these factors also contribute to the efficacy of botulinum toxin therapy.

Botulinum toxin therapy requires anesthesia and as such it is invasive. Therefore, there is need to find predictive factors that enable us to distinguish between patients who will respond to the treatment and those who will not; the latter should subsequently be offered a different type of treatment (18–20).

Based on our clinical experience, we hypothesize that anal basal pressure measured before injection of botulinum toxin may be one of the factors that determines the response of the anal sphincter to this neurotoxin. In this study, we aimed to investigate factors that contribute to the decrease of anal basal pressure in pediatric patients whom we treated with botulinum toxin for chronic constipation.

MATERIALS AND METHODS

Patients and Data Collection

This was a retrospective observational study. We included pediatric patients who received at least one botulinum toxin injection for severe chronic constipation and who underwent anorectal physiology tests at the Anorectal Physiology Laboratory at the University Medical Center of Groningen before and after treatment between March 2013 and November 2020. The patients were diagnosed with chronic constipation and failed to respond to conservative treatment. This included laxatives, enemas, and finally, rectal washouts if their defecation remained troublesome even after all the conservative treatments had been tried. Some patients were treated with botulinum toxin more than once (**Figure 1**). We defined each injection as a separate case. We excluded those cases in which anal basal pressure was measured longer than 12 months before the botulinum toxin injection or more than 3 months afterwards. We also excluded the cases of patients who received anal surgery, which may influence anal function, between the botulinum toxin injection and manometry (**Figure 1**). This study was performed in accordance with the Ethical standards of our Institutional Research Committee and registered as M19.235067.

Treatment Procedure

All the patients referred for botulinum toxin therapy for chronic constipation were given injections in the anal sphincter according to the same protocol. We administered the injection with the patient in supine position. The patients were treated under general anesthesia, without locoregional anesthesia. A rectal speculum was used for clear vision. We administered the same dose of 100 IU of botulinum toxin (Botox, Allergen, the Netherlands) with each injection. We inserted a 27-guage needle into the anal sphincter parallel to the anal canal axis by penetrating the skin outside the anal verge and injected the botulinum toxin in four quadrants, at 3, 6, 9, 12 o'clock (**Supplementary Figure 1**). The injections were all administered by the same group of experienced pediatric surgeons.

The laxative treatments that had already been initiated before referring the patients for botulinum toxin therapy were continued for approximately 6 months after administering the botulinum toxin injections. In case patients were treated with rectal washouts before the botulinum toxin treatment, they used NaCl 0.9% once or twice a day. This procedure was continued during the first week after injection. The volume of NaCl was adjusted according to patients' age and weight. After the first week, depending on the severity of the constipation symptoms at that moment, the frequency of rectal washouts was gradually reduced. Instead of following a standardized protocol for the gradual reduction of bowel management, reduction of washouts was strictly personalized in that it was based on each patient's individual symptoms.

Measuring Anal Basal Pressure

We performed the anal basal pressure test within at most 12 months before the injection and within 3 months after the injection, thereby considering the 3–6 months' effect duration of botulinum toxin (15, 20, 21). We measured anal basal pressure with a Laborie/Unisensor K12981solid-state (Boston type) circumferential catheter (Laborie Portsmouth, NH, USA) with an outer diameter of 12F (**Supplementary Figure 1C**). After placing the catheter, time was allowed for the child to become

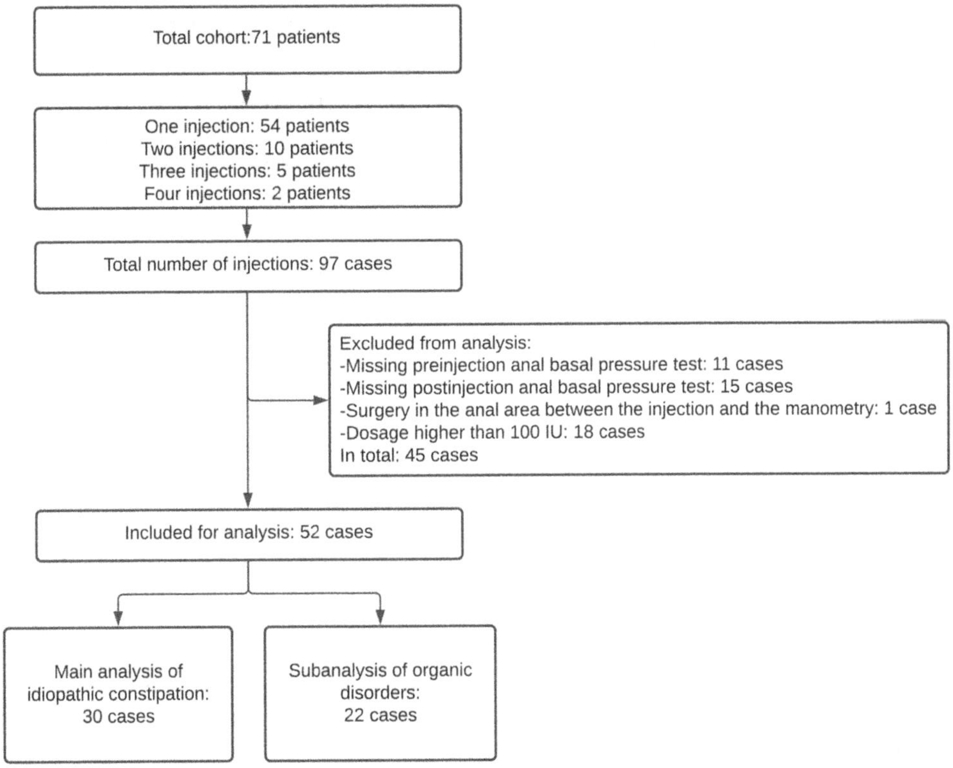

FIGURE 1 | Flowchart illustrating patients' inclusion and exclusion steps.

used to the catheter and for us to measure the resting pressure correctly. We defined a change in anal basal pressure as the value after injection minus the value before injection. We used the gastrointestinal, high-resolution manometry system Solar GI HRAM, Version 8.23 (Laborie/Medical Measurement Systems, Enschede, the Netherlands) to record and analyse the data. The measurements were performed without anesthesia.

Evaluation of Symptomatic Improvement

We based symptomatic improvement on the interviews held by medical specialists with the pediatric patients' parents during postoperative consultations. Symptomatic improvement was achieved if parents reported that their children were able to defecate without bowel management and/or without pain and/or effort after receiving botulinum toxin therapy. For analysis, the cut-off value of a 30% decrease in anal basal pressure after injection was considered as effective. We based this value on the report by Minkes and Langer (6).

Statistical Analysis

All statistical analyses were performed using IBM SPSS Statistics, Version 23.0 (IBM Corp, Armonk, NY, USA). The continuous variables were reported as means ± standard deviations and compared with *t*-tests. Relation between categorical variables was analyzed with Fisher exact test. The Pearson test was used to analyse the correlation between the basal pressure changes after injecting botulinum toxin and other continuous variables. Univariable analysis was used to search for possible predictors of the change in the basal pressure. The multivariable linear regression analysis was used to adjust for any possible cofactors and to find independent factors that may predict the change in basal pressure. The receiver operating characteristic (ROC) curve and Youden index were utilized to determine the optimal cut-off value. A P-value < 0.05 was accepted as significant. Figures were generated using GraphPad Prism 8.2.0 (GraphPad Software Inc, San Diego, CA, USA).

RESULTS

Demographics and Clinical Characteristics

We included 43 pediatric patients who were subjected to botulinum toxin treatment for chronic constipation, 35 (81%) of whom received 1 injection, 7 (16%) received 2 injections and 1 patient (2%) received 3 injections, which resulted in 52 cases (**Figure 1**). In 30 cases (57.7%) the patients suffered idiopathic constipation, that is they had no organic disorders that could be associated with chronic constipation. In 20 cases (38.5%) the patients had Hirschsprung disease and in 2 (3.8%) cases the patients had congenital anorectal malformation. For the main analysis we included the cases with idiopathic constipation, and for the subanalysis we included the patients with organic disorders. The clinical characteristics of the cases included in this study are summarized in **Table 1**.

TABLE 1 | Clinical characteristics of cases included in this study.

Variables	Idiopathic constipation	Organic disorder
Total number of cases:	30	22
Age (months; median)	20.5 (7.75–53.25)	29.5 (20.5–108.5)
Sex (boys/girls)	19/11 (63%/37%)	15/7 (68%/32%)
Weight (kg; median)	11.1 (8.39–17.03)	13.55 (11.58–27.95)
Rectal washout		
Yes	9 (30%)	15 (68%)
No	21 (70%)	7 (32%)
Time between pre-treatment manometry and injection (days)	101.47 ± 61.81	68.23 ± 60.85
Time interval between the injection and manometry after injection (days)	21.3 ±10	27.68 ±15.26
Number of patients		
Single injection	25 (93%)	10 (63%)
Two injections	1 (4%)	6 (38%)
Three injections	1 (4%)	0

The Change in Anal Basal Pressure After Botulinum Toxin Therapy in Patients With Idiopathic Constipation

In cases with idiopathic constipation, the anal canal basal pressure was 91.33 ± 28.25 mmHg before the botulinum toxin injection and 73.17 ± 22.49 mmHg after the injection (P = 0.008, **Figure 2A**, **Table 2**). The time between the injection and measurement after injection was 21.3 ± 10 days. In 20 cases (66.7%), anal basal pressure after injecting botulinum toxin had decreased when compared to the pressure before the injection. A graphical representation of the anal basal pressure change is presented as a 2D map in **Supplementary Figure 2**. No changes were observed in 3 (10%) cases, while pressure increased in 7 cases (23.3%). In these 7 cases the mean value of anal basal pressure before injection was significantly lower than in the other 20 cases whose anal basal pressure decreased after injection (77.14 ± 24.3 mmHg vs. 100.75 ± 26.12 mmHg, P = 0.047) (**Table 2**).

Anal basal pressure before injection and the changes in pressure observed after injection were significantly correlated (R^2 = 0.593, $P < 0.001$, **Figure 2B**). Using the ROC curve analysis, we found that the preinjection anal basal pressure was 67.5 mmHg when reaching the highest Youden index of 0.50 (**Figure 2C**). When we rounded off the cut-off value to 70 mmHg, we observed that sensitivity was 100%, specificity was 50%, the positive prediction value was 80% and the negative prediction value was 100%. Consequently, we used 70 mmHg as a cut-off value to distinguish two subgroups: cases with anal basal pressure ≤70 mmHg and cases whose anal basal pressure was >70 mmHg. Anal basal pressure decreased significantly after injection in cases whose anal basal pressure before injection was >70 mmHg (P = 0.005, **Figure 2D**). In contrast, in cases whose anal basal pressure before injection was ≤70 mmHg, we observed no significant decrease of anal basal pressure (P = 0.07, **Figure 2D**).

Factors That May Influence Changes in Anal Basal Pressure in Patients With Idiopathic Constipation After the Botulinum Toxin Injection

Using the univariable linear regression analysis we found that in cases with idiopathic constipation the change in anal basal pressure was negatively associated with basal pressure before injection (β = −0.960, $P < 0.001$, **Table 3**). The change in anal basal pressure was not significantly associated with age at the time of injection (β = 0.179, P = 0.163), the time interval between injection and testing postinjection anal basal pressure (β = 0.441, P = 0.510), weight (β = 0.652, P = 0.177), number of injections (β =13.293, P = 0.387), rectal washouts (β = −16.111, P = 0.258) and sex (β = 25.144, P = 0.058).

Weight was significantly correlated with the age (r = 0.951, $P < 0.001$). When analyzing correlation of anal basal pressure changes with weight and with age using Pearson' correlation, we found that the r and P-values were comparable for age and weight (r = 0.261, P = 0.163 and r = 0.253, P = 0.177, respectively). Because weight can differ between patients of the same age and based on our clinical experience, we think that it is weight itself rather than age that contributes to the efficacy of botulinum toxin therapy. Therefore, to investigate the predictive value of anal basal pressure before injection for anal basal pressure change, we chose to adjust only for weight in the multivariable analysis. The four variables included in the multivariate analysis, that is anal basal pressure before injection, rectal washout and weight and sex, were independent of each other (**Supplementary Table 1**). Using multivariable analysis, we found that the anal basal pressure change after injection was negatively associated with anal basal pressure before injection (β = −0.913, $P < 0.001$) and rectal washout (β = −21.015, P = 0.007). Furthermore, change in anal basal pressure was positively associated with weight (β = 0.512, P = 0.046) and with being a boy (β = 22.971, P = 0.002) (**Table 3**).

Clinical Symptomatic Improvement in Patients With Idiopathic Constipation

Information regarding symptomatic improvement was available in 29 cases of patients with idiopathic constipation. We found that 23 (79%) cases experienced symptom improvement and that the symptomatic improvement was associated with neither preinjection anal basal pressure nor decrease of the anal basal pressure (P = 0.553 and 1.00, respectively, **Figure 3**).

The Change in Anal Basal Pressure After Botulinum Toxin Injection in Patients With Organic Constipation

In cases with organic constipation, the anal canal basal pressure was 88.86 ± 15.81 mmHg before the botulinum toxin injection and 73.64 ± 17.54 mmHg after the injection ($P < 0.001$ **Figure 4A**, **Table 2**). The time between the injection and measurement after injection was 27.68 ± 15.26 days. In 19 cases (86.4%), anal basal pressure after injecting botulinum toxin had decreased when compared to the pressure before the injection. No change was observed in none of the cases. Pressure increased

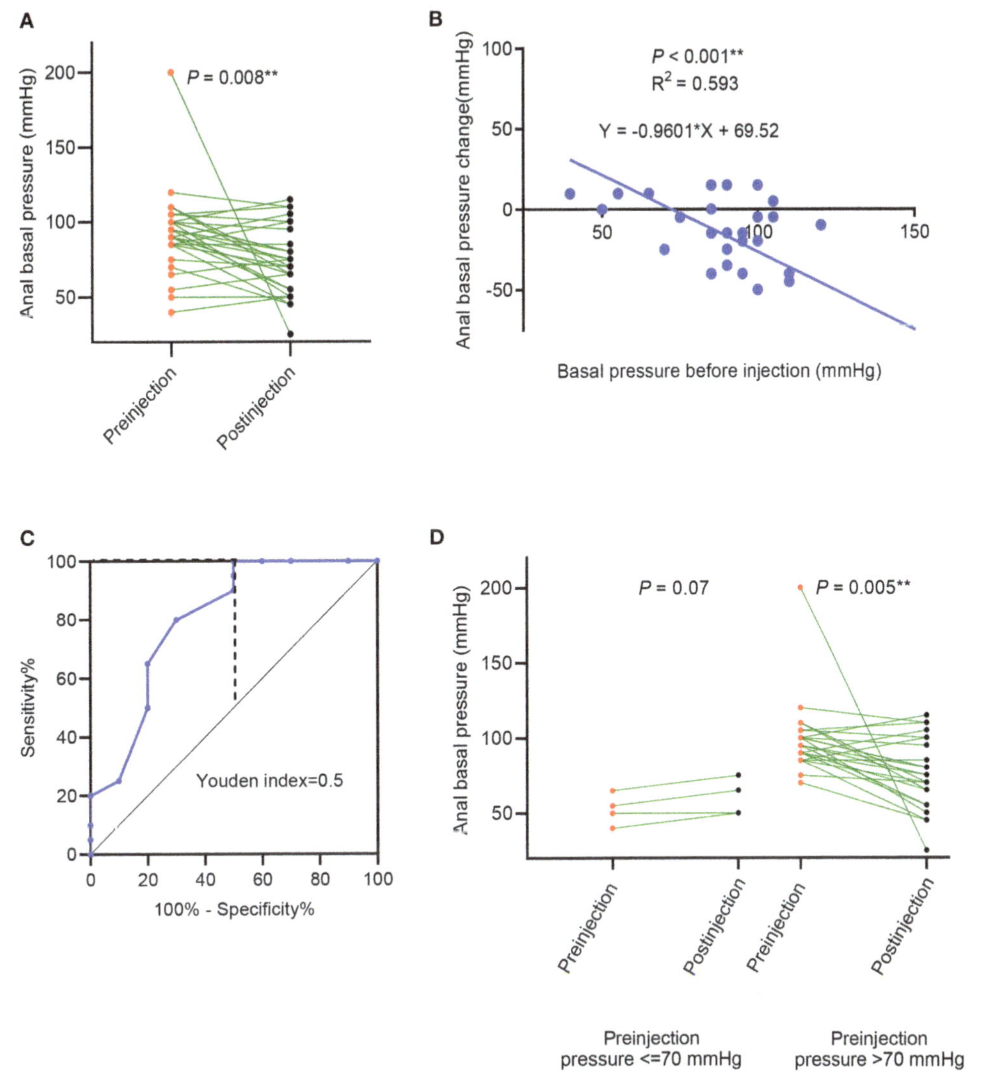

FIGURE 2 | Anal basal pressure change, after botulinum toxin injection in patients with idiopathic constipation. **(A)** The change in anal basal pressure after the botulinum toxin; **(B)** linear correlation between preinjection anal basal pressure and change in anal basal pressure; **(C)** receiver operating characteristic (ROC) curve using preinjection anal basal pressure to predict the decrease of anal basal pressure; **(D)** comparison of anal basal pressure before and after the botulinum toxin injection in patients whose anal basal pressure before injection was ≤70 mmHg and >70 mmHg.

in 3 cases (13.6%). In these 3 cases, the mean value of anal basal pressure before injection was lower than in the other 19 cases whose anal basal pressure decreased after injection. The difference, however, was not statistically significant (75 ± 13.23 mmHg vs. 91.05 ± 15.33 mmHg, $P = 0.103$).

Anal basal pressure before injection and the change in pressure observed after injection were correlated ($R^2 = 0.167$, $P = 0.059$). Using the ROC curve analysis, we found that preinjection anal basal pressure was 72.5 mmHg when reaching the highest Youden index of 0.562 (**Figure 4B**). When we rounded off the cut-off value to 70 mmHg, we observed that sensitivity was 89.5%, specificity was 33.3%, the positive prediction value was 89.47% and the negative prediction value was 33.3%. Consequently, we used 70 mmHg as a cut-off value to distinguish two subgroups: cases with anal basal pressure ≤70 mmHg and cases whose anal basal pressure was >70 mmHg. Anal basal pressure decreased significantly after injection in cases whose anal basal pressure before injection was >70 mmHg ($P < 0.001$, **Figure 4C**). In contrast, in cases whose anal basal pressure before injection was ≤70 mmHg, we observed no significant decrease of anal basal pressure ($P = 1.00$, **Figure 4C**).

Factors That May Influence Change in Anal Basal Pressure After the Botulinum Toxin Injection in Cases With Organic Disorders

Using univariable linear regression analysis we found that also in cases with organic disorders the change in anal basal pressure

TABLE 2 | Anal basal pressure before and after botulinum toxin injection.

Variables	Number of cases *n* (%)	Basal pressure before injection† (mmHg)	*P**	Basal pressure after injection† (mmHg)
Patients with idiopathic constipation				
Overall	30	91.33 ± 28.25	0.008	73.17 ± 22.49
Pressure change				
Decreased	20 (66.7%)	100.75 ± 26.12	0.001	69.5 ± 20.19
Unchanged	3 (10%)	61.67 ± 20.21	-	61.67 ± 20.21
Increased	7 (23.3%)	77.14 ± 24.3	<0.001	88.57 ± 25.12
Sex				
Boys	19 (63.3%)	90 ± 16.83	0.045	81.05 ± 17.04
Girls	11 (36.7%)	93.64 ± 42.37	0.05	59.55 ± 24.95
Rectal washout				
Yes	9 (30%)	90 ± 45	0.165	60.56 ± 19.44
No	21 (70%)	91.90 ± 18.61	0.005	78.57 ± 21.92
Patients with organic disorder				
Overall	22	88.86 ± 15.81	<0.001	73.64 ± 17.54
Pressure change				
Decreased	19 (86.4%)	91.05 ± 15.33	<0.001	72.11 ± 17.82
Unchanged	0	-	-	-
Increased	3 (13.6%)	75 ± 13.23	0.038	83.33 ± 14.43
Sex				
Boys	15 (68.2%)	91 ± 17.03	0.002	73.67 ± 18.94
Girls	7 (31.8%)	84.29 ± 12.72	0.094	73.57 ± 15.47
Rectal washout				
Yes	15 (68.2%)	85.67 ± 14.86	0.001	67 ± 13.73
No	7 (31.8%)	95.71 ± 16.69	0.091	87.86 ± 17.04

†*Data are presented as mean ± standard deviation.*
P, paired t-test between anal basal pressure before injection and anal basal pressure after injection.*

was negatively associated with basal pressure before injection ($\beta = -0.425$, $P = 0.059$). The change in anal basal pressure was not significantly associated with age at the time of the injection ($\beta = 0.058$, $P = 0.488$), the time interval between injection and testing postinjection anal basal pressure ($\beta = 0.048$, $P = 0.845$), weight ($\beta = 0.157$, $P = 0.671$), number of injections ($\beta = -6.563$, $P = 0.418$), rectal washout ($\beta = -10.81$, $P = 0.155$) and sex ($\beta = -6.619$, $P = 0.392$).

Using multivariable analysis, we found that the anal basal pressure change after injection was negatively associated with anal basal pressure before injection ($\beta = -0.577$, $P = 0.009$), and rectal washout ($\beta = -16.607$, $P = 0.02$), but it was not statistically associated with weight (**Table 4**).

Clinical Symptomatic Improvement in Patients With Organic Disorders Constipation

Information regarding symptomatic improvement was available for 20 cases with organic disorders constipation. We found that 16 (80%) cases experienced symptom improvement and that symptomatic improvement was associated with neither preinjection anal basal pressure nor decrease of the anal basal pressure ($P = 0.368$ and 1.00, respectively, **Figures 3C,D**).

DISCUSSION

With this study we demonstrated that preinjection anal basal pressure and rectal washouts contribute to the decrease of anal basal pressure after botulinum toxin therapy. In patients with idiopathic constipation, weight and sex were also associated with the changes in anal basal pressure after treatment with botulinum toxin.

It is known that approximately 66% of patients treated with botulinum toxin for chronic constipation do not respond or show a suboptimal response to this treatment, but the reasons for this observation remain unclear (16). Although botulinum toxin therapy in patients with chronic constipation is intended to decrease the pathophysiologically elevated anal basal pressure, patients are usually referred for treatment without first measuring the pressure. Chumpitazi et al., suggested measuring anal basal pressure before the botulinum toxin injection (18). They proposed that only patients with high anal canal pressure would benefit from botulinum toxin therapy for functional

TABLE 3 | Univariable linear regression analyses of factors that could influence changes in anal basal pressure change in cases with idiopathic constipation ($n = 30$).

Univariable analysis					
Independent variables	**Beta coefficient**[†]	**95% CI**		**Standard error**	***P***
		Lower bound	**Upper bound**		
Basal pressure before injection (mmHg)	−0.960	−1.268	−0.652	0.150	<0.001
Age at injection[§] (months)	0.179	−0.077	0.435	0.125	0.163
Time interval (days)[¶]	0.441	−0.912	1.793	0.660	0.510
Weight (kg)	0.652	−0.313	1.617	0.471	0.177
Number of injections	13.293	−17.686	44.271	15.123	0.387
Rectal washout					
Yes	−16.111	−44.691	12.469	13.952	0.258
No	0[‡]				
Sex					
Boys	25.144	−0.916	51.203	12.722	0.058
Girls	0[‡]				
Multivariable analysis					
Basal pressure before injection (mmHg)	−0.913	−1.153	−0.672	0.117	<0.001
Weight (kg)	0.512	0.011	1.013	0.243	0.046
Rectal washout	−21.015	−35.598	−6.432	7.081	0.007
Sex					
Boys	22.971	9.205	36.736	6.684	0.002
Girls	0[‡]				

[†]*Unstandardised beta coefficient;* [‡]*Reference category.*
[§]*Age and weight were significantly correlated and therefore, for multivariable analysis, age was not taken as a cofactor.*
[¶]*Time interval between injection and anal basal pressure measurement after injection.*

obstruction. They did not, however, provide the cut-off value. Consequently, in clinical practice the definition for high pressure is a subjective matter. Our finding that anal basal pressure had only decreased significantly in patients whose anal basal pressure before injection of botulinum toxin was higher than approximately 70 mmHg, provides such a cut-off value. This finding is supported by the fact that the change in anal basal pressure after injection of botulinum toxin showed a negative linear correlation with the anal basal pressure observed before injection. A ROC analysis also confirmed that sensitivity and specificity regarding prediction of anal basal pressure was highest when the cut-off value was set at 70 mmHg. Interestingly, is seemed that the cut-off value we established could be used independently of the cause of increased anal basal pressure. We base this conclusion on the fact that we found that patients without organic disorders as well as patients with Hirschsprung's disease or patients with anorectal malformations responded to botulinum toxin therapy provided their anal basal pressure was >70 mmHg.

Like Minkes and Langer (6), we too found no relation between changes of anal basal pressure and clinical outcomes in terms of constipation-related symptoms. One might therefore question the value of manometric tests to assess anal basal pressure. With this study, however, we showed that manometry in constipated patients is useful because it can confirm or exclude the presence of increased anal basal pressure—one of the causes of constipation (22). Furthermore, in case of increased anal basal pressure, manometric tests can indicate whether botulinum toxin therapy could be profitable. Nevertheless, manometric assessment should not be considered the only diagnostic tool with which to diagnose the causes of constipation. Moreover, particularly in children, monitoring anal basal pressure both prior to as well as after injecting botulinum toxin may have additional value. It provides a quantitative and objective outcome, viz. the magnitude of decrease of anal basal pressure, which can be used to follow the patient. Currently, treatment efficacy is based mostly on symptomatic improvement, which is extremely subjective, especially in case of young pediatric patients. A recent systematic review by Roorda et al., showed that the prevalence of symptomatic improvement of pediatric patients varies between 17 to 91% (16). Such a wide range might result from the fact that the youngest patients often cannot describe their symptoms themselves, while their parents are unable to provide objective information concerning the severity of certain symptoms.

Even though we were unable to pinpoint the exact reason why decreased anal basal pressure was not associated with symptomatic improvement in our study, we think it might be due to one or more of the following reasons. First, for this study the information regarding the symptoms was neither collected objectively nor investigated systematically. This was a result of the retrospective study design and because at

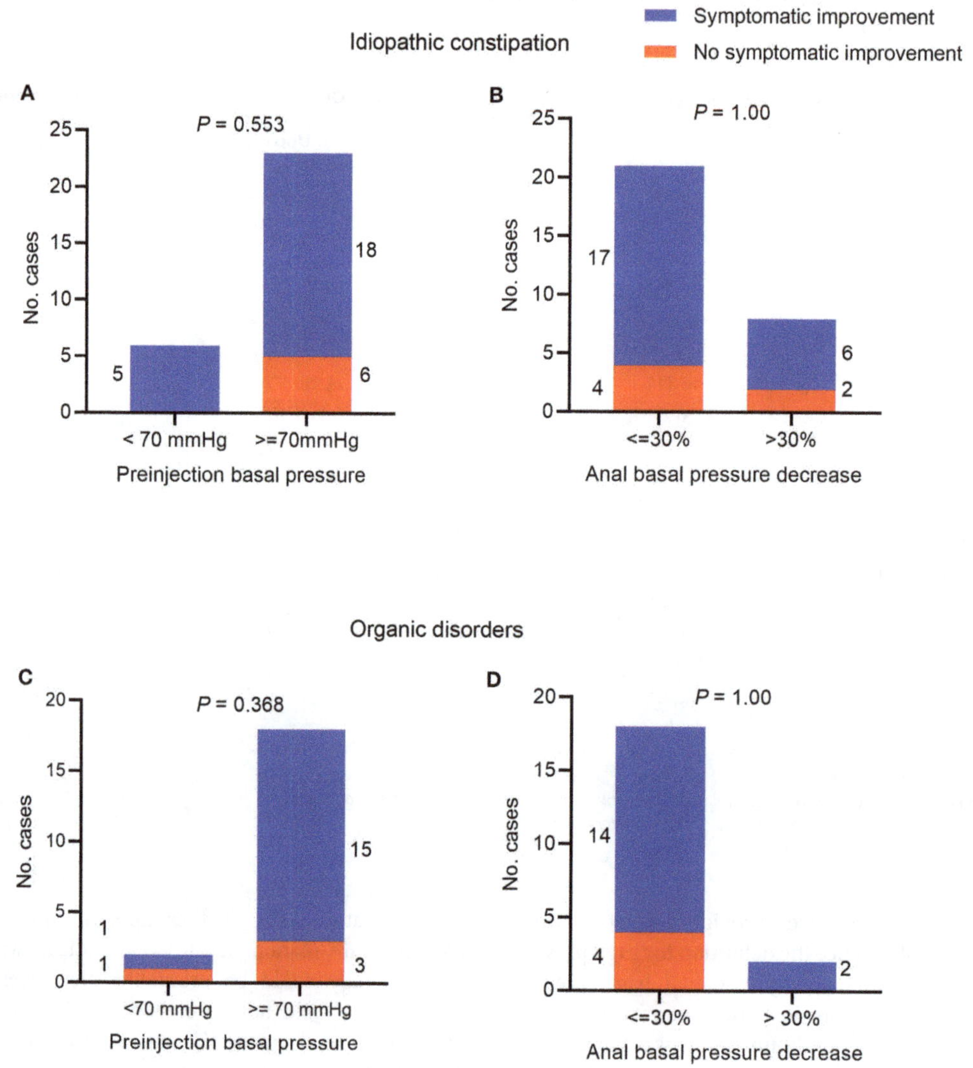

FIGURE 3 | Symptomatic improvement after botulinum toxin injection. In patients with idiopathic constipation and Chi-square test between symptom improvement and **(A)** preinjection anal basal pressure <70 mmHg/≥70 mmHg; **(B)** decrease of anal basal pressure ≤30/>30% post-injection. In patients with organic disorders and Chi-square test between symptom improvement and **(C)** preinjection anal basal pressure <70 mmHg/≥70 mmHg; **(D)** decrease of anal basal pressure ≤30%/>30% post-injection.

our hospital medical specialists do not use a validated tool routinely during control visits. Second, although increased anal basal pressure is frequently considered to be the sole cause of constipation, other causes might coexist with increased pressure and, as a consequence reducing anal basal pressure alone may not be sufficient to lead to symptomatic improvement. There are also causes that could lead to constipation independent of anal basal pressure, for instance, decreased colon motility (23), in which case decreased anal basal pressure will also not result in symptomatic improvement. Finally, the reason that symptoms persist in congenital cases such as Hirschsprung's disease may reside in retained aganglionic segments or other dysganglionoses in the proximal colon, events that may explain postoperative enterocolitis, but constipation as well (24, 25). A noteworthy finding by Meunier et al., is that among children with chronic constipation over 50% have low or normal anal basal pressure (12). This information, taken together with our finding, explains why not all patients respond positively to botulinum toxin therapy. Apparently, anal basal pressure needs to be sufficiently elevated in order to decrease after botulinum toxin injection. This finding indicates the importance of monitoring anal basal pressure prior to injecting botulinum toxin. However, currently such monitoring does not occur frequently according to the literature. Perhaps this is because anorectal manometry is not routinely available at all hospitals where botulinum toxin injections are administered. Moreover, the current criteria

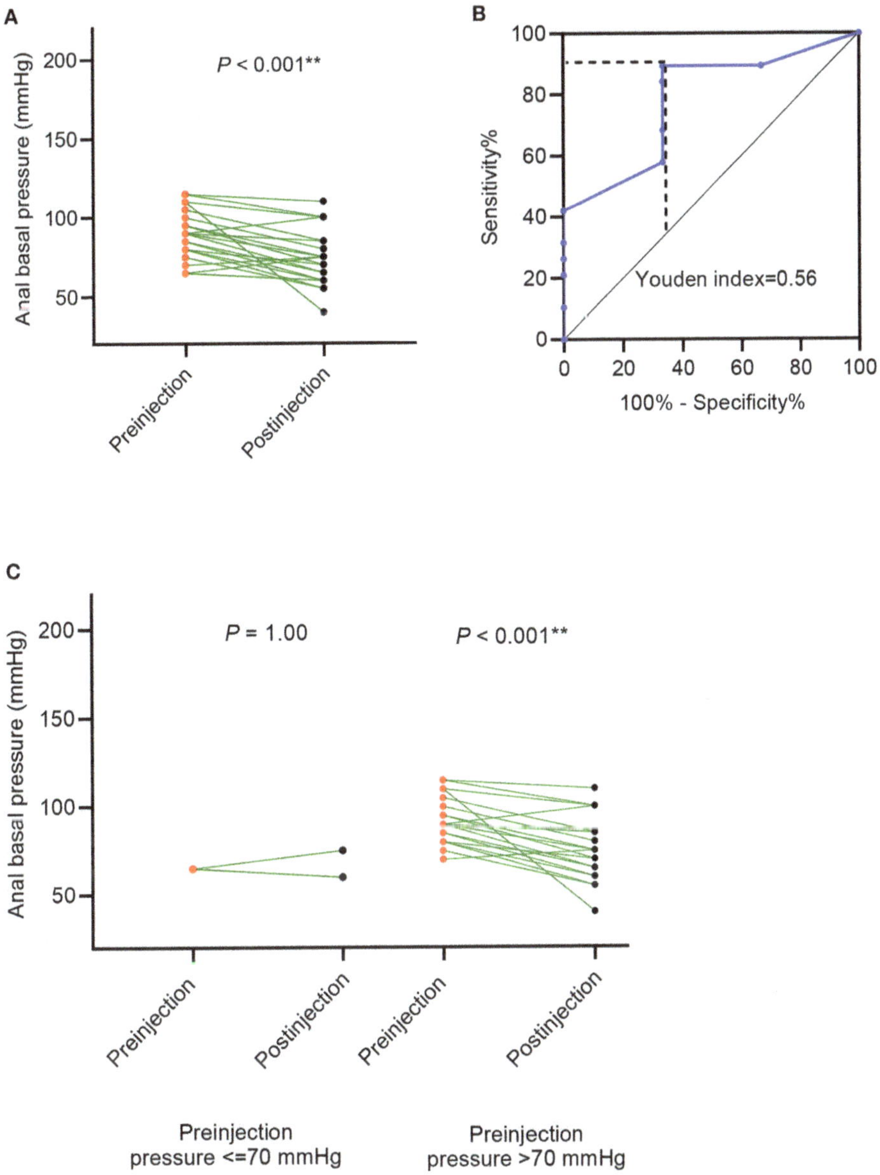

FIGURE 4 | Anal basal pressure change after botulinum toxin injection in patients with organic disorders, such as Hirschsprung's disease (HD) and congenital anorectal malformations (CARM). **(A)** The change in anal basal pressure after botulinum toxin injection; **(B)** receiver operating characteristic (ROC) curve using preinjection anal basal pressure to predict the decrease of anal basal pressure decrease; **(C)** comparison of anal basal pressure before and after the botulinum toxin injection in patients whose anal basal pressure before injection was ≤70 mmHg and >70 mmHg.

for referring a patient for botulinum toxin therapy has been undefined on account of the lack of a cut-off value. Thus, little could be gained by measuring the pressure before the injection. Now, the insight that injecting botulinum toxin into the anal sphincter when its pressure is lower than 70 mmHg does not decrease anal basal pressure, provides a clear indication which patients should not be referred for this treatment if the aim is to decrease anal basal pressure. Noteworthy, this value is valid only if the anal basal pressure is measured with a solid-state catheter. For other systems, such as a water perfused system, follow-up studies should be performed to determine such a cut-off value. Our finding partially corroborates the study of Lindsay et al., who also found an association between the response of anal sphincter to botulinum toxin and anal basal pressure before the botulinum toxin injection (26).

In the group of patients with idiopathic constipation we found that patients' ages and weights both correlated with the changes in basal pressure. It is natural that as children grow older, their weight and musculature increases. Weight, however, may vary greatly even between the children of the same age. In clinical practice a medical specialist should therefore adjust the dose according to children's weights rather than to their ages. For the

TABLE 4 | Univariable linear regression analyses of factors which possibly influence changes in the anal basal pressure change in cases with organic disorders ($n = 22$).

Independent variables	Beta coefficient†	95% CI		Standard error	P
		Lower bound	Upper bound		
Univariable analysis					
Basal pressure before injection (mmHg)	−0.425	−0.868	0.017	0.212	0.059
Age at injection§ (months)	0.058	−0.112	0.228	0.082	0.488
Time interval (days)¶	0.048	−0.454	0.550	0.241	0.845
Weight (kg)	0.157	−0.601	0.914	0.363	0.671
Number of injections	−6.563	−23.101	9.976	7.928	0.418
Rectal washout					
Yes	−10.810	−26.081	4.462	7.321	0.155
No	0‡				
Sex					
Boys	−6.619	−22.402	9.164	7.566	0.392
Girls	0‡				
Multivariable analysis					
Basal pressure before injection (mmHg)	−0.577	−0.990	−0.164	0.197	0.009
Rectal washout	−16.607	−30.310	−2.903	6.547	0.02

†Unstandardised beta coefficient; ‡Reference category.
§Age and weight were significantly correlated and therefore, for multivariable analysis, age was not taken as a cofactor.
¶Time interval between injection and anal basal pressure measurement after injection.

same dosage of botulinum toxin, the higher the child's weight, the less obvious the decrease in anal basal pressure. Moreover, male sex seems to contribute negatively to treatment outcomes when measured in terms of decrease in anal basal pressure. We explain this observation by the fact that male patients usually have a longer anal canal and that the volume of their anal sphincter muscle is larger (27). We did not confirm the correlation between the change in basal pressure and either age or weight in the group with organic constipation. This might have been caused by the smaller size of this group.

In our study the time interval between injection and the postinjection test was not correlated with changes in anal basal pressure. According to the literature, the effect duration of botulinum toxin varies between 3 to 6 months. To avoid any bias caused by the diminishing effect of botulinum toxin, we excluded all the cases with a time interval of more than 3 months between injection and the postinjection test. Additionally, we took the time interval between the injection and the postinjection anal basal pressure measurement as a cofactor in regression analysis to correct for it statistically (15, 20, 21).

Finally, we demonstrated that rectal washouts also contribute significantly to the magnitude of decrease of anal basal pressure after botulinum toxin therapy. This finding is corroborated by the study of Chan et al., who showed that rectal washouts are an useful tool to manage chronic constipation in adults (9). Some physicians consider rectal washouts to be relatively invasive in the sense that repeated washouts might irritate the rectum, damage the mucosa (28) and increase anal canal pressure and that, consequently, resulting in even more severe constipation. Our study showed that such concerns are unjustified. Regarding the relation between bowel washouts and the decrease of anal basal pressure, we think that this relation might be caused by the fact that there are receptors of the anal external sphincter continence reflex (AESCR) in the mucosa of anal canal (29). In healthy subjects the AESCR controls fecal continence by involuntary contraction of the external anal sphincter. In constipated patients, hard feces passing the anal canal during defecation may irritate and damage the mucosa of the anal canal and make the AESCR receptors hypersensitive. In turn, this could lead to overactivation of the AESCR, causing the spasm of the anal sphincter, and thus lead to chronically increased anal basal pressure. We have described this hypothesis before (30). Bowel management softens the feces. This supports regeneration of anal mucosa and prevents it from damaging, which stops the AESCR from overreacting, and allows the anal basal pressure to decrease to its physiological level.

This study has several limitations. First, on account of its retrospective design, some information such as the frequency and duration of rectal washouts, is missing. Second, we were unable to analyse detailed symptomatic improvement in order to compare it to physiological changes. It is not a standard procedure in our hospital to use validated tools to assess constipation symptoms during control visits, which in case of this retrospective study disabled consistent collection of outcomes.

CONCLUSION

In summary, botulinum toxin therapy significantly decreases anal basal pressure when the preinjection pressure is higher than 70 mmHg. In our opinion, patients suffering from severely elevated anal canal pressure should be advised to use rectal washouts in combination with botulinum toxin therapy to increase treatment efficacy.

AUTHOR CONTRIBUTIONS

GS: conducting the study, collecting, analyzing interpreting data, and drafting the manuscript. MT: conceptual design of the study, interpreting data, and critical revision of the manuscript. PB: conceptual design of the study, interpreting data, and critical revision of the manuscript. All authors contributed to the article and approved submitted version.

ACKNOWLEDGMENTS

We thank Steffie Gerritsen, specialized nurse at the Anorectal Physiology Laboratory, for her excellent technical support. We also thank T. van Wulfften Palthe, Ph.D. for correcting the English manuscript.

SUPPLEMENTARY MATERIAL

Supplementary Figure 1 | The administration of the botulinum toxin injections. **(A)** Injections were administered in four quadrants; **(B)** injection migratory direction and distance; **(C)** measurement of anal canal pressure with manometry.

Supplementary Figure 2 | The 2D map representing graphical outcome of anal canal pressure measured with manometry from one patient. **(A)** Before injection, the anal canal pressure was high; **(B)** after injection anal canal pressure has decreased.

Supplementary Table 1 | Correlation analysis[†] between the variables taken into the multivariable linear regression analysis in cases with idiopathic constipation (n=30).

REFERENCES

1. Rubin G, Dale A. Clinical review:chronic constipation in children. *BMJ.* (2006) 333:1051–5. doi: 10.1136/bmj.39007.760174.47
2. Keshtgar AS, Ward HC, Sanei A, Clayden GS. Botulinum toxin, a new treatment modality for chronic idiopathic constipation in children: long-term follow-up of a double-blind randomized trial. *J Pediatr Surg.* (2007) 42:672–80. doi: 10.1016/j.jpedsurg.2006.12.045
3. Basson S, Charlesworth P, Healy C, Phelps S, Cleeve S. Botulinum toxin use in paediatric colorectal surgery. *Pediatr Surg Int.* (2014) 30:833–8. doi: 10.1007/s00383-014-3536-4
4. Langer JC. Persistent obstructive symptoms after surgery for Hirschsprung's disease: development of a diagnostic and therapeutic algorithm. *J Pediatr Surg.* (2004) 39:1458–62. doi: 10.1016/j.jpedsurg.2004.06.008
5. Liu LWC. Chronic constipation: current treatment options. *Can J Gastroenterol.* (2011) 25 (Suppl. B):22B–8B. doi: 10.1155/2011/930108
6. Minkes RK, Langer JC, A prospective study of botulinum toxin for internal anal sphincter hypertonicity in children with Hirschsprung's disease. *J Pediatr Surg.* (2000) 35:1733–6. doi: 10.1053/jpsu.2000.19234
7. Langer JC, Birnbaum E. Preliminary experience with intrasphincteric botulinum toxin for persistent constipation after pull-through for Hirschsprung's disease. *J Pediatr Surg.* (1997) 32:1059–62. doi: 10.1016/S0022-3468(97)90399-7
8. Patrus B, Nasr A, Langer JC, Gerstle JT. Intrasphincteric botulinum toxin decreases the rate of hospitalization for postoperative obstructive symptoms in children with Hirschsprung disease. *J Pediatr Surg.* (2011) 46:184–7. doi: 10.1016/j.jpedsurg.2010.09.089
9. Chan D, Saklani A, Shah P, Lewis M, Haray P. Rectal irrigation: a useful tool in the armamentarium for functional bowel disorders. *Colorectal Disease.* (2012) 14:748–52. doi: 10.1111/j.1463-1318.2011.02797.x
10. Andromanakos N, Skandalakis P, Troupis T, Filippou D. Constipation of anorectal outlet obstruction: pathophysiology, evaluation and management. *J Gastroenterol Hepatol.* (2006) 21:638–46. doi: 10.1111/j.1440-1746.2006.04333.x
11. Duthie G, Bartolo D. Anismus: the cause of constipation? Results of investigation and treatment. *World J surg.* (1992) 16:831–5. doi: 10.1007/BF02066978
12. Meunier P, Marechal JM, De Beaujeu MJ. Rectoanal pressures and rectal sensitivity studies in chronic childhood constipation. *Gastroenterology.* (1979) 77:330–6. doi: 10.1016/0016-5085(79)90287-7
13. Molnar D, Taitz L, Urwin O, Wales J. Anorectal manometry results in defecation disorders. *Arch Dis Child.* (1983) 58:257–61. doi: 10.1136/adc.58.4.257
14. Hallan R, Melling J, Womack N, Williams N, Waldron D, Morrison J. Treatment of anismus in intractable constipation with botulinum A toxin. *Lancet.* (1988) 332:714–7. doi: 10.1016/S0140-6736(88)90188-2
15. Dressler D, Saberi FA. Botulinum toxin: mechanisms of action. *Eur Neurol.* (2005) 53:3–9. doi: 10.1159/000083259
16. Roorda D, Abeln ZA, Oosterlaan J, van Heurn LW, Derikx JP. Botulinum toxin injections after surgery for Hirschsprung disease: Systematic review and meta-analysis. *World J Gastroenterol.* (2019) 25:3268. doi: 10.3748/wjg.v25.i25.3268
17. Sonnenberg A, Koch TR. Epidemiology of constipation in the United-States. *Dis Colon Rectum.* (1989) 32:1–8. doi: 10.1007/BF02554713
18. Chumpitazi BP, Fishman SJ, Nurko S. Long-term clinical outcome after botulinum toxin injection in children with nonrelaxing internal anal sphincter. *Am J Gastroenterol.* (2009) 104:976–83. doi: 10.1038/ajg.2008.110
19. Irani K, Rodriguez L, Doody DP, Goldstein AM. Botulinum toxin for the treatment of chronic constipation in children with internal anal sphincter dysfunction. *Pediatr Surg Int.* (2008) 24:779–83. doi: 10.1007/s00383-008-2171-3
20. Ciamarra P, Nurko S, Barksdale E, Fishman S, Di Lorenzo C. Internal anal sphincter achalasia in children: clinical characteristics and treatment with Clostridium botulinum toxin. *J Pediatr Gastroenterol Nutr.* (2003) 37:315–9. doi: 10.1097/00005176-200309000-00020
21. Flynn TC. Botulinum toxin: examining duration of effect in facial aesthetic applications. *Am J Clin Dermatol.* (2010) 11:183–99. doi: 10.2165/11530110-000000000-00000
22. Staller K, Barshop K, Kuo B, Ananthakrishnan AN. Resting anal pressure, not outlet obstruction or transit, predicts healthcare utilization in chronic constipation: a retrospective cohort analysis. *Neurogastroenterol Motil.* (2015) 27:1378–88. doi: 10.1111/nmo.12628
23. Andrews CN, Storr M. The pathophysiology of chronic constipation. *Can J Gastroenterol.* (2011) 25 (Suppl. B):16B–21B. doi: 10.1155/2011/715858
24. Carvalho JL, Campos M, Soares-Oliveira M, Estevao-Costa J. Laparoscopic colonic mapping of dysganglionosis. *Pediatr Surg Int.* (2001) 17:493–5. doi: 10.1007/s003830000577
25. Estevao-Costa J, Fragoso AC, Campos M, Soares-Oliveira M, Carvalho JL. An approach to minimize postoperative enterocolitis in Hirschsprung's

disease. *J Pediatr Surg.* (2006) 41:1704–7. doi: 10.1016/j.jpedsurg.2006.05.041
26. Lindsey I, Jones OM, Cunningham C. A contraction response of the internal anal sphincter to Botulinum toxin: does low-pressure chronic anal fissure have a different pathophysiology? *Colorectal Dis.* (2011) 13:1014–8. doi: 10.1111/j.1463-1318.2010.02318.x
27. Carrington EV, Brokjaer A, Craven H, Zarate N, Horrocks EJ, Palit S, et al. Traditional measures of normal anal sphincter function using high- resolution anorectal manometry (HRAM) in 115 healthy volunteers. *Neurogastroenterol Motil.* (2014) 26:625–35. doi: 10.1111/nmo.12307
28. Podzemny V, Pescatori LC, Pescatori M. Management of obstructed defecation. *World J Gastroenterol.* (2015) 21:1053–60. doi: 10.3748/wjg.v21.i4.1053
29. Broens PM, Penninckx FM, Ochoa JB. Fecal continence revisited: the anal external sphincter continence reflex. *Dis Colon Rectum.* (2013) 56:1273–81. doi: 10.1097/DCR.0b013e3182a42d16
30. van Meegdenburg MM, Trzpis M, Heineman E, Broens PM. Increased anal basal pressure in chronic anal fissures may be caused by overreaction of the anal-external sphincter continence reflex. *Med Hypotheses.* (2016) 94:25–9. doi: 10.1016/j.mehy.2016.06.005

14

Efficacy Analysis of Day Surgery A1 Pulley Release for Pediatric Trigger Thumb

*Yan Linhua, Jiang Linjun, Qu Xiangyang, Liu Xing, Li Ming and Wu Jun**

Department of Orthopedics, Children's Hospital of Chongqing Medical University, Ministry of Education Key Laboratory of Child Development and Disorders, Chongqing Key Laboratory of Pediatrics, National Clinical Research Center for Child Health and Disorders, Chongqing, China

Correspondence:
Wu Jun
doctorwujun@hospital.cqmu.edu.cn

Objective: To investigate clinical application of day surgery A1 pulley release for pediatric trigger thumb.

Methods: We retrospectively analyzed the clinical data of 1,642 children with trigger thumb who were treated with day surgery A1 pulley release at our hospital, including satisfaction surveys, functional recovery, and complications.

Results: The operative time for unilateral and bilateral tenolysis was 4.8 ± 3.1 and 9.2 ± 3.8 min, respectively. Three children had postoperative fever and were discharged on the 2nd day after surgery. The rest of the children were discharged on the day of surgery. All incisions healed primarily, and no complications of vascular and nerve injury were reported. The patients' degree of satisfaction with the medical treatment process, diagnosis and treatment workflow, treatment effectiveness, length of hospital stay and hospitalization cost, and discharge guidance were 97.9, 96.1, 99.3, 91.1, and 98.5%, respectively. The follow-up period was between 5 months and 3 years and 1 month. Four children experienced symptom relapse after the operation, and re-tenolysis was performed in one of them. At the final follow-up, the appearance and function of the thumb had recovered well in all cases.

Conclusion: Day surgery A1 pulley release can effectively release tendon sheaths and has a short operative time, no complications of vascular and nerve injury, and good recovery of thumb function. It is a safe and reliable procedure with high patient satisfaction, and it is worthy of clinical promotion.

Keywords: children, patient satisfaction, pulley release, surgical complications, thumb

INTRODUCTION

Trigger thumb is a commonly encountered disease in pediatric practice, accounting for 87–93% of finger-stenosing tenosynovitis. It is most common in children aged 1–4 years, with an incidence of 1–3% (1). The main pathological changes are collagen degeneration of the flexor pollicis longus muscle tendon and thickening and narrowing of the tendon sheath (2). To date, non-surgical and surgical treatments for pediatric trigger thumbs are available (3, 4). Non-surgical treatments include local hot compress, massage, medicine fumigation, and intrathecal injection of medicine (5). The success rate of non-surgical treatment may vary, and the treatment duration is long (6). Open A1 pulley release is currently considered to be a safe and effective treatment for pediatric trigger thumb (7).

Day surgery refers to a procedure that requires the participation of an anesthesiologist and the completion of admission, operation, and discharge in a single working day (8). A large number of clinical studies have shown that the day surgery model has the advantages of safety and efficiency. Day surgery is safer than outpatient surgery (9, 10). Compared with traditional inpatient surgery, day surgery can effectively shorten the length of hospital stay, reduce hospitalization costs, and optimize the allocation of medical resources (11). In developed countries such as Europe and the US, most common surgical indications are treated with day surgery, which accounts for ~40–70% of all surgeries (12). In the 1960's, day surgery for indirect inguinal hernia in children was performed in China (13). With the development of medical technology and the continuous advancement of anesthesia technology, the types of diseases indicated for day surgery and the amount of day surgeries performed in the field of pediatric surgery have increased yearly (14). Nonetheless, day surgery for pediatric trigger thumb has not been reported.

Day surgery has been performed since 2014 at the Children's Hospital of Chongqing Medical University, China. With the aim of ensuring the safety of clinical medical care and the continuous improvement of the medical management system and standards, we improved the day medical services workflow and gradually created a day medical service system for pediatric patients (15). This article retrospectively analyzes the clinical data of 1,642 children who underwent tenolysis of the thumb under the day surgery model at our hospital and explores the clinical experience of day surgery A1 pulley release for the treatment of pediatric trigger thumb.

TABLE 1 | Demographics of the pediatric patients.

		Numbers (n)	Ratio (%)
Age			
	≤3 years	1,381	84.1
	>3, ≤6 years	194	11.8
	>6 years	67	4.1
Sex			
	Male	644	39.2
	Female	998	60.8
Hand involvement			
	Left	604	36.8
	Right	750	45.7
	Biolateral	288	17.5
Stage of triggers*			
	Stage I (tumor type-pretriggering)	0	0
	Stage II (active triggering)	135	8.2
	Stage III (passive triggering)	281	17.1
	Stage IV (rigid type-contracture)	1,226	74.7

According to modified Green DP classification.

METHODS

Study Subjects

We retrospectively analyzed the clinical data of children who underwent day surgery tenolysis of the thumb at Children's Hospital of Chongqing Medical University from April 2014 to December 2019. Patients who were lost to follow-up or had incomplete clinical data were excluded. A total of 1,642 children were included in this study, including 644 males and 998 females. Their average age was 3.17 ± 1.92 years (range: 1 year 3 months to 8 years 1 month). From all the subjects, 1,381 patients were under 3 years old, 194 patients were between 3 and 6 years old, and 67 were over 6 years old. Unilateral trigger thumb was diagnosed in 1,354 patients (on the left side in 604 patients and on the right side in 750 patients), and bilateral trigger thumb was diagnosed in 288 patients. The general data of the children is shown in **Table 1**.

Diagnostic and Treatment Workflow for Day Surgery

The diagnostic and treatment workflow for day surgery in our hospital is shown in **Figure 1**. The thumb A1 pulley release is performed. Vital signs, the incision condition and the blood supply of the fingertip are observed after the surgery. The child is evaluated for discharge. The dressing is changed 2 days after the operation, and finger function training begins. The child is followed up at the Pediatric Orthopedic Specialty Clinic regularly after the surgery.

Surgical Procedure

After successful intravenous induction of anesthesia, median nerve block anesthesia is performed under ultrasound guidance (16). An 0.5–1.0-cm incision is made along the transverse lines at Notta's nodule on the palm side of the metacarpophalangeal joint to incise the skin layer by layer and separate the subcutaneous tissue. Attention is paid not to injure the blood vessels and nerves. The flaps and neurovascular tissue are retracted to opposite sides to expose the flexor pollicis longus muscle tendon sheath, and the fibrous layer of the hyperplastic tendon sheath is incised along the longitudinal axis of the tendon sheath. The synovial layer is not opened. After pulley release, the ROM of the interphalangeal joint of the thumb is examined. If the ROM is normal, with smooth motion of the tendon, and the tendon is not entrapped, the incision is closed. The incision is dressed, and the thumb is immobilized in the dorsal extension position (open position of the thumb-index web space) (17).

Postoperative Observation and Discharge Evaluation

The vital signs and incision condition are observed carefully after the operation. The discharge criteria are based on the Aldrete and Marshall Chung scoring system (18) and are as follows: ① Vital signs are stable for more than 2 h; ② The child can drink water and urinate; ③ No frequent nausea and vomiting; ④ Good orientation ability; ⑤ No bleeding in the incision and good blood supply at the fingertips.

With reference to relevant domestic and foreign literature regarding day surgery and based on the 8-dimensional Hospital Consumer Assessment of Healthcare Providers and Systems (HCAHPS) scale covering the core experience of patients during

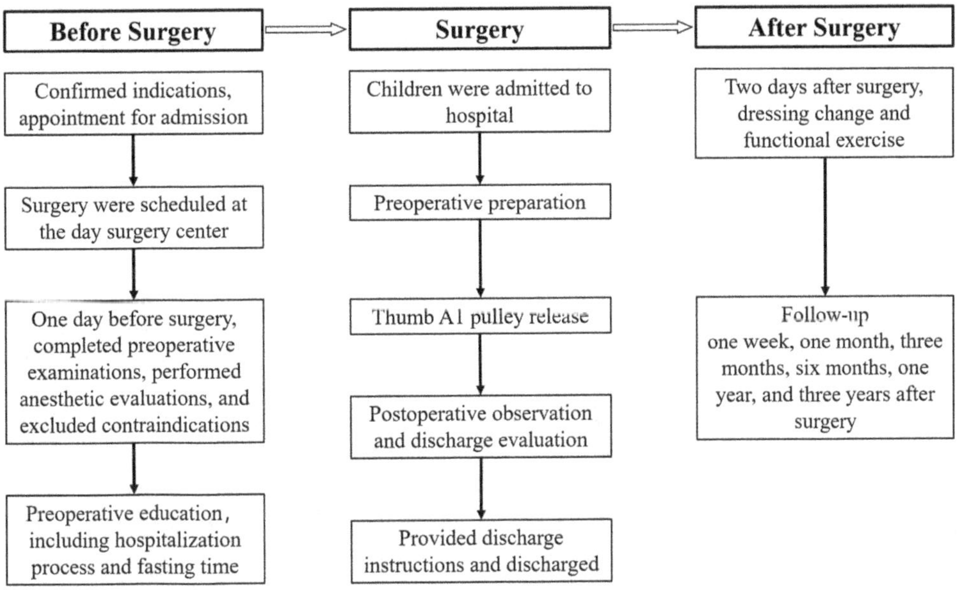

FIGURE 1 | Diagnostic and treatment workflow for day surgery.

hospitalization (19), the "Child Satisfaction Questionnaire" was designed. The satisfaction evaluation includes satisfaction with the medical treatment process, treatment effectiveness, service of the medical staff, and discharge guidance. Before a child is discharged from the hospital, the surveyors distribute and retrieve this questionnaire at bedside.

RESULTS

The wait time for day surgery was 1–13 days in pediatric patients. The operative time for unilateral or bilateral injury was 4.8 ± 3.1 min and 9.2 ± 3.8, respectively. After the release of the tendon sheath, unrestricted passive movement of the interphalangeal joint of the thumb was observed. No complications of vascular or nerve injury occurred during or after the operation. None of the children had frequent nausea, vomiting, severe pain, and no serious complications, such as death, occurred after the operation. Three children developed postoperative fever and were transferred to a specialty ward. After symptomatic treatment, they were discharged the next day. All of the children were discharged on the day of surgery except for the three who had delayed discharge. All incisions were free of infection and healed primarily. The sutures were removed 12–14 days after surgery.

In terms of the patients' satisfaction with the service of the medical staff, the satisfaction with the doctor was 97.8%, the satisfaction with the nursing staff and anesthesiologist was 99.6%, and the satisfaction with the laboratory service staff and the operating room staff was 96.2%. The patients' satisfaction with the medical treatment process, diagnostic and treatment workflow, treatment effectiveness, length of hospital stay and hospitalization cost, and discharge guidance were 97.9, 96.1, 99.3, 91.1, and 98.5%, respectively (**Table 2**).

The follow-up period was ranged from 5 months to 3 years and 1 month. Relapse occurred in 4 children after the operation. Repeat tenolysis was performed in one of them due to incomplete release. The other 3 patients were cured after conservative treatment, and their recurrence might be related to postoperative tendon adhesion. At the final follow-up, the Notta's nodules at the metacarpophalangeal joints disappeared in 1,341 cases but were still palpable in 301 cases. There was no significant difference in the range of flexion and extension of the interphalangeal joint of the affected thumb compared with that of the healthy thumb, and the thumb had good functions of abduction, adduction, and thumb opposition. The appearance of the thumb was normal, and no sympathetic muscle atrophy occurred in the hand. A typical case is shown in **Figure 2**.

DISCUSSION

The following principles apply to diseases indicated for pediatric day surgery: (1) The disease is common in children, the identical procedure is performed in a number of patients, and the operation can be implemented according to clinical pathway specifications; (2) the surgical technique is mature and minimally invasive, with a short operative time; and (3) the procedures are associated with mild postoperative pain, quick recovery, few complications, and no requirements for special care (20). Han et al. used A1 pulley release to treat trigger thumb in children and achieved good outcome of complete tendon release and well-recovered joint function, without postoperative pain or complications such as vascular or nerve damage (21). Dinham et al. reported the use of A1 pulley release to treat 105 patients with trigger thumb (131 thumbs). The range of motion (ROM) of the interphalangeal joints of the thumb was recovered completely in 100 thumbs. Reoperation was required in one thumb due to incomplete release. Incision infection was reported in one patient. Three patients had more than 15° flexion deformity of the interphalangeal joints for unknown reasons. The surgical remission rate was 95.2% (22). McAdams et al. retrospectively

TABLE 2 | Patient satisfaction [n(%)].

	Very Satisfied	Satisfied	Somewhat satisfied	Dissatisfied
Environment of the medical facility	704 (42.9)	713 (43.4)	190 (11.6)	35 (2.1)
Diagnostic and treatment workflow	594 (36.2)	698 (42.5)	286 (17.4)	64 (3.9)
Treatment effectiveness	553 (33.7)	880 (53.6)	197 (12.0)	12 (0.7)
Length of hospital stay and expenses	682 (41.5)	642 (39.1)	172 (10.5)	146 (8.9)
Discharge guidance	499 (30.4)	965 (58.8)	153 (9.3)	25 (1.5)

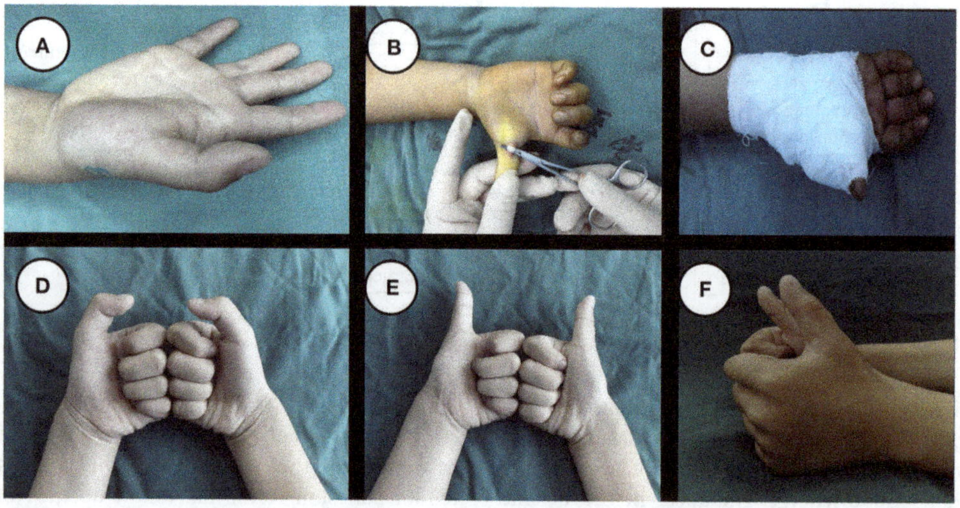

FIGURE 2 | A 3-year and 5-month-old boy presented with inability to extend his right thumb for 4 months. Before the operation, extension of the interphalangeal joint of the thumb was limited **(A)**. A1 pulley release was performed. After the tendon sheath was released, the motion of the interphalangeal joint of the thumb returned. The tendon glided well without entrapment and with a normal ROM **(B)**. The incision was closed with sutures, and the thumb was immobilized in the dorsal extension position **(C)**. A follow-up visit at 1 year and 9 months after the operation showed a well-healed incision, no obvious scar formation, normal appearance of the thumb, and unrestricted movement of the interphalangeal joint of the thumb, frontal view of the thumb in flexion **(D)**, frontal view of the thumb in straight position **(E)** and side view of the thumb in straight position **(F)**.

analyzed the clinical data of 21 patients with trigger thumb (30 thumbs) with an average of 15 years of follow-up and reported no recurrence or interdigital dysfunction. They concluded that A1 pulley release is an effective treatment for pediatric trigger thumb (23). In this study, 1,642 patients with thumb-stenosing tenosynovitis (1,930 thumbs) were included. The operative time was only a few minutes, and no complications such as vascular or nerve damage or severe pain after the operation were reported. This study shows that as a procedure for the treatment of pediatric trigger thumb, A1 pulley release is appropriate for day surgery.

The quality and safety of day surgery have become important factors in its development. Therefore, day surgery must implement a perioperative management system that is same as that used in traditional inpatient surgery (12, 13). Ma et al. analyzed the clinical data of 129,869 pediatric patients undergoing day surgery under the centralized admission management model and found that strict adherence to the "three requirements" and "three evaluations" standards, a reasonable hospital observation time, standardized discharge education and follow-up, and a sound day surgery safety system can effectively reduce the rates of delayed discharge and postoperative complications. Therefore, the quality, safety, and overall management of day surgery are the same as or even higher than those of traditional surgery (14). In this study, day surgery A1 pulley release for pediatric trigger thumb was selected as the research object. The patient admission and chief surgeon privilege systems were strictly implemented, and a standardized preoperative evaluation, anesthesia evaluation, and discharge evaluation were carried out. Postoperative follow-up showed complete release of the tendon sheath, well-recovered thumb function, and no complications such as vascular or nerve injury. The results suggest that day surgery A1 pulley release for pediatric trigger thumb is a safe and reliable procedure.

In this study, the wait time for scheduled surgery was between 1 and 13 days. Three children had postoperative fever and were discharged on the 2nd day after surgery. The other children were discharged on the day of surgery. The patient satisfaction survey showed a high degree of satisfaction with the medical treatment process, diagnostic and treatment workflow, treatment effectiveness, length of hospital stay, hospitalization cost, and discharge guidance.

CONCLUSION

A1 pulley release is a procedure for the treatment of pediatric trigger thumb that offers a short operative time, minimal trauma, quick recovery, and reduced complications. It is appropriate for completion as a day surgery. Standardized perioperative management is an important guarantee of the safety and quality of day surgery. Reasonable surgical workflow management provides considerable support for the promotion of day surgery. Day surgery A1 pulley release can effectively release tendon sheaths, with good recovery of thumb function and no complications, such as vascular nerve damage. It is safe and reliable procedure with high patient satisfaction, and it is worthy of clinical promotion.

ETHICS STATEMENT

The studies involving human participants were reviewed and approved by Children's Hospital of Chongqing Medical University. Written informed consent to participate in this study was provided by the participants' legal guardian/next of kin. Written informed consent was obtained from the individual(s) legal guardian/next of kin for the publication of any potentially identifiable images or data included in this article.

AUTHOR CONTRIBUTIONS

WJ, QX, LX, and LM were involved in the design of the project and participated in the surgery and follow-up. YL and JL participated in the preoperative preparation and discharge education. YL, JL, and QX collected the data and conducted the analysis. WJ, YL, and QX drafted the manuscript. LX and LM made the critical revisions. All of the authors read and approved the final manuscript.

ACKNOWLEDGMENTS

We thank the Department of Anesthesiology of the Children's Hospital of Chongqing Medical University for providing excellent preoperative anesthesia assessment, intraoperative anesthesia management, and postoperative resuscitation.

REFERENCES

1. Hutchinson DT, Rane AA, Montanez A. The natural history of pediatric trigger thumb in the United States. *J Hand Surg Am.* (2021) 46:424.e1–7. doi: 10.1016/j.jhsa.2020.10.016
2. Venkatadass K, Bhardwaj P, Sabapathy SR. Pediatric trigger thumb: congenital or developmental? A unique case report. *J Hand Microsurg.* (2020) 12(Suppl 1):S75–7. doi: 10.1055/s-0040-1701166
3. Amster KH, Terletzky S, Netser N, David Y, Oron A. The congential trigger thumb-clinical presentation and treatment. *Harefuah.* (2019) 158:799–801.
4. Matthews A, Smith K, Read L, Nicholas J, Schmidt E. Trigger finger: An overview of the treatment options. *JAAPA.* (2019) 32:17–21. doi: 10.1097/01.JAA.0000550281.42592.97
5. Jung HJ, Lee JS, Song KS, Yang JJ. Conservative treatment of pediatric trigger thumb: follow-up for over 4 years. *J Hand Surg Eur Vol.* (2012) 37:220–4. doi: 10.1177/1753193411422333
6. Farr S, Grill F, Ganger R, Girsch W. Open surgery versus nonoperative treatments for paediatric trigger thumb: a systematic review. *J Hand Surg Eur Vol.* (2014) 39:719–26. doi: 10.1177/1753193414523245
7. Dautel G. Management strategy for congenital thumb differences in paediatric patients. *Orthop Traumatol Surg Res.* (2017) 103:S125–33. doi: 10.1016/j.otsr.2016.04.016
8. Jarrett P. The International Association for Ambulatory Surgery (IAAS). *Ambul. Surg.* (2003) 10:113. doi: 10.1016/j.ambsur.2003.10.001
9. Castoro C. Ambulatory surgery: current status and future trends. *East Centr Afric J Surg.* (2006) 11:67–8.
10. Marij Z, Aurangzeb Q, Rizwan HR, Haroon R, Pervaiz MH. Outpatient percutaneous release of trigger finger: a cost effective and safe procedure. *Malays Orthop J.* (2017) 11:52–6. doi: 10.5704/MOJ.1703.021
11. Jacqui W. ENT surgery: increasing day cases could save money, release beds, and benefit patients. *BMJ.* (2019) 367:l6440. doi: 10.1136/bmj.l6440
12. Anderson T, Walls M, Canelo R. Day case surgery guidelines[J]. *Surgery Oxford.* (2017) 35:85–91. doi: 10.1016/j.mpsur.2016.11.013
13. Endoscopic Surgery Group, Chinese Society of Pediatric Surgery, Chinses Medical Association. Expert consensus on pediatric ambulatory surgery. *Chin J Pediatric Surg.* (2020). 41:676–82. doi: 10.3760/cma.j.cn421158-20200221-00106
14. Ma J, Bian H, Duan X, Wang J, Liu X. Safety analysis of pediatric day surgery. *Chin J Pediatr Surg.* (2020) 41:704–9. doi: 10.3760/cma.j.cn421158-20200330-00222
15. Yang C, Zhang X, Liu J, Ao W, Lv K, Wang Y. Clinical practice of day care mode at a children's specialist hospital. *Chin J Hosp Admin.* (2019) 35:324–7. doi: 10.3760/cma.j.issn.1000-6672.2019.04.013
16. Liu W, Liu J, Tan X, Wang S. Ultrasound-guided lower forearm median nerve block in open surgery for trigger thumb in 1- to 3-year-old children: A randomized trial. *Paediatr Anaesth.* (2018) 28:134–41. doi: 10.1111/pan.13296
17. Bauer AS, Bae DS. Pediatric trigger digits. *J Hand Surg.* (2015) 40:2304–9. doi: 10.1016/j.jhsa.2015.04.041
18. Robert C, Soulier A, Sciard D, Dufour G, Alberti C, Boizeau P, et al. Cognitive status of patients judged fit for discharge from the post-anaesthesia care unit after general anaesthesia: a randomized comparison between desflurane and propofol. *BMC Anesthesiol.* (2021) 21:76. doi: 10.1186/s12871-021-01287-9
19. Khan I, Tripathi S, Read C, Mischler M. 334: US healthcare customers rank most HCAHPS questions as mandatory: a kano analysis of HCAHPS survey. *Crit Care Med.* (2021) 49:155. doi: 10.1097/01.ccm.0000727224.31184.43
20. Criss CN, Brown J, Gish JS, Gadepalli SK, Hirschl RB. Clinic-day surgery for children: a patient and staff perspective. *Pediatr Surg Int.* (2018) 34:755–61. doi: 10.1007/s00383-018-4288-3
21. Han SH, Yoon HK, Shin DE, Song DG. Trigger thumb in children: results of surgical treatment in children above 5 years of age. *J Pediatr Orthop.* (2010) 30:710–4. doi: 10.1097/BPO.0b013e3181edef8d
22. Dinham JM, Meggitt BF. Trigger thumbs in children. A review of the natural history and indications for treatment in 105 patients. *J Bone Joint Surg Br.* (1974) 56:153–5.
23. McAdams TR, Moneim MS, Omer GE. Long-term follow-up of surgical release of the A(1) pulley in childhood trigger thumb. *J Pediatr Orthop.* (2002) 22:41–3. doi: 10.1097/00004694-200201000-00010

15

A Randomized Controlled Study of Caudal Dexmedetomidine for the Prevention of Postoperative Agitation in Children Undergoing Urethroplasty

Weichao Zhu[1†]*, Jie Sun*[2†]*, Jianhua He*[1,3*]*, Wangping Zhang*[4*] *and Meng Shi*[5]

[1] Department of Pediatric Surgery, The Affiliated Hospital of Medical School, Ningbo University, Ningbo, China, [2] Department of Urology, Shanghai Children's Medical Center, Shanghai Jiao Tong University School of Medicine, Shanghai, China, [3] Diagnosis and Treatment Center of Pelvic Floor, The Affiliated Hospital of Medical School, Ningbo University, Ningbo, China, [4] Department of Anesthesiology, Women and Children's Hospital of Jiaxing University, Jiaxing, China, [5] Department of Anesthesiology, Xuzhou Medical University, Xuzhou, China

***Correspondence:**
Wangping Zhang
zhang650679@163.com
Jianhua He
hejhdr@163.com*

Background: Postoperative agitation is a common complication in children undergoing general anesthesia. This study aimed to investigate the effect of caudal dexmedetomidine for the prevention of postoperative agitation in children undergoing urethroplasty.

Materials and Methods: Eighty children were prospectively recruited to this study and randomized to two groups (40 cases in each group), specifically, a dexmedetomidine group (group D) who received 0.2% ropivacaine + 0.5 μg/kg dexmedetomidine for caudal block, and a control group who received 0.2% ropivacaine alone. The time to wake up, the time to discharge from the postanesthesia care unit (PACU), the duration of the caudal block, and the Ramsay sedation scale (RSS) were evaluated in the patients. Adverse events such as postoperative agitation, respiratory depression, bradycardia, hypotension, excessive sedation, nausea, and vomiting were also recorded during the first postoperative 24 h.

Results: The incidence of postoperative agitation was lower in group D compared with patients in the control group (2.5 vs. 22.5%, $p = 0.007$). The time to wake up and the time to discharge from PACU were longer in group D than in the control group (15.2 ± 2.6 vs. 13.4 ± 1.3 min, 48.2 ± 7.7 vs. 41.5 ± 8.0 min, respectively, $p < 0.001$). However, the extubation times were similar between the two groups. The duration of the caudal block was longer in group D compared with the control group (8.8 ± 1.6 vs. 4.6 ± 0.7 h, $p < 0.001$).

Conclusions: Caudal dexmedetomidine prolongs the duration of caudal block and decreases the incidence of postoperative agitation in children undergoing urethroplasty.

Clinical Trial Registration: ChiCTR1800016828.

Keywords: dexmedetomidine, caudal block, postoperative agitation, children, general anesthesia

INTRODUCTION

Postoperative agitation is one of the common complications in pediatric patients after general anesthesia (1, 2). It is characterized by crying, shouting, screaming, non-purposeful restlessness, and disorientation (3). The rate of postoperative agitation has been reported to range from 10 to 80% in pediatric patients (4).

Dexmedetomidine is an α_2 adrenergic agonist that is used for sedation by intravenous infusion. Studies have shown that intravenous dexmedetomidine can reduce the incidence of postoperative agitation in pediatric patients receiving general anesthesia (5, 6). Also, venous infusion of dexmedetomidine may lead to delayed discharge from the hospital (7). Ropivacaine (0.2%) with or without adjuvants is usually used for the caudal block in children. However, studies on the use of caudal dexmedetomidine to prevent postoperative agitation are yet to be reported in the literature. The purpose of this study was to investigate the efficacy of caudal dexmedetomidine in reducing postoperative agitation in children undergoing urethroplasty.

MATERIALS AND METHODS

This study was conducted in accordance with the Declaration of Helsinki and approved by the Ethical Committee of the Jiaxing Children's Hospital (approval number: 2018-36, Chairman: Prof L. Xia). Written informed consent was obtained from the parents or guardians of the children recruited to the study (www.chictr.org.cn, registration number: ChiCTR1800016828).

From July 2018 to July 2019, a total of 80 children undergoing urethroplasty with ASA I–II who weighed between 10 and 30 kg and were aged 1 to 6 years were recruited to this study. Children with cardiopulmonary diseases, body mass index (BMI) >29 kg/m^2, and contradictions to caudal block were excluded from the study. Children were randomized to the control group or the dexmedetomidine group (the group D) with 40 patients in each group. The anesthesiologists, nurses, investigators, and children were blinded to the allocated groups.

All children were fasted for 6–8 h before treatment and had no premedications. Upon arrival in the operating room, venous access was established. Routine monitoring included an electrocardiogram, pulse oxygen saturation (S_PO_2), noninvasive systolic blood pressure (SBP), diastolic blood pressure (DBP), and heart rate (HR). After the induction of anesthesia with intravenous fentanyl (3 μg/kg) and propofol (3 mg/kg), a laryngeal mask airway (LMA) (classical type, Tuoren Company, Changyuan, China) was inserted. Subsequently, the lungs were mechanically ventilated with pressure-controlled ventilation. The ventilation parameters were set as a driving pressure of 12–15 cmH_2O, a respiratory frequency of 14–20 breaths/min, an oxygen flow rate of 2 L/min, the fraction of inspired oxygen was 0.5, an I:E ratio of 1:1.5, and a positive end-expiratory pressure of zero.

The caudal block was performed under general anesthesia in the left lateral position. The D group received 1 ml/kg of analgesic solution that consisted of 0.2% ropivacaine (AstraZeneca Pharmaceutical Company, Beijing, China) and 0.5 μg/kg dexmedetomidine (Jiangsu Hengrui Pharmaceutical Company, Lianyungang, China) for the caudal block. The control group received 0.2% ropivacaine 1 ml/kg alone. The analgesic medications were prepared by the nurses. The driving pressure was adjusted to keep the end-tidal carbon dioxide partial pressure ($P_{ET}CO_2$) between 35 and 50 mmHg. Anesthesia was maintained with 2%–3% end-tidal sevoflurane to keep the blood pressure within a 20% range of baseline. Anesthetic agents were stopped 5 min before the end of the operation and the children were transferred to the postanesthesia care unit (PACU) at the end of the operation.

The SBP, DBP, and HR were recorded at 5-min intervals during the operation. The time to remove the LMA (extubation time), wake-up time, time to discharge from the PACU, the duration of the caudal block, and the Ramsay sedation scale (RSS) during the first postoperative 24 h were also noted. The adverse events (postoperative agitation, respiratory depression, bradycardia, hypotension, excessive sedation, nausea, and vomiting) were recorded. The LMA was removed when the tidal volumes were >6 ml/kg, the S_PO_2 was >96%, and the $P_{ET}CO_2$ was <50 mmHg during inhalation. The children were discharged from the PACU when the modified Aldrete score was >9. The standards for the modified Aldrete scores were as follows:

a. Movements: 2 = spontaneous movement of the arms, legs, and head; 1 = spontaneous movement of the arms or legs with restricted spontaneous head movements; and 0 = no movement of the limbs or head.
b. Breathing: 2 = Deep breathing and effective coughing with a normal respiratory rate; 1 = Difficult or restricted breathing but spontaneous breathing is shallow and slow. 0 = Paused or weak breathing that requires assisted breathing.
c. Blood pressure: 2 = Within ±20% before anesthesia; 1 = ±20%−49% before anesthesia; and 0 = > ±50% before anesthesia.
d. Consciousness: 2 = Completely awake and can answer questions accurately; 1 = the patient can wake up but is drowsy; and 0 = nonresponsive.
e. SpO_2: 2 = air breathing SpO_2 >92%; 1 = oxygen breathing SpO_2 >92%; and 0 = oxygen breathing SpO_2 <92%.

The duration of the caudal block was defined as the time from the caudal injection to the first occasion when the children complained of incisional pain. Respiratory depression was defined as SpO_2 levels <94% while receiving oxygen and a respiratory frequency of <10 times/min. Hypotension was defined as SBP reduction to >20% from the baseline values and bradycardia was defined as a HR <60 beats/min or reduction to >20% from the baseline values. Children were treated with propofol (1 mg/kg) if postoperative agitation occurred.

The level of sedation was assessed using the Ramsay sedation scale (RSS) (1 indicated that the patient was anxious, agitated, or restless, 2 indicated that the patient was cooperative, oriented, and alert, 3 indicated that the patient was responsive to commands, 4 indicated that the patient was asleep but had a brisk response to a light glabellar tap or loud auditory stimulus, 5 indicated that the patient was asleep with a sluggish response to a light glabellar tap or loud auditory stimulus, and 6 that the patient was asleep and not responsive) (8). The RSS values were recorded at intervals of 1 h during the first

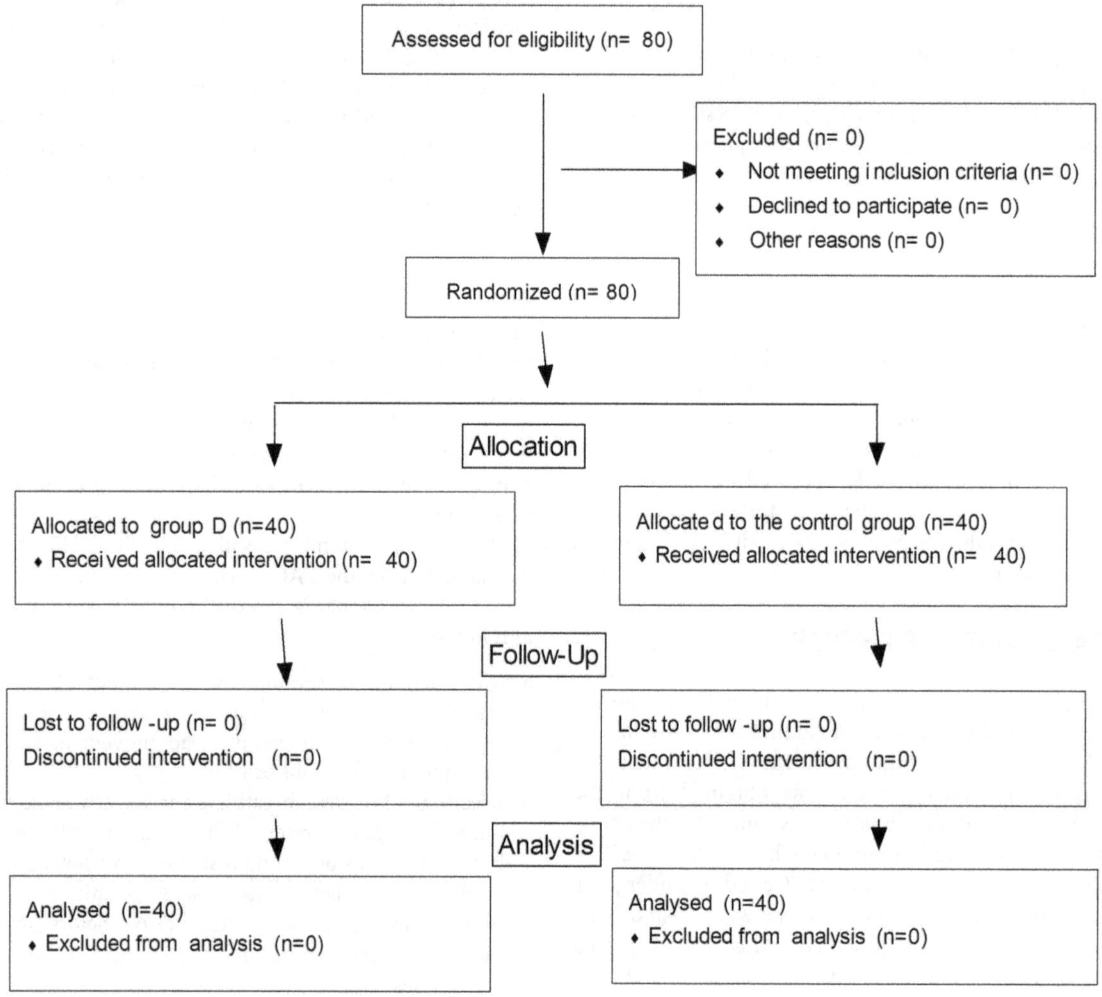

FIGURE 1 | A flow diagram of the study.

TABLE 1 | Data of children ($n = 40$).

Index	Group D	Control group	*P*-value
Age (year)	3.7 ± 0.9	3.5 ± 1.2	0.466
Weight (kg)	15.2 ± 2.0	14.7 ± 2.2	0.305
BMI (kg/m^2)	23.6 ± 3.5	23.5 ± 3.2	0.869
Duration of anesthesia (min)	97.6 ± 6.3	98.4 ± 6.3	0.447
Duration of surgery (min)	83.4 ± 7.7	84.3 ± 8.2	0.586
Duration of caudal block (h)	9.7 ± 1.6	4.5 ± 0.7	<0.001
Extubation time (min)	8.1 ± 2.0	8.5 ± 2.1	0.447
Wake-up time (min)	15.2 ± 2.5	13.4 ± 1.3	<0.001
Time to discharge from PACU (min)	48.2 ± 7.7	41.5 ± 8.0	<0.001

Data are expressed as the mean + standard deviation or number. BMI, body mass index; LMA, laryngeal mask airway; PACU, post-anesthesia care unit.

postoperative 24 h. Excessive sedation was defined as when the RSS value was >4. Postoperative agitation was defined as an RSS value of 1.

Statistical Analysis

In this study, the primary outcome was the incidence of postoperative agitation and the secondary outcome was the duration of the caudal block. According to our pilot study, 40 samples in each group were required to allow for dropouts using a two-sided Chi-square test at a significance level of 0.05 with a power of 80%. Data analysis was performed with the SPSS 20.0 statistical software (SPSS Inc., Chicago, IL, USA). Data are presented with mean ± standard deviation. Comparison of the numerical variables between the two groups was performed using a Student's *t*-test for independent samples. The categorical data were compared using a Chi-square test. *P*-values < 0.05 were considered statistically significant.

RESULTS

Eighty children were recruited to and completed the study (**Figure 1**). No significant differences in age, weight, BMI, the duration of operation, and the duration of anesthesia were observed between the two groups ($p > 0.05$) (**Table 1**). The extubation time was similar between the two groups (8.1 ± 2.0 vs. 8.5 ± 2.1 min, $p = 0.447$), while the time to wake up and discharge from PACU were significantly longer in group D compared with the control group (15.2 ± 2.5 vs. 13.4 ± 1.3 min, 48.2 ± 7.7 vs. 41.5 ± 8.0 min, respectively, $p < 0.001$) (**Table 1**). The duration of the caudal block was significantly longer in group D compared with the control group (8.8 ± 1.6 vs. 4.6 ± 0.7 h, $p < 0.001$). The postoperative RSS was higher in group D compared with the control group within the first postoperative 4 h but was similar between the two groups during 5–24 h after the operation (**Figure 2**).

There was one case of postoperative agitation in group D, while nine cases were reported in the control group (2.5 vs. 22.5%, $p = 0.007$). There were no significant differences in the incidence of respiratory depression, bradycardia, hypotension, nausea, and vomiting between the two groups. Postoperative hypoxemia and excessive sedation were not observed in either of the groups during the study period (**Table 2**).

DISCUSSION

Emergence agitation may cause injury to patients and may also result in the accidental removal of intravenous catheters, dislodgement of urinary catheters, postoperative wound bleeding, and increases in the nursing requirements in PACU. This study indicated that caudal dexmedetomidine prolonged the duration of analgesia and reduced the incidence of postoperative agitation in children undergoing urethroplasty.

The duration of the caudal block was longer in group D compared with the control group. These data indicated that dexmedetomidine prolonged the duration of the caudal block and maintained long-term effective analgesia. Dexmedetomidine can produce analgesia by activating the spinal α_2 adrenergic receptor (9). In our study, the RSS in the first postoperative 4 h was higher in group D than in the control group, but the RSS was similar between the two groups at 4–24 h after the operation suggesting that dexmedetomidine could increase the sedative effect of the caudal block. Dexmedetomidine can produce a sedative effect by activating the α_2 adrenergic receptor (10–12). As the sedative effect of dexmedetomidine gradually disappeared, the RSS after dexmedetomidine administration decreased. Hassan et al. (13) reported that caudal bupivacaine combined with dexmedetomidine prolonged the analgesic time of bupivacaine and increased the sedation scores in pediatrics undergoing hypospadias surgery. These observations are in agreement with our findings.

The extubation time (time to remove LMA) was similar between the two groups, but the wake-up time and discharge time from PACU were longer in group D than in the control

TABLE 2 | Adverse events of children ($n = 40$).

Index	Group D	Control group	*P*-value
Postoperative agitation (*n*)	1(2.5)	9(22.5%)	0.007
Respiratory depression (*n*)	0	0	0.999
Bradycardia (*n*)	2	0	0.494
Hypotension (*n*)	1	0	0.999
Nausea and vomiting (*n*)	1	2	0.999
Excessive sedation (*n*)	0	0	0.999
Postoperative hypoxemia (*n*)	0	0	0.999

Data are expressed as number (percent).

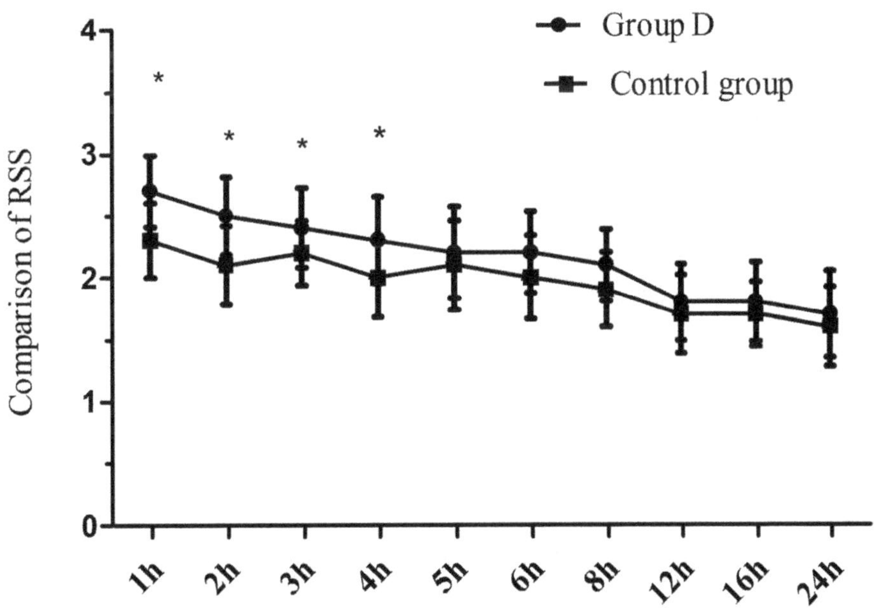

FIGURE 2 | A comparison of the postoperative RSS at different time points, $^*p < 0.05$.

group. Dexmedetomidine did not cause respiratory depression when used for sedation (14), so it did not result in prolongation of the time to remove LMA. Dexmedetomidine provided lasting sedation and affected the Aldrete score and led to prolongation of the wake-up time and delaying discharge from PACU.

In the present study, the incidence of postoperative agitation was decreased in group D compared with the control group (2.5 vs. 22.5%, $p = 0.007$). It indicated that a single bolus dose of caudal dexmedetomidine 0.5 μg/kg decreased the incidence of postoperative agitation in children undergoing urethroplasty. Postoperative agitation is related to many factors including postoperative pain, the use of inhalant anesthetics, anoxia, the types of surgical procedures, and airway obstruction (15). Postoperative pain and discomfort are the main causes of postoperative agitation. In our study, dexmedetomidine prolonged the duration of the caudal block and maintained long-term analgesia. Excellent analgesia would reduce the incidence of postoperative agitation in pediatric patients. Hence, we concluded that the use of caudal dexmedetomidine at a dose of 0.5 μg/kg reduced the incidence of postoperative agitation in children undergoing urethroplasty. In agreement with our findings, previous studies have shown that the venous infusion of dexmedetomidine decreases the incidence of postoperative agitation in children (1–3).

No significant differences in the incidence of respiratory depression, bradycardia, hypotension, excess sedation, nausea, and vomiting between the two groups in this study were found. Two patients developed bradycardia in group D, but no patients required treatment with atropine. Hypotension and bradycardia are common side effects of neuraxial dexmedetomidine administration. Konakci et al. (16) reported that the hemodynamic adverse events are less pronounced in children compared with adults and may be dose dependent.

LIMITATIONS

Our study has several limitations. Currently, the FDA has no approved the use of neuraxial dexmedetomidine and the levels of pain cannot be accurately assessed in young children (age <6 years). Further studies are needed to assess the side effects of caudal dexmedetomidine.

CONCLUSIONS

This study showed that caudal dexmedetomidine is effective in the prevention of postoperative agitation in children undergoing urethroplasty and prolongs the duration of the caudal block without excessive sedation.

AUTHOR CONTRIBUTIONS

WeZ, JH, and MS: study design and data analysis. WaZ: patient recruitment and data collection. JS and WaZ: writing of the paper. All authors contributed to the article and approved the submitted version.

ACKNOWLEDGMENTS

We would like to thank our colleagues at Xuzhou University for their valuable contributions.

REFERENCES

1. Cao JL, Pei YP, Wei JQ, Zhang YY. Effects of intraoperative dexmedetomidine with intravenous anesthesia on postoperative emergence agitation/delirium in pediatric patients undergoing tonsillectomy with or without adenoidectomy: a CONSORT-prospective, randomized, controlled clinical trial. *Medicine.* (2016) 95:e5566. doi: 10.1097/MD.0000000000005566
2. Mohkamkar M, Farhoudi F, Alam-Sahebpour A, Mousavi SA, Khani S, Shahmohammadi S. Postanesthetic emergence agitation in pediatric patients under general anesthesia. *Iran J Pediatr.* (2014) 24:184–90.
3. Ni J, Wei J, Yao Y, Jiang X, Luo L, Luo D. Effect of dexmedetomidine on preventing postoperative agitation in children: a meta-analysis. *PLoS ONE.* (2015) 10:e0128450. doi: 10.1371/journal.pone.0128450
4. Acar HV, Yilmaz A, Demir G, Eruyar SG, Dikmen B. Capsicum plasters on acupoints decrease the incidence of emergence agitation in pediatric patients. *Paediatr Anaesth.* (2012) 22:1105–9. doi: 10.1111/j.1460-9592.2012.03876.x
5. Kim J, Kim SY, Lee JH, Kang YR, Koo BN. Low-dose dexmedetomidine reduces emergence agitation after desflurane anaesthesia in children undergoing strabismus surgery. *Yonsei Med J.* (2014) 55:508–16. doi: 10.3349/ymj.2014.55.2.508
6. Sun Y, Li Y, Sun Y, Wang X, Ye H, Yuan X. Dexmedetomidine effect on emergence agitation and delirium in children undergoing laparoscopic hernia repair: a preliminary study. *J Int Med Res.* (2017) 45:973–83. doi: 10.1177/0300060517699467
7. Edokpolo LU, Mastriano DJ, Serafin J, Weedon JC, Siddiqui MT, Dimaculangan DP. Discharge readiness after propofol with or without dexmedetomidine for colonoscopy: a randomized controlled trial. *Anesthesiology.* (2019) 131:279–86. doi: 10.1097/ALN.0000000000002809
8. Zhang W, Li C. EC50 of Epidural ropivacaine combined with dexmedetomidine for labor analgesia. *Clin J Pain.* (2018) 34:950–3. doi: 10.1097/AJP.0000000000000613
9. Al-Mustafa MM, Badran IZ, Abu Ali HM, Al-Barazangi BA, Massad IM, Al-Ghanem SM. Intravenous dexmedetomidine prolongs bupivacaine spinal analgesia. *Middle East J Anesthesiol.* (2009) 20:225–231.
10. Luo K, Xu JM, Cao L, Gao J. Effect of dexmedetomidine combined with sufentanil on preventing emergence agitation in children receiving sevoflurane anesthesia for cleft palate repair surgery. *Exp Ther Med.* (2017) 14:1775–82. doi: 10.3892/etm.2017.4660
11. Rao Y, Zeng R, Jiang X, Li J, Wang X. The effect of dexmedetomidine on emergence agitation or delirium in children after anesthesia. a systematic review and meta-analysis of clinical studies. *Front Pediatr.* (2020) 8:329. doi: 10.3389/fped.2020.00329
12. Shi M, Miao S, Gu T, Wang D, Zhang H, Liu J. Dexmedetomidine for the prevention of emergence delirium and postoperative behavioral changes in pediatric patients with sevoflurane anesthesia: a double-blind, randomized trial. *Drug Des Devel Ther.* (2019) 13:897–905. doi: 10.2147/DDDT.S196075
13. Hassan PF, Hassan AS, Elmetwally SA. Caudal analgesia for hypospadias in pediatrics: comparative evaluation of adjuvants dexamethasone and dexmedetomidine combination versus dexamethasone or dexmedetomidine to bupivacaine: a prospective, double-blinded, randomized comparative study. *Anesth Essays Res.* (2018) 12:644–50. doi: 10.4103/aer.AER_77_18

14. Yan MJ, Wang T, Wu XM, Zhang W. Comparison of dexmedetomidine or sufentanil combined with ropivacaine for epidural analgesia after thoracotomy: a randomized controlled study. *J Pain Res.* (2019) 12:2673–8. doi: 10.2147/JPR.S208014
15. Kim HJ, Kim DK, Kim HY, Kim JK, Choi SW. Risk factors of emergence agitation in adults undergoing general anesthesia for nasal surgery. *Clin Exp Otorhinolaryngol.* (2015) 8:46–51. doi: 10.3342/ceo.2015.8.1.46
16. Konakci S, Adanir T, Yilmaz G, Rezanko T. The efficacy and neurotoxicity of dexmedetomidine administered via the epidural route. *Eur J Anaesthesiol.* (2008). 25:403–9. doi: 10.1017/S0265021507003079

Micro-CT Imaging of Pediatric Thyroglossal Duct Cysts

Claire Frauenfelder[1,2]*, *Susan C. Shelmerdine*[1,3,4], *Ian C. Simcock*[1,3,4], *Andrew Hall*[1], *John Ciaran Hutchinson*[1,3,4,5], *Michael T. Ashworth*[1], *Owen J. Arthurs*[1,3,4] *and Colin R. Butler*[1,3]

[1] Great Ormond Street Hospital for Children NHS Foundation Trust, London, United Kingdom, [2] Discipline of Surgery, School of Medicine, University of Adelaide, Adelaide, SA, Australia, [3] UCL Great Ormond Street Institute of Child Health, Great Ormond Street Hospital for Children, London, United Kingdom, [4] National Institute for Health Research Great Ormond Street Hospital Biomedical Research Centre, London, United Kingdom, [5] Department of Histopathology, St Thomas' Hospital, London, United Kingdom

Correspondence:
Claire Frauenfelder
claire.frauenfelder@adelaide.edu.au

Objectives: To determine the feasibility of micro-CT as a high-resolution 3D imaging tool for thyroglossal duct cysts and to evaluate its role augmenting traditional histopathological examination of resected specimens.

Methods: A single centre, prospective case series of consecutive children undergoing excision of a thyroglossal duct cyst was performed at a quaternary paediatric referral hospital in the United Kingdom. Consecutive children listed for excision of a thyroglossal duct cyst whose parents agreed to participate were included and there were no exclusion criteria.

Results: Surgically excised thyroglossal duct cyst or remnant specimens from five patients (two males, three females) were examined using micro-CT alongside traditional histopathological examination. In all cases, micro-CT imaging was able to demonstrate 3D imaging datasets of the specimens successfully and direct radio-pathological comparisons were made (**Figures 1–5**, **Supplementary Video 1**).

Conclusions: The study has shown the feasibility and utility of post-operative micro-CT imaging of thyroglossal duct cysts specimens as a visual aid to traditional histopathological examination. It better informs the pathological specimen sectioning using multi-planar reconstruction and volume rendering tools without tissue destruction. In the complex, often arborised relationship between a thyroglossal duct cyst and the hyoid, micro-CT provides valuable image plane orientation and indicates proximity of the duct to the surgical margins. This is the first case series to explore the use of micro-CT imaging for pediatric thyroglossal duct specimens and it informs future work investigating the generalizability of micro-CT imaging methods for other lesions, particularly those from the head and neck region where precisely defining margins of excision may be challenging.

Keywords: diagnosis, radiology/imaging, thyroglossal duct cyst, head and neck, pathology

INTRODUCTION

Thyroglossal duct cysts account for up to 70% of pediatric neck masses encountered in clinical practice (1, 2). A clear understanding of the embryological path of the thyroid gland and its relationship to the hyoid bone, tongue base musculature, and anterior neck tissue are key to successful surgery. As far back as 1893, Schlange described excision of the mid-portion of the hyoid bone during thyroglossal duct cyst surgery (3), while Sistrunk in his eponymous procedure for excision of thyroglossal duct cysts expanded the operation to include a block of midline tissue (4, 5). Removing the entirety of the remnant tract along the path of the primitive thyroid descending confers higher likelihood of complete excision of the lesion and significantly decreases recurrence, which occurs in up to 10% of patients following primary surgical excision and over 20% following revision procedures (6–8).

Histopathological assessment of the removed tissue is the current standard in confirming the diagnosis and complete surgical excision of the tract. One of the main drawbacks of this traditional approach is that sectioning is only possible in a single plane (typically longitudinal) as the tissue is destroyed during sectioning. In the past, imaging methods for reviewing surgical specimens were unable to provide the magnification and resolution required for detailed assessment, however novel strategies are now emerging.

Micro-focus computed tomography (micro-CT) imaging is being increasingly used as a non-destructive method for digital specimen analysis. It uses multiple X-rays to create a high-resolution 3D volume imaging dataset at a spatial resolution comparable to light microscopy (voxel size down to 1 micron) (9). At our institution, we currently provide a post-mortem fetal micro-CT clinical imaging service (10–12), however only a few publications have reported using this technology for excised human surgical specimens (13–16) and the utility of this imaging modality for pediatric thyroglossal duct cyst specimens is unknown, but clearly has appeal in providing high resolution 3D imaging of complex neck structures to aid pathological dissection.

The objectives of this study were two-fold: to determine whether micro-CT can provide high resolution imaging datasets to diagnose thyroglossal duct cysts and tracts, and, to evaluate the role for micro-CT imaging in aiding histopathological evaluation in this setting.

MATERIALS AND METHODS

Setting and Participants

In this single center, prospective study we recruited consecutive children undergoing excision of a thyroglossal duct cyst over 11 months whose parents agreed to participate (5 November 2019–5 October 2020). Only those with written parental consent for micro-CT imaging of the post-operative specimen were included in the final study cohort. There were no exclusion criteria.

All patients underwent a routine extended Sistrunk's procedure (17). A midline neck skin incision was made with subplatysmal flaps elevated. A comprehensive block of midline neck tissue was excised, including infrahyoid tissue to the level of the thyroid isthmus, the medial adjacent strap muscles, the mid-portion of the hyoid bone, and the submucosal tongue base musculature superiorly. The cyst and any remnant thyroglossal duct tract are contained within the specimen block and may not be separately visualized if not active or previously ruptured during infection (or unsuccessful primary surgery). Where previous infection had ruptured through skin, the scarred overlying skin was excised as well.

Tissue Preparation

All specimens were immersed in a solution of 10% formalin and potassium triiodide (I_2KI; total iodine content of 63.25 mg/mL). Specimens were stored at room temperature for 72 h until fully iodinated then rinsed and dried before micro-CT imaging.

Micro-Focus Computed Tomography Examination

Imaging of the specimens were acquired using 1 of 2 micro-CT scanners located on-site (XTH 225 ST or Med-X Alpha; Nikon Metrology, Tring, United Kingdom), both equipped with a multi-metal target. All imaging was undertaken by trained researchers (I.C.S or S.C.S). Specimens were secured within the scanner using foam supports, moisture absorbent wrapping material, and Parafilm M (Bemis Company, Inc., Oshkosh, WI) to ensure mechanical stability.

Imaging parameters varied according to specimen size, with X-ray energies and beam current ranging between 100 and 120 kV and 133 and 180 mA, respectively. Exposure times ranged from 354 to 500 ms, with 2 X-ray frames per projection and total number of projections varying between 2,301 and 3,141. Projection images acquired by the scanner were reconstructed using modified Feldkamp filtered back-projection algorithms with proprietary software (CTPro3D; Nikon Metrology, United Kingdom) and post-processed using VGStudio MAX 3.0 (Volume Graphics GmbH, Heidelberg, Germany). Isotropic voxel sizes varied according to specimen size and magnification, ranging from 8.18 to 22.19 microns.

Histopathological Examination

After imaging samples were embedded in paraffin and processed by standard protocols, including staining with Haematoxylin and Eosin (H&E). The histopathological sections were reviewed by a pediatric pathologist (M.T.A) with >30 years of experience.

Image Analysis

All micro-CT images were evaluated side by side with the histopathology results by two pediatric radiologists (O.J.A. and S.C.S.) with 4 years of micro-CT imaging reporting experience and a pediatric pathologist (M.T.A.). The radiologists and pathologist were not blinded to the clinical history. Images were evaluated to gain comparative radiological-pathological views, and contribution to diagnosis was discussed.

Reporting

This case series has been reported in line with the PROCESS Guideline (18).

RESULTS

Patient and Specimen Details

Over the 11-month study period, five patients who underwent primary excision of presumed thyroglossal duct cysts were recruited. The patient demographics, abbreviated clinical histories, and histopathological results are presented in **Table 1**. Lesions were excised from two male and three female patients aged 16 months to 14 years old.

In two cases, a primary extended Sistrunk's procedure was performed (i.e., no previous infection or rupture of the thyroglossal duct cyst, nor surgical intervention). In three cases, the surgery was performed due to recurrent cyst infections, which had led to discharge through the skin on at least one occasion prior to the surgery. For these cases, the overlying skin incorporating the scar was also excised in continuity with the routine operative specimen. Post-operative recovery for all patients was unremarkable. There was no evidence of recurrence in the 12 months following surgery.

Radio-Pathological Correlation

In three cases, a thyroglossal duct cyst was identified, and in two cases a thyroglossal duct remnant (without cyst) was found. In all cases, micro-CT imaging was able to demonstrate 3D imaging datasets of the specimens, which were reformatted to create the same macroscopic appearances as histopathology on low magnification, light microscopy assessment. There were no additional structural features seen at histological assessment that were not visible on the micro-CT imaging. Direct radio-pathological comparisons between the micro-CT imaging and histopathological specimen appearances are provided in **Figures 1–5**, **Supplementary Video 1**. There were no cases of malignancy or cellular atypia in the specimens.

Surgeons were able to subjectively understand the Micro CT images more easily than the histopathology sections, and in combination they provided an excellent guide to interpreting complete surgical excision in these cases. Micro-CT also allowed for a 3D imaging "stack" to be stored in a digital format, which was particularly helpful for one of the cases (**Figure 3**, **Supplementary Video 1**) where the thyroglossal duct was not included in the pathological section but could be clearly delineated by reconstructing the micro-CT images.

Cellular appearances from high magnification, histopathological review (for ruling out cellular atypia or malignancy) were beyond the image resolution and magnification for the micro-CT imaging technology, however having a global overview of the specimen appearances allowed the pathologist to have a more informed approach when sectioning the specimens for subsequent histopathological assessment and for multidisciplinary discussions with the surgeons regarding completeness of the excision margins.

DISCUSSION

In this case series, we demonstrate the feasibility of micro-CT for imaging thyroglossal duct cyst specimens and reveal how high-resolution 3D imaging datasets can aid pathological dissection and demonstrate surgical excision, using histopathology results as a comparator/comparison.

The main advantages therefore conferred by using the micro-CT technique over traditional histopathological sectioning included the ability to review internal structures using multi-planar reconstruction and volume rendering tools without tissue destruction or sectioning. This was of particular relevance in this particular context because it helped to provide a detailed overview of the anatomical appearances of the thyroglossal duct, relationship to the hyoid bone and information on proximity of the duct to the surgical margins in a variety of planes. Post-excision recurrence is often attributed to the complex structure of the thyroglossal duct and incomplete excision of the arborised tract. Micro-CT enabled the pathologist to understand the optimal plane for tissue sectioning to display the key findings. The visualization of the micro-CT images, from a surgical perspective, were also subjectively easier to understand than those of the histopathology sections, and provided a useful adjunct in clinicians' interpretation of the cases.

To our knowledge, this is the first case series to explore the use of micro-CT imaging for pediatric thyroglossal duct specimens. Previous work has already discussed the benefits of this technique for other uses, such as for imaging excised whole organs [e.g., cardiac (19), brain (20)] as well as assessing cartilage rings in a pediatric case of tracheal stenosis (13). Micro-CT is becoming a more widely accepted tool for non-invasive post-mortem whole body fetal imaging (10, 12), as it allows internal visualization without surgical dissection. These studies have also demonstrated that iodine based micro-CT does not affect the histologic or immunohistochemical phenotype of normal tissues [skin biopsies and blood vessels (21) or diseased tissues, including cardiomyopathic cardiac tissue (22), cystic kidneys (23), and in neoplastic lesions of the heart (24), and brain (20)]. It has also been extensively used in mouse studies (25) and in human fetal autopsy (10) with subsequent histological examination, without reported alteration in subsequent tissue phenotype.

However, micro-CT availability is currently limited to specialist centres, and requires technological expertise for image acquisition and interpretation. It also cannot achieve imaging resolution to provide detailed cellular assessment, thus not replacing traditional histopathological assessment in its entirety. Through multi-disciplinary collaboration and comparison with histopathological sectioning, our centre has rapidly built experience in interpreting these radio-pathological appearances.

Micro-CT has the drawback of requiring exogenous contrast for surgical specimen imaging, necessitating a 72-h delay in our study. This was not an issue in this specific indication but could limit the usage of this technique where more urgent histopathology feedback is required. It is also currently unknown whether this iodination staining would affect more specialized pathology techniques (e.g., DNA extraction methods) downstream, if later required. For most thyroglossal duct cysts this may not be relevant but may impact the rare clinical situations where deposition of thyroid malignant tissue may be present within the excised cyst (26, 27). A recent study of micro-CT in thyroid cancer successfully evaluated capsular and vascular invasion and metastatic lymph node volume in

TABLE 1 | Patient demographics and clinical details.

Case	Age/Gender	Primary/Previous infections	Clinical and procedural details	Specimen size (cm)	Outcome
1	4 years, Female	Primary	18-month history of recurrent midline neck swelling. No previous infections or surgery. Extended Sistrunk's procedure performed.	3.0 × 0.6 × 1.0	Completely excised cystic tract, consistent with thyroglossal duct cyst. No atypia or malignancy.
2	5 years, Male	Primary	4-month history soft midline neck swelling. No previous infections or surgery. Extended Sistrunk's procedure performed.	3.5 × 2.5 × 1.5	Completely excised thyroglossal duct cyst. No atypia or malignancy.
3	6 years, Male	Previous infections with discharge through skin	Recurrent midline neck mass from 6 months of age. Multiple infections and discharge through skin. Overlying scarred skin excised during extended Sistrunk's procedure.	3.0 × 2.5 × 1.5	Completely excised thyroglossal duct cyst with overlying skin. No atypia or malignancy.
4	16 months, Female	Previous infections with discharge through skin	Recurrent midline neck swelling from 8 months of age. Multiple infections and discharge through skin. Overlying scarred skin excised during extended Sistrunk's procedure.	1.0 × 0.4 × 2.0	Completely excised thyroglossal duct remnant with overlying skin. No cyst identified. No atypia or malignancy.
5	14 months, Female	Previous infections with discharge through skin	6-year history of recurrent neck swelling right of midline with multiple infection. Small scar present. Overlying scarred skin excised during extended Sistrunk's procedure.	4.0 × 2.0 × 1.2	Completely excised thyroglossal duct remnant. No atypia or malignancy.

Case number assigned in chronological order by date of operative procedure. Patient age denotes the age at time of the operation.

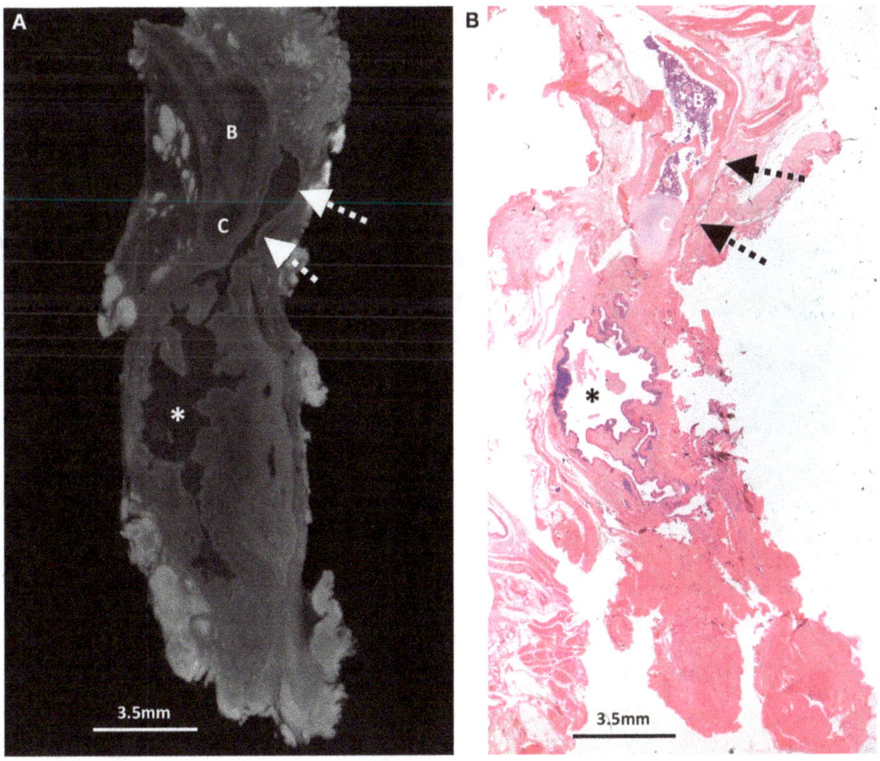

FIGURE 1 | Excised thyroglossal duct cyst specimen from a 4-year-old female patient (case 1). **(A)** Paired iodinated micro-CT imaging at 17.3 micron resolution and **(B)** histopathological section with H&E staining in sagittal section demonstrate the thick-walled thyroglossal duct cyst (*) and the thyroglossal duct (dashed arrows) anterior to the hyoid bone (B) and hyoid cartilage (C).

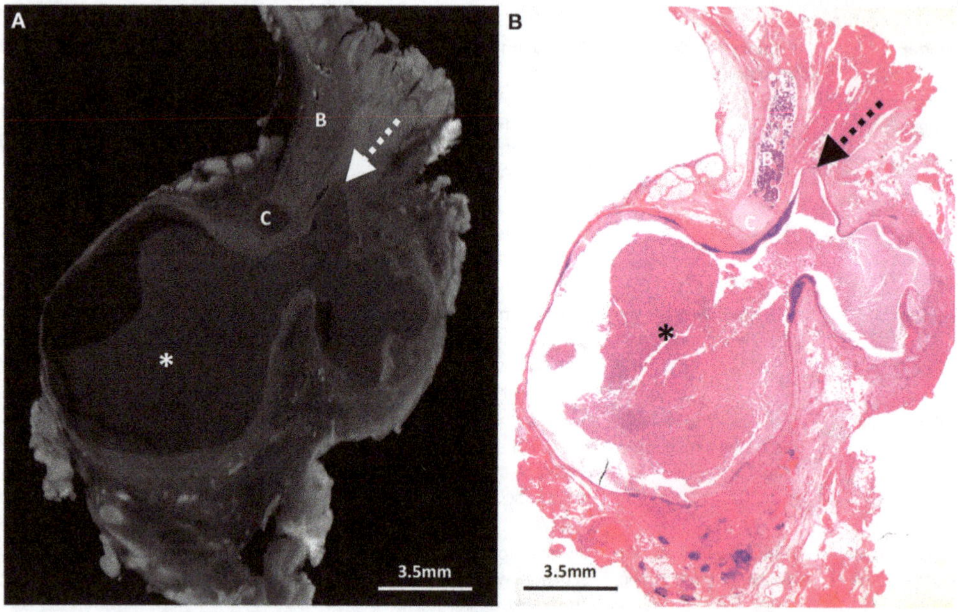

FIGURE 2 | Excised thyroglossal duct cyst specimen from a 5-year-old male patient (case 2). **(A)** Paired iodinated micro-CT imaging at 20.0 micron resolution and **(B)** histopathological section with H&E staining in sagittal section demonstrate a large bilobed thyroglossal duct cyst (*) with mixed internal contents containing blood and pus, leading to a blind ending thyroglossal duct (dashed arrows) anterior to the hyoid bone (B) and hyoid cartilage (C).

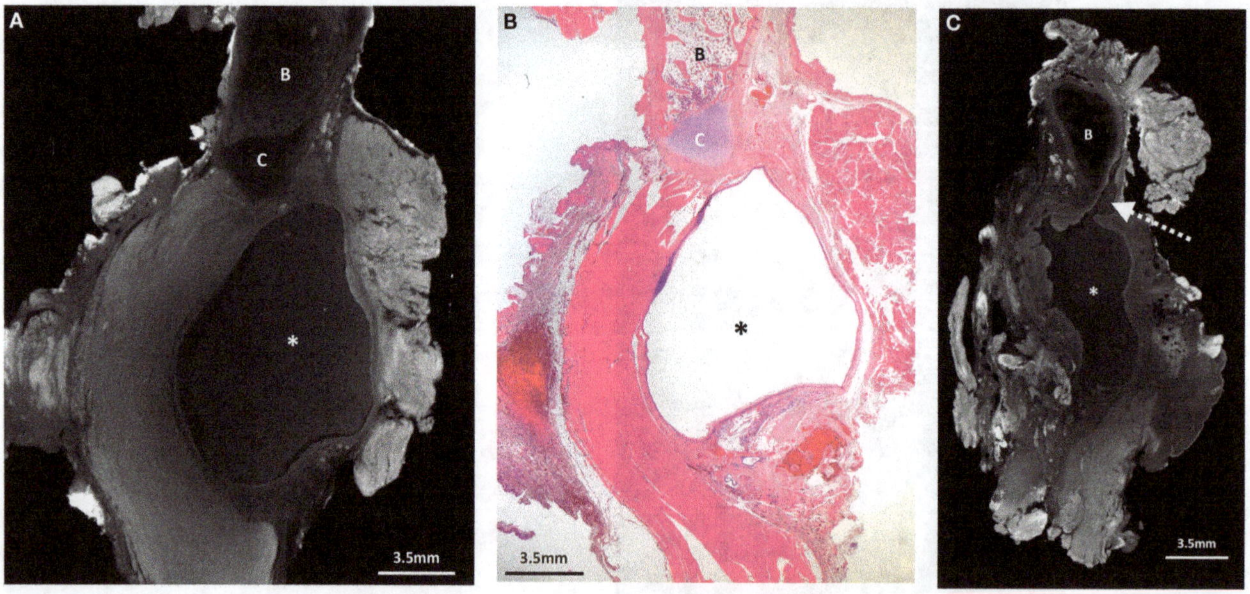

FIGURE 3 | Excised thyroglossal duct cyst specimen from a 6-year-old male patient (case 3). **(A)** Paired iodinated micro-CT imaging at 19.9 micron resolution, and **(B)** histopathological section with H&E staining in sagittal section demonstrate a well encapsulated thyroglossal duct cyst (*), just anterior to the hyoid cartilage (C). The hyoid bone is demonstrated by the "B." Although the thyroglossal duct was not present in the histopathological section, it was possible from the 3D imaging dataset to reconstruct the **(C)** sagittal viewing plane for better duct visualisation (dashed arrow).

specimens and was incorporated into pathology department workflow (28).

Limitations to our study include the small sample size and single centre design, although we have included a range of patient ages with varying clinical history including previously infected cysts, those which have been decompressed and primary surgical cases with an intact cyst. Pre-iodination contrast enhancement of our specimens could have caused a small amount of tissue shrinkage secondary to dehydration of the specimen [as previously reported (28)], and although we did not assess this in detail, no specimen degradation or significant impact on the histopathological diagnosis was found. Even at the highest

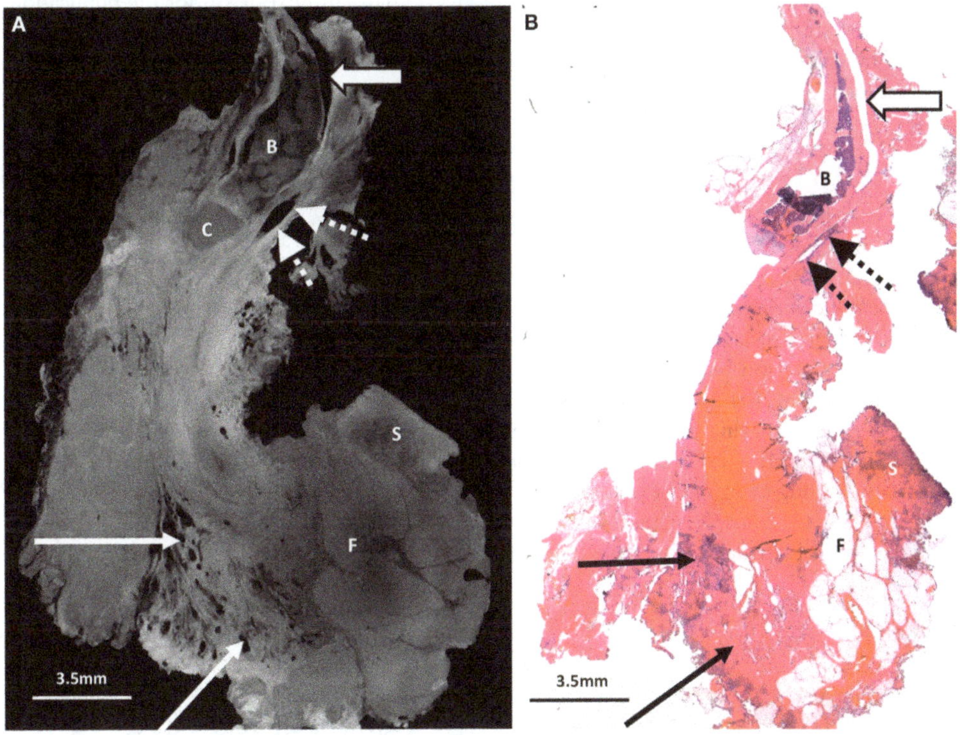

FIGURE 4 | Excised thyroglossal duct cyst specimen from a 16-month old female patient (case 4). **(A)** Paired iodinated micro-CT imaging at 14.2 micron resolution and **(B)** histopathological section with H&E staining demonstrate the thyroglossal duct (dashed arrows) anterior to the hyoid bone (B) and hyoid cartilage (C). An artefactual cleft is demonstrated with the open arrow. There is no cystic structure on this image. Some skin (S) and fatty tissue (F) from the neck was removed at surgery, and areas of chronic inflammation with tethering of the adjacent musculature and surrounding tissues (solid arrows) are shown.

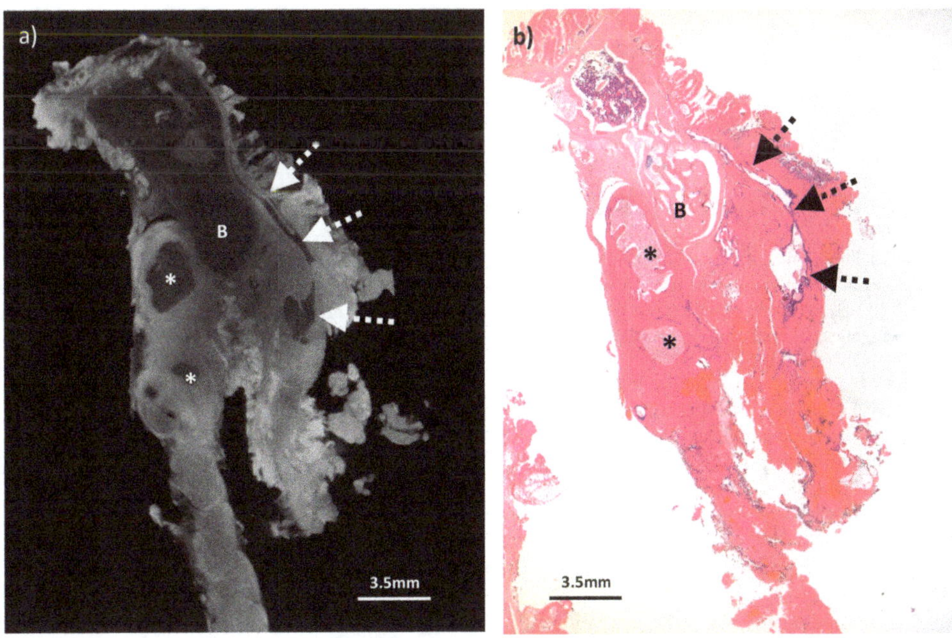

FIGURE 5 | Excised thyroglossal duct cyst specimen from a 14-year old female patient (case 5). **(a)** Paired iodinated micro-CT imaging at 22.2 micron resolution and **(b)** histopathological section with H&E staining demonstrate the thyroglossal duct (dashed arrows) anterior to the hyoid bone (B) with areas of cystic change (remnants) from a previously infected and ruptured cyst (*).

possible micro-CT image magnification, microscopic cellular detail was not possible. Future studies could investigate whether micro-CT imaging could be undertaken to a similar effect and quality across a larger case load.

CONCLUSION

In conclusion, we have shown the feasibility and utility of post-operative micro-CT imaging of thyroglossal duct cysts specimens, particularly in allowing for 3-D reconstruction in different planes without tissue destruction, and ability to store the specimen data in a digital format. It appears to be a helpful adjunct in specimen evaluation but does not currently replace histopathological assessment. Future work will focus on the generalizability of micro-CT imaging methods for other paediatric ENT specimens particularly those from the head and neck region where precisely defining margins of excision may be challenging (e.g., malignancies close to key structures) as well as investigating techniques to reduce time delays for tissue staining.

ETHICS STATEMENT

The studies involving human participants were reviewed and approved by the National Health Service (NHS) Health Research Authority (HRA) (Research Ethics Committee Reference 17/WS/0089, awarded April 2017; IRAS ID: 222334). All samples were handled in accordance with the Human Tissue Act 2004. Written informed consent to participate in this study was provided by the participants' legal guardian/next of kin. Written informed consent was obtained from the minor(s)' legal guardian/next of kin for the publication of any potentially identifiable images or data included in this article.

AUTHOR CONTRIBUTIONS

CF, SS, AH, CB, and IS contributed to conception and design of the study. CF wrote the first draft of the manuscript. SS, AH, CB, IS, JH, MA, and OA wrote sections of the manuscript. All authors contributed to manuscript revision, read, and approved the submitted version.

FUNDING

SS was supported by a RCUK/UKRI Innovation Fellowship and Medical Research Council (MRC) Clinical Research Training Fellowship (grant no. MR/R002118/1). This award was jointly funded by the Royal College of Radiologists (RCR). IS was funded by a National Institute for Health Research (NIHR) Clinical Doctoral Research Fellowship (ICA-CDRF-2017-03-53). OA was funded by an National Institute for Health Research (NIHR) Career Development Fellowship (NIHR-CDF-2017-10-037).

ACKNOWLEDGMENTS

This article presents independent research funded by the MRC, RCR, and NIHR, and the views expressed in this article are those of the authors and do not necessarily reflect the views of the NHS, MRC, RCR, NIHR, or the Department of Health, United Kingdom.

REFERENCES

1. Foley DS, Fallat ME. Thyroglossal duct and other congenital midline cervical anomalies. *Semin Pediatr Surg.* (2006) 15:70–5. doi: 10.1053/j.sempedsurg.2006.02.003
2. Allard RHB. The thyroglossal cyst. *Head Neck Surg.* (1982) 5:134–46. doi: 10.1002/hed.2890050209
3. Schlange H. Uber die fistula colli congentia. *Arch Kin Chir.* (1893) 46:390–2.
4. Sistrunk WE. The surgical treatment of cysts of the thyroglossal tract. *Ann Surg.* (1920) 71:121–2. doi: 10.1097/00000658-192002000-00002
5. Sistrunk WE. Technique of removal of cysts and sinuses of the thyroglossal duct. *Surg Gynecol Obstetr.* (1928) 46:109–12.
6. Galluzzi F, Pignataro L, Gaini RM, Hartley B, Garavello W. Risk of recurrence in children operated for thyroglossal duct cysts: a systematic review. *J Pediatr Surg.* (2013) 48:222–7. doi: 10.1016/j.jpedsurg.2012.10.060
7. Isaacson G. Sistrunk centennial: evolution of a classic operation. *Laryngoscope.* (2020) 130:E45–7. doi: 10.1002/lary.27914
8. Marianowski R, Amer JLA, Morisseau-Durand M-P, Manach Y, Rassi S. Risk factors for thyroglossal duct remnants after Sistrunk procedure in a pediatric population. *Int J Pediatr Otorhi.* (2003) 67:19–23. doi: 10.1016/s0165-5876(02)00287-2
9. Hutchinson JC, Shelmerdine SC, Simcock IC, Sebire NJ, Arthurs OJ. Early clinical applications for imaging at microscopic detail: microfocus computed tomography (micro-CT). *Br J Radiol.* (2017) 90:20170113. doi: 10.1259/bjr.20170113
10. Hutchinson JC, Kang X, Shelmerdine SC, Segers V, Lombardi CM, Cannie MM, et al. Postmortem microfocus computed tomography for early gestation fetuses: a validation study against conventional autopsy. *Am J Obstet Gynecol.* (2018) 218:445.e1–12. doi: 10.1016/j.ajog.2018.01.040
11. Shelmerdine SC, Hutchinson JC, Kang X, Suich JD, Ashworth M, Cannie MM, et al. Novel usage of microfocus computed tomography (micro-CT) for visualisation of human embryonic development—Implications for future non-invasive post-mortem investigation. *Prenatal Diag.* (2018) 38:538–42. doi: 10.1002/pd.5281
12. Shelmerdine SC, Simcock IC, Hutchinson JC, Guy A, Ashworth MT, Sebire NJ, et al. Postmortem microfocus computed tomography for noninvasive autopsies: experience in >250 human fetuses. *Am J Obstet Gynecol.* (2020) 224: 103.e1–15. doi: 10.1016/j.ajog.2020.07.019
13. Shelmerdine SC, Ashworth MT, Calder AD, Muthialu N, Arthurs OJ. Micro-CT of tracheal stenosis in trisomy 21. *Thorax.* (2019) 74:419. doi: 10.1136/thoraxjnl-2018-212966
14. Scott AE, Vasilescu DM, Seal KAD, Keyes SD, Mavrogordato MN, Hogg JC, et al. Three dimensional imaging of paraffin embedded human lung tissue samples by micro-computed tomography. *PLoS ONE.* (2015) 10:e0126230. doi: 10.1371/journal.pone.0126230
15. DiCorpo D, Tiwari A, Tang R, Griffin M, Aftreth O, Bautista P, et al. The role of Micro-CT in imaging breast cancer specimens. *Breast Cancer Res Treat.* (2020) 180:343–57. doi: 10.1007/s10549-020-05547-z
16. Shelmerdine SC, Simcock IC, Hutchinson JC, Aughwane R, Melbourne A, Nikitichev DI, et al. 3D printing from microfocus computed tomography (micro-CT) in human specimens: education and future implications. *Br J Radiol.* (2018) 91:20180306. doi: 10.1259/bjr.20180306

17. Ahmed J, Leong A, Jonas N, Grainger J, Hartley B. The extended Sistrunk procedure for the management of thyroglossal duct cysts in children: how we do it. *Clin Otolaryngol.* (2011) 36:271–5. doi: 10.1111/j.1749-4486.2011.02277.x
18. Agha RA, Sohrabi C, Mathew G, Franchi T, Kerwan A, O'Neill N, et al. The PROCESS 2020 guideline: updating consensus preferred reporting of case series in surgery (PROCESS) guidelines. *Int J Surg.* (2020) 84:231–5. doi: 10.1016/j.ijsu.2020.11.005
19. Hutchinson JC, Arthurs OJ, Ashworth MT, Ramsey AT, Mifsud W, Lombardi CM, et al. Clinical utility of postmortem microcomputed tomography of the fetal heart: diagnostic imaging vs. macroscopic dissection. *Ultrasound Obst Gyn.* (2016) 47:58–64. doi: 10.1002/uog.15764
20. Apps JR, Hutchinson JC, Arthurs OJ, Virasami A, Joshi A, Zeller-Plumhoff B, et al. Imaging Invasion: Micro-CT imaging of adamantinomatous craniopharyngioma highlights cell type specific spatial relationships of tissue invasion. *Acta Neuropathol Commun.* (2016) 4:57. doi: 10.1186/s40478-016-0321-8
21. Walton LA, Bradley RS, Withers PJ, Newton VL, Watson REB, Austin C, et al. Morphological characterisation of unstained and intact tissue micro-architecture by x-ray computed micro- and nano-tomography. *Sci Rep.* (2015) 5:10074. doi: 10.1038/srep10074
22. Matos JN, Garcia-Canadilla P, Simcock IC, Hutchinson JC, Dobromylskyj M, Guy A, et al. Micro-computed tomography (micro-CT) for the assessment of myocardial disarray, fibrosis and ventricular mass in a feline model of hypertrophic cardiomyopathy. *Sci Rep.* (2020) 10:20169. doi: 10.1038/s41598-020-76809-5
23. Hutchinson JC, Barrett H, Ramsey AT, Haig IG, Guy A, Sebire NJ, et al. Virtual pathological examination of the human fetal kidney using micro-CT. *Ultrasound Obst Gyn.* (2016) 48:663–5. doi: 10.1002/uog.15859
24. Hutchinson JC, Ashworth MT, Sebire NJ, Arthurs OJ. Multiple cardiac rhabdomyomas visualised using micro-CT in a case of tuberous sclerosis. *Fetal Diagn Ther.* (2017) 41:157–60. doi: 10.1159/000448708
25. Peltzer N, Darding M, Montinaro A, Draber P, Draberova H, Kupka S, et al. LUBAC is essential for embryogenesis by preventing cell death and enabling haematopoiesis. *Nature.* (2018) 557:112–7. doi: 10.1038/s41586-018-0064-8
26. Thompson LDR, Herrera HB, Lau SK. Thyroglossal duct cyst carcinomas: a clinicopathologic series of 22 cases with staging recommendations. *Head Neck Pathol.* (2017) 11:175–85. doi: 10.1007/s12105-016-0757-y
27. Kwon JK, Lee SM, Lee HM, Lee JC. Papillary thyroid carcinoma arising from a primary thyroglossal duct cyst with cervical node metastases. *Thyroid.* (2012) 22:330–1. doi: 10.1089/thy.2011.0283
28. Vickerton P, Jarvis J, Jeffery N. Concentration-dependent specimen shrinkage in iodine-enhanced microCT. *J Anat.* (2013) 223:185–93. doi: 10.1111/joa.12068

17

Midterm Outcomes of Cross-Linked Acellular Bovine Jugular Vein Conduit for Right Ventricular Outflow Tract Reconstruction

Tao Qian [1,2], Zhong-Shi Wu [1,2], Jian-Guo Hu [1], Yi-Feng Yang [1], Qin Wu [1], Ting Lu [1,2], Can Huang [1,2] and Jia Li [3,4*]*

[1] Department of Cardiovascular Surgery, The Second Xiangya Hospital, Central South University, Changsha, China, [2] Engineering Laboratory of Hunan Province for Cardiovascular Biomaterials, Changsha, China, [3] Clinical Physiology Laboratory, Guangzhou Women and Children's Medical Center, Institute of Pediatrics, Guangzhou Medical University, Guangzhou, China, [4] Guangdong Provincial Key Laboratory of Research in Structural Birth Defect Disease, Guangzhou Women and Children's Medical Center, Guangzhou Medical University, Guangzhou, China

***Correspondence:**
Zhong-Shi Wu
owenzswu@csu.edu.cn
Jia Li
jiali_beijing@126.com

Objectives: Conduits for reconstructing right ventricular outflow tract (RVOT) in children with congenital heart disease have evolved for better durability over the past decades, but conduits failure remains common. We designed decellularized and photooxidatively crosslinked bovine jugular vein conduit (DP-BJVC) and now aim to evaluate the midterm results of DP-BJVC for RVOT reconstruction.

Methods: Ninety patients (median age: 4.2 years) undergoing RVOT reconstruction using DP-BJVC were prospectively followed for median of 4.7 years (range: 0.2–16.1 years). Kaplan–Meier analysis was used to examine the survival, freedom from conduit explantation and catheter-based reintervention. Risk factors were analyzed with Cox regression analysis.

Results: Follow-up was completed in 92% of patients. There were five (5.6%) early deaths. The 10-year survival rate was 85.2%, with palliative procedure at DP-BJVC implantation as the risk factor. The 10-year freedom from conduit explantation and reintervention were 84.4 and 67.3% respectively, with previous cardiac operation as the only risk factor for explantation. Complications during the follow-up included conduit stenosis (peak gradient $\geq$50 mmHg) in 12 (12.9%), severe regurgitation in 2 (2.4%), and infective endocarditis in 2 (2.4%). The annual increase in gradient was highest in the first year ($P = 0.003$), but not appreciably afterwards. The echo-measured annulus diameter trends to increase by an average of 0.37 mm per year. Calcification appeared mild in the failed conduits.

Conclusions: DP-BJVC provides satisfactory durability and functionality for RVOT reconstruction for children, with low morbidity of stenosis and endocarditis, as well as increase in diameter mildly with age in midterm follow-ups.

Keywords: bovine jugular vein conduit, decellularized and photooxidatively crosslink, right ventricular outflow tract reconstruction, congenital heart disease, outcomes

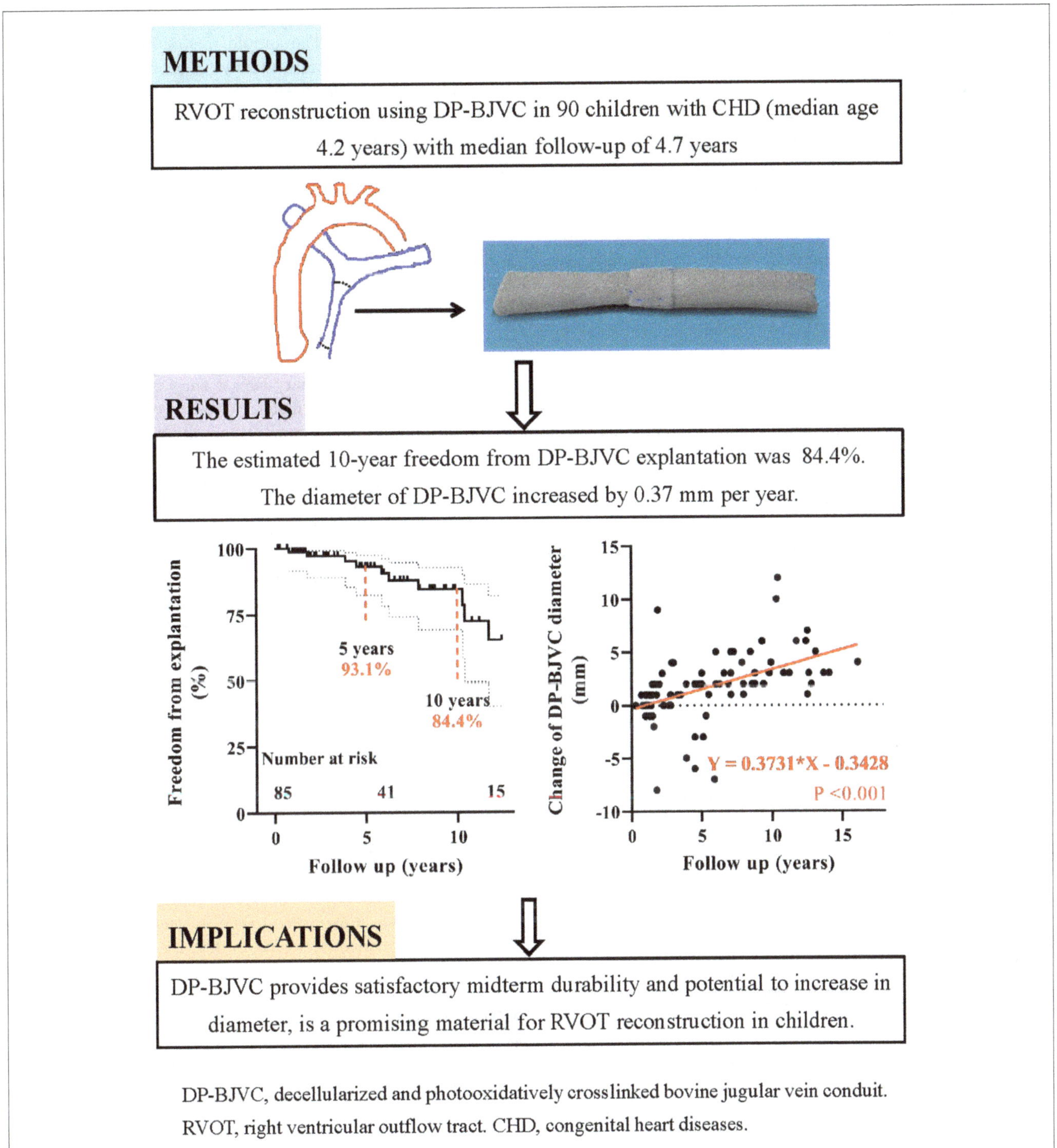

Graphical Abstract | Midterm performance of DP-BJVC for RVOT reconstruction in 90 patients with median follow-up of 4.7 years showed good durability and the potential to increase in diameter.

INTRODUCTION

The surgical reconstruction of right ventricular outflow tract (RVOT) with valved conduit remains a common cardiac procedure for patients with congenital heart diseases (CHD) (1). However, explantation remains common for the currently available conduits, thus improving the durability of RVOT conduits in young children remains a challenge. Younger age at implantation was the leading adverse factor of the valved conduits failure (2–4), mainly as the result of fast somatic growth.

The durability of RVOT conduit in young children remains to be improved yet challenging.

Historically, cryopreserved pulmonary homograft was the "gold standard" from the mid-1980s through the late 1990s. Due to concerns of limited durability, availability and costs of homografts, attention has turned to xenograft and artificial material as alternatives. The Contegra conduit (Medtronic Inc., Minneapolis, Minnesota, USA), a glutaraldehyde-treated bovine jugular vein conduit (BJVC) developed in 1990s, is one of the most successful alternates. It makes up the shortage of homograft and costs less. Its hemodynamic performance and durability have been found comparable to homograft (5–8). Nonetheless, <25% of infants receiving the glutaraldehyde-treated BJVC were free from replacement at 10 years (4, 5, 9). The glutaraldehyde brings unpredictable cytotoxicity and possibility of early calcification (10). Moreover, the graft-related immune response induced by residual donor cells and cell debris plays an important role in the failure of glutaraldehyde-treated xenografts (11). The latter factor may be avoided by decellularization, which has been adopted in cardiovascular biomaterials over 30 years (12). The decellularized homografts have significantly improved functionality compared with standard cryopreserved homograft used for RVOT reconstruction (13). Recently, the Japanese approach of hand-sewn expanded polytetrafluoroethylene (ePTFE) valved conduit has attracted attention, with satisfactory long-term outcomes from Japanese multi-center studies (14). But its application was limited largely within Japan by the inconsistent quality control of hand-sewn valve until recent years.

Our team started working on the non-glutaraldehyde-treatment of BJVC combined with decellularization and photooxidatively crosslinking (DP-BJVC) since 2002 (15). We hypothesized that DP-BJVC prevents the immunogenicity from xenogeneic cells and avoids the toxic effects of glutaraldehyde. In a series of animal experiments in rats or dogs, DP-BJVC was shown to have favorable biocompatibility and tissue structure stability, and greater calcification resistance than glutaraldehyde-treated BJVC (16, 17). In the past 16 years, DP-BJVC has been used clinically in our center. The aim of this study was to evaluate the outcomes of our cohort.

PATIENTS AND METHODS

Patients

After approved by the Institutional Ethics Committee (reference number: LYF2004011) and written informed consent obtained from patients or their guardians, 122 patients were prospectively enrolled for DP-BJVC implantation. The study protocol was also approved (reference number: LYF2020097). Among 122 patients, 32 were excluded from this study. Two patients underwent superior vena cava reconstruction using DP-BJVC, and 30 received DP-BJVC implantation in the form of valved patch.

DP-BJVC Preparation

The conduit was prepared with the multi-step detergent-enzymatic decellularization and dye-mediated photooxidation procedures as previously reported (16, 17). The DP-BJVC (Yaxin Medical Technology Co., Ltd., Wuhan, Hubei, China.) consists of natural tri-leaflet valve with size ranging from 12 to 20 mm with 1 mm as spacing. The annulus restraining device located at the level of valve annulus mainly fixed on the outer wall of the conduit, was made to enhance the conduit stability since 2013. The device was a rectangular Dacron patch wrapped loosely around the conduit, and gently held together circumferentially by several 6-0 Prolene sutures (Ethicon, Inc., Somerville, New Jersey, USA).

Surgical Techniques

Written informed consent was obtained from parents or guardians before surgery. Conduit size was determined by age and the body surface area and converted to z-score. A conduit with z-score over +1 was preferred up to 20 mm of the conduit diameter.

Standard cardiopulmonary bypass surgical procedures were performed. Intra-cardiac malformations were corrected. The end-to-end distal anastomosis was made away from the pulmonary artery bifurcation and leaving about 5 mm conduit above the valve. When the left pulmonary artery (LPA) and/or right pulmonary artery (RPA) were hypoplasia, extra bovine jugular vein patch was used for angioplasty before the implantation of DP-BJVC. Following the distal anastomosis, probes were used to measure the dimension of anastomosis and orifices of LPA and RPA. Next, the proximal orifice of DP-BJVC was anastomosed to the right ventricular infundibulum. All anastomoses were sutured continuously with single 6-0 or 5-0 Prolene suture.

Before discontinuation of cardiopulmonary bypass, transesophageal echocardiogram was performed to assess the hemodynamics of the neo-pulmonary arterial trunk. Before chest closure, the GORE® Pericardial Membrane (W.L. Gore and Associates, Arizona, USA) was used to keep the conduit and right atrium from adhering to the sternum in order to reduce the potential risks in any future sternotomy.

Postoperatively, antibiotics covering gram-negative and gram-positive bacteria were used for 3 days and then adjusted according to clinical assessment. The International Normalized Ratio was maintained between 1.6 and 2.0 with warfarin for 6 months.

Follow-Ups

Follow-ups were made via clinic visits at the 1, 6, 12 months after operation and then annually, including physical examination, transthoracic echocardiography, and cardiac MRI or CT when appropriate. Last follow-up was completed between January to June, 2020. Echocardiography was performed to measure conduit diameter at the level of annulus and hemodynamics. The peak gradient across the conduit (PG) was the sum pressure gradients at the proximal, valvular, and distal levels. Conduit stenosis was defined as PG ≥50 mmHg (18). Conduit valve regurgitation was graded as none, trivial, mild, moderate and severe mainly according to the strength and size of the regurgitant jet (19). Patients with conduit stenosis or over moderate regurgitation received catheter based reintervention or surgical replacement.

The primary outcomes included patient death, conduit reintervention, and conduit explantation. Early mortality was defined as death within 30 postoperative days. The time from the date of the conduit implantation to the date of the conduit replacement or the last follow-up was defined as the time of freedom from conduit explantation. The time from the date of the conduit implantation to the date of first catheter-based reintervention or the last follow-up was defined as the time of freedom from reintervention.

Other demographic and clinical variables were collected, including gender, age, weight, height, diagnosis of CHD, diameter and z-score of the conduit, preoperative SpO_2, previous cardiac corrective or palliative procedures, LPA and/or RPA angioplasty, cardiopulmonary bypass time and aortic cross clamp time.

Statistical Analysis

Data were described as mean ± SD, median (range) or frequency (%) when appropriate. Early deaths were censored for analysis of freedom from conduit explantation and reintervention and the associated factors. The Kaplan-Meier method was used to estimate the survival, freedom from conduit explantation, and freedom from conduit first reintervention which was further compared between groups using Log-rank (Mantel-Cox) test. Stepwise forward Cox multivariable analyses were performed to assess the risk factors for mortality, conduit explantation, and conduit reintervention. Variables were retained when $P < 0.10$. Results were reported as corresponding hazard ratios (HR) with 95% confidence intervals (CI). The PG across the conduit in different follow-up time were compared using mixed-effects analysis with the Geisser-Greenhouse correction and Sidak's multiple comparisons test for *post-hoc* analysis. Spearman correlation coefficient was used to analyze the correlations between the change of conduit diameter (defined as the diameter of pulmonary artery measured at the latest echocardiography minus that at implantation) and hemodynamics. $P < 0.05$ was considered significant. Data analysis was performed using IBM SPSS Statistics 23.0 (SPSS Inc., Chicago, Illinois, USA) and GraphPad Prism 8.0 software (GraphPad Software, San Diego, California, USA).

RESULTS

Demographics and Operative Data

Ninety patients (median age: 4.2 years, range: 0.2–20.0) were enrolled in this study, including 35 (38.9%) patients ≤3 years old. Detailed demographic data, diagnosis of CHD, previous cardiac operations and operative data of RVOT reconstruction using DP-BJVC are presented in **Table 1**. Fourteen (15.6%) patients underwent DP-BJVC implantation as part of palliative operation, including VSD closure and pulmonary artery reconstruction (classic repair) for patients with congenitally corrected transposition of the great arteries ($n = 4$), operation with Glenn shunt ($n = 3$) or without taking-down of previous Glenn shunt ($n = 2$), and operation without closure of ventricular septal defect ($n = 5$).

The distribution of DP-BJVC size with age is shown in **Figure 1A**. The conduit diameter ranged from 12 to 20 mm (median 16), with mean z-score of +1.95. The conduit z-score trended to be lower with older age (**Figure 1B**). Specifically, four

TABLE 1 | Demographic and operative data of the cohort using DP-BJVC.

Variables	$n = 90$
Demographics	
Age (years)	4.2 (0.2–20.0)
Gender (male: female)	48:42
Height (cm)	95.5 (55–172)
Weight (kg)	13.3 (3.5–51.0)
Body surface area (m^2)	0.58 (0.23–1.56)
McGoon ratio	1.7 (1.0–3.3)
Preoperative SpO_2 (%)	82 (34–98)
Anatomic diagnoses	
PA/VSD	41 (45.6%)
DORV/PS or DORV/PA	12 (13.3%)
AV diseases	11 (12.2%)
Truncus arteriosus	7 (7.8%)
TGA/PS or TGA/PA	6 (6.7%)
ccTGA/PS or ccTGA/PA	5 (5.6%)
PR with repaired TOF	5 (5.6%)
TOF/APV	2 (2.2%)
MV diseases	1 (1.1%)
Previous cardiac operations	
Systemic-to-pulmonary shunt	13 (14.4%)
TOF repair	5 (5.6%)
Bidirectional Glenn shunt	3 (3.3%)
SAV	2 (2.2%)
PDA stenting	2 (2.2%)
Intraoperative characteristics	
Cardiopulmonary bypass time (min)	173 (72–563)
Aortic cross-clamp time (min)	92 (0–239)
DP-BJVC diameter (mm)	16 (12–20)
DP-BJVC z-score	1.95 ± 0.11
Reinforced conduit	52 (57.8%)
Major combined procedures	
LPA angioplasty	16 (17.8%)
RPA angioplasty	6 (6.7%)
ncVSD management	8 (8.9%)
ECMO	5 (5.6%)

AV, aortic valve; ccTGA, corrected transposition of the great arteries; DORV/PS, double-outlet right ventricle with pulmonary stenosis; ECMO, extracorporeal membrane oxygenation; LPA, left pulmonary artery; ncVSD, non-committed ventricular septal defect; PA/VSD, pulmonary atresia with ventricular septal defect; PR, pulmonary regurgitation; PDA, patent ductus arteriosus; RPA, right pulmonary artery; SAV, surgical aortic valvoplasty; TOF, tetralogy of Fallot; TOF/APV, TOF with absent pulmonary valve; TGA, transposition of the great arteries.

(11.4%) patients ≤3 years old and 42 (76.4%) aged 3 to 20 years received a conduit with z-score < +2.

Follow-Up Results

Follow-up was completed in 83 (92%) patients. In the remaining seven (8%) patients, follow-up was lost at 1 ($n = 3$), 5 ($n = 2$), 6 ($n = 1$) and 8 ($n = 1$) years after DP-BJVC implantation. The duration of follow-up ranged 0.2 to 16.1 years (median 4.7).

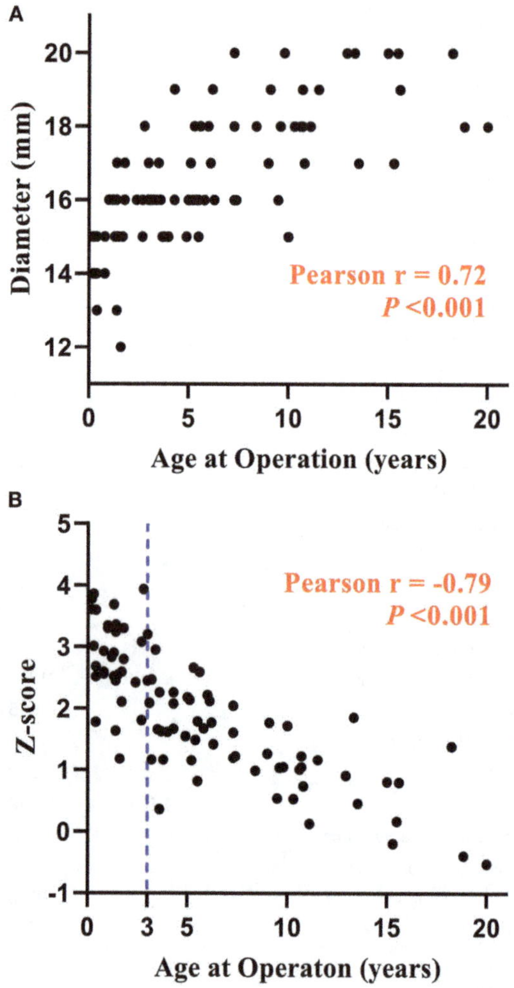

FIGURE 1 | Distribution of the diameter **(A)** and z-score **(B)** of DP-BJVC at implantation. The conduit diameter (range from 12 to 20 mm) is significant positive corrected with patients' age (*P* <0.001), while the conduit z-score is significant negative corrected with patients' age (*P* <0.001). Particularly, four patients ≤3 years, as well as most of the older patients, received a conduit with z-score < +2.

Mortality

There were five (5.6%) early deaths and five (5.6%) late deaths (**Table 2**) due to cardiac, pulmonary or cerebral events, and none from any DP-BJVC complications. One late death occurred on 65th days after operation while staying in the hospital, making the in-hospital mortality 6.7%. The Kaplan-Meier estimated overall survival was 89.1 and 85.2% at 5 and 10 years, respectively, for the entire cohort (**Figure 2A**). It was 91.4 and 81.3%, respectively, at 5 and 10 years in children ≤ 3 years old, similar to the older patients (87.4% both at 5 and 10 years) (P = 0.970, **Figure 2B**). Palliative procedure at the DP-BJVC implantation was the only risk factor for overall mortality both on univariate analysis (P = 0.028, **Supplementary Tables 1, 2**) and multivariate analysis (HR: 3.64, 95% CI: 1.03-12.93, P = 0.045).

Explantation

Ten patients required DP-BJVC explantation at median of 6.1 years (range: 0.8 to 11.7) follow-up, including four (40%) with previous shunt operations (**Table 3**). The indications for explantation included conduit stenosis in five patients, among whom it was the distal anastomotic level in four and the middle of the conduit due to sternal compression in one; conduit aneurysmal dilatation with severe regurgitation in two patients and moderate regurgitation in 1, all being over 10 years after implantation without the annulus restraining device; infective endocarditis in two patients, with one at 2 months after catheter-based intervention resulting in severe regurgitation and the other with conduit valvular stenosis. **Supplementary Figure 1** showed three examples of the failed DP-BJVCs with mild calcification and degeneration that was easily handled with tissue scissors.

The Kaplan-Meier estimated freedom from conduit explantation was 93.1 and 84.4% at 5 and 10 years, respectively, for the entire cohort (**Figure 2C**). It was 94.7% at 5 and 10 years in children ≤ 3 years old, similar to the older patients (91.9% at 5 years and 78.1% at 10 years) (P = 0.264, **Figure 2D**). On univariable analysis, lower preoperative SpO_2 (P = 0.032) and previous cardiac operation (P = 0.018) were significantly associated with explantation (**Supplementary Tables 1, 2**). On multivariate analysis, previous cardiac operation was the only significant risk factor for conduit explantation(HR: 6.31, 95% CI: 1.12–35.66, P = 0.037).

Reintervention

Fifteen (16.7%) patients required 18 catheter-based reintervention during the follow-ups, including 16 (89%) balloon dilations, 7 for LPA, 6 for distal anastomosis, 2 for RPA, and 1 for conduit valve; and 2 (11%) stent placements in LPA.

The first reintervention occurs at median of 4.1 years (range: 0.8 to 10.5) follow-up. The Kaplan–Meier estimated freedom from first reintervention was 83.4 and 67.3% at 5 and 10 years respectively (**Figure 2E**). It was 78.3 and 52.9%, respectively, at 5 and 10 years in children ≤3 years old, which was not significantly different compared to older patients (87.0% at 5 years and 75.1% at 10 years) (P = 0.076, **Figure 2F**). On univariate analysis, PG before discharge (P = 0.008), previous cardiac operation (P = 0.091) and non-Ross operation (P = 0.084) were associated with increased reintervention rate (**Supplementary Tables 1, 2**). None of these were significant on multivariate analysis.

Conduit Hemodynamics

Before hospital discharge after the initial implantation, the median PG across the conduit was 23.0 mmHg (range: 2.0 to 40.0 mmHg). It became significantly higher during follow-ups (P < 0.001). The annual increase in PG was highest in the first postoperative year (P = 0.003), but without any significant annual difference in the subsequent consecutive year-to-year comparisons (Ps >0.30, **Figure 3A** and **Supplementary Figure 2**).

Eleven (12.9%) patients had conduit stenosis during follow-up with median PG of 68.0 mmHg (ranging 52.0 to 92.0), including 8 at the distal anastomosis level, 2 at the valvular level, and 1 at the middle of the conduit. Six of them were alleviated by

TABLE 2 | Operative data and the main causes for the early and late deaths ($n = 10$).

	Age (years)	Diagnosis	Surgical strategy*	Conduit's hemodynamics			Survival time	Cause of death
				Post-op. time**	PG (mmHg)	PR		
Early deaths								
Case 1	3.0	Truncus arteriosus	Rastelli	1 day	12	Trivial	2 days	Pulmonary hypertension crisis
Case 2	10.7	IE/AVS	Ross	1 day	8	None	9 days	Intracranial hemorrhage
Case 3	6.3	PA/VSD	Rastelli	1 day	10	None	11 days	LCOS
			ECMO					Multiple organs failure
Case 4	3.6	PA/VSD	RVOT reconstruction	10 day	26	Trivial	14 days	LCOS
			LPA angioplasty					
Case 5	7.3	AVS	Ross	20 days	6	None	24 days	Right heart failure
		Post- SAV	CABG (RCA)					LCOS
			Glenn shunt					
			ECMO					
Late deaths								
Case 6	1.4	DORV/PA	RVOT reconstruction	1 month	23	None	65 days	Sepsis
		Post-PDA stenting						Choking and asphyxia
								Intracranial hemorrhage after CPR
Case 7	0.3	PA/VSD	Rastelli	3 months	12	None	4 months	Choking and asphyxia
Case 8	10.3	ccTGA/PS	Senning	1 year	21	Trivial	13 months	Heart failure
			Rastelli					
Case 9	5.1	DORV/PS	Rastelli	4 years	8	Trivial	4.5 years	Sudden death (unknown reason)
Case 10	1.3	PA/VSD	RVOT reconstruction	7 years	18	Mild	8.5 years	Heart failure

AVS, aortic valve stenosis; CPR, cardiopulmonary resuscitation; CABG, coronary artery bypass grafting; ccTGA/PS, corrected transposition of the great arteries with pulmonary stenosis; DORV/PA, double-outlet right ventricle with pulmonary atresia; DORV/PS, double-outlet right ventricle with pulmonary stenosis; ECMO, extracorporeal membrane oxygenation; IE, infective endocarditis; LPA, left pulmonary artery; LCOS, low cardiac output syndrome; PG, peak gradient (across the conduit); PR, pulmonary regurgitation; PA/VSD, pulmonary atresia with ventricular septal defect; PDA, patent ductus arteriosus; RVOT, right ventricular outflow tract; RCA, right coronary artery; SAV, surgical aortic valvoplasty; VSD, ventricular septal defect.

**Rastelli operation, including all Rastelli-type operations for patients with Truncus arteriosus, PA/VSD, and DORV/PS et al.*

***Post-op. time, means the time from the date of operation to the date of last echocardiography examination.*

balloon dilation, and 5 ultimately received conduit explantation as described above.

Before hospital discharge, conduit valve regurgitation was described as trivial in 27 patients and none in the remaining. Conduit regurgitation measured at the last echocardiography was graded as trivial in 48 patients, mild in 6, moderate in 3, severe in 2, and none in the remaining. Both the two patients with severe regurgitation received conduit explantation as described above.

No serious thrombotic events were found during follow-up. **Supplementary Figures 3, 4** provided the follow-up echocardiography, CT, and MRI examples for DP-BJVC, and the example of aneurysmal dilatation.

Change in Conduit Diameter

The overall change of conduit diameter significantly and positively correlated with follow-up time ($P < 0.001$), with regression coefficient of 0.37 (**Figure 3B**). The change of conduit diameter did not significantly correlate with the change of PG (defined as the PG measured at the last echocardiography minus that before discharge. $P = 0.940$), or the change of regurgitation grade (defined as the grade of regurgitation measured at the last echocardiography minus that before discharge. $P = 0.680$). The diameter change of reinforced conduit has similar regression coefficient with the non-reinforced conduit ($P = 0.806$. **Supplementary Figure 5**). Of note, four conduits had a diameter decrease over 5 mm after implantation (marked by arrows in **Figure 3B**) due to stenosis mainly at the distal anastomosis, which had been replaced (case 2 to 5 in **Table 3**).

DISCUSSION

We examined the midterm outcomes of our novel designed DP-BJVC for RVOT reconstruction in children with CHD (**Graphical Abstract**). The overall survival rate was 85.2% at 10 years. The 10-year freedom from conduit explantation and reintervention was 84.4 and 67.3%, respectively. These figures were largely comparable between children ≤ 3 years old and the older patients.

The early mortality in our cohort was 5.6%, which was higher compared to previous reports up to 4.1% (3, 4, 20). This reflects the developing course in our center. Two of them received the Ross operation that was being implemented as learning curve. The other three deaths were due to the much older age at operation resulting in poorer cardiac and pulmonary vascular function. Indeed, the age at operation in children with CHD is generally older in our cohort (**Table 1**), representing the current situation in China and other developing countries.

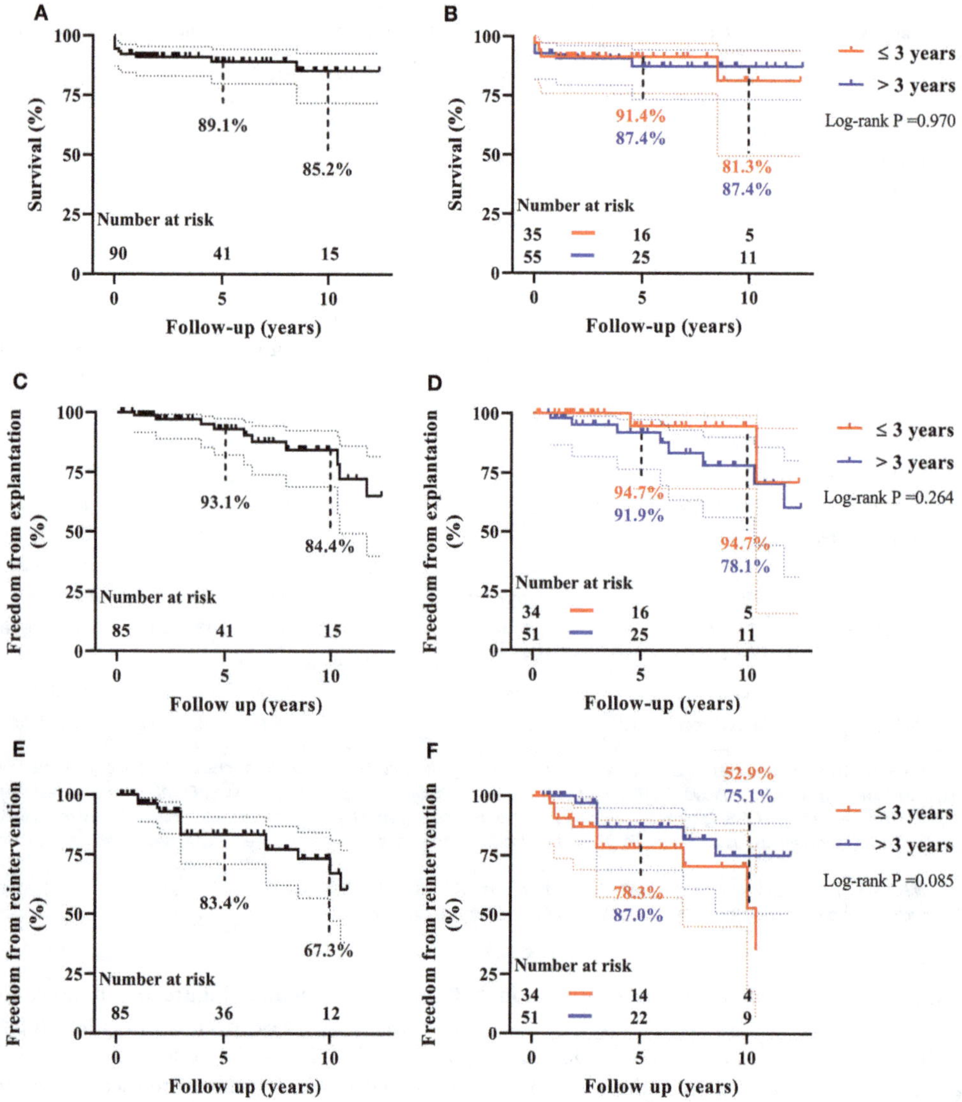

FIGURE 2 | The Kaplan–Meier estimates of overall survival, freedom from DP-BJVC explantation, and freedom from first catheter-based reintervention for the entire cohort are shown in **(A)**, **(C)**, and **(E)**, respectively. The comparisons of these estimated values between children ≤3 years and older patients are shown in **(B)**, **(D)**, and **(F)**, respectively. Dashed lines represent 95% CIs. In summary, the performance of DP-BJVC in young children (≤3 years) is similar with that in larger patients.

Nonetheless, midterm survival of our cohort is comparable to previous reports on RVOT reconstruction in children with CHD (3, 4, 9, 20). The significant risk factor for overall mortality was palliative procedures, which are usually associated with more complex structural deformities and un-physiological postoperative hemodynamics.

The notion for us to design DP-BJVC included the followings: (1) It is a cell-free xenogeneic scaffold, thus preventing the immunogenicity from donor cells (21); (2) It is a non-glutaraldehyde-treated BJVC, thus avoiding the toxic effects of glutaraldehyde (11); (3) the structure and composition of the extracellular matrix are preserved by photooxidation and its effective crosslink with the collagen proteins (22). The hypothesized advantages were demonstrated in a series of experimental studies *in vitro* and *in vivo* by our team (15–17, 23, 24). The tissue structure of DP-BJVC was stable after 12-week subcutaneous implantation in rats, with all-layer host cells repopulation and neo-capillaries formation (16). The conduit showed good valvular function without calcification after 6-month implantation in dogs, with the host cells infiltrated and migrated from outer layer to the middle layer of the conduits' walls (17).

These advantages are further demonstrated in the present cohort. The midterm durability of DP-BJVC is satisfactory and comparable with that of glutaraldehyde-treated BJVC, in which the 10-year freedom rate from replacement ranged from 59 to 90% (4, 7, 20, 25). Previous cardiac operation was the only risk factor for conduit explantation as most of those procedures

TABLE 3 | Operative data and the causes for explantations ($n = 10$).

	Age (y)	Diagnosis	Surgical strategy	Conduit diameter (mm)	Conduit durability (years)	Causes of failure	Replacement material
Case 1	15.0	PR Post TOF repair	RVOT reconstruction	20	0.8	IE PS (valvular)	Homograft
Case 2	9.8	AVS Post SAV	Ross	20	1.8	PS (distal)	ePTFE conduit*
Case 3	9.5	Truncus arteriosus	Truncus repair	16	3.9	PS (distal) PR	DP-BJV patch**
Case 4	2.7	PA/VSD Post B-T shunt	Rastelli	15	4.5	IE PR	ePTFE conduit
Case 5	9.1	DORV/PA/ncVSD Post B-T shunt	Rastelli (intra-ventricular conduit***)	19	5.9	PS (distal)	DP-BJVC
Case 6	13.5	PA/VSD Post Melb. shunt	Rastelli	17	6.3	PS (distal) PR	DP-BJVC
Case 7	5.2	TGA/PS/VSD	Rastelli Glenn shunt	16	7.9	PS (middle)	DP-BJVC
Case 8	3.5	Truncus arteriosus	Truncus repair	17	10.3	PR Aneurysmal dilatation	DP-BJVC
Case 9	0.4	TGA/PA/VSD Post B-T shunt	Rastelli	14	10.4	PR Aneurysmal dilatation	DP-BJVC
Case 10	3.2	TOF/APV	TOF repair	16	11.7	PR Aneurysmal dilatation	DP-BJVC

DORV/PA, double-outlet right ventricle with pulmonary atresia; ePTFE, expanded polytetrafluoroethylene; IE, infective endocarditis; ncVSD, non-committed ventricular septal defect; PR, pulmonary regurgitation; PS, pulmonary stenosis; PA/VSD, pulmonary atresia with ventricular septal defect; RVOT, right ventricular outflow tract; TGA/PA, transposition of the great arteries with pulmonary atresia; TOF/APV, tetralogy of Fallot with absent of pulmonary valve.

**ePTFE conduit, Gore-Tex vessel (W.L. Gore and Associates, Arizona, USA) equipped with hand-sewn 0.1 mm thick ePTFE valve.*

***DP-BJV patch, valved decellularized-and-photooxidated bovine jugular vein patch.*

****Intra-ventricular conduit repair of DORV/ncVSD previous reported by our team (1).*

were for pulmonary vascular dysplasia, which limits the size of distal anastomosis with heavier afterload for the conduit. More importantly, DP-BJVC appeared to do equally well in younger children, that is, ≤3 years old, which is, in other words, better than previously reported cohorts. Younger age has been identified as the independent risk factor for conduit failure (2–4). The Congenital Heart Surgeons Society in 2006 year reported that 58% of children ≤2 years old required reintervention within 3 years of implantation using glutaraldehyde-treated BJVC for RVOT reconstruction (26). Another single-center reports by Ugaki et al. demonstrated the 10-years freedom from BJVC replacement rate of 37.1%, with age <3 years as an independent risk factor (27).

Several factors may be attributable to the good durability of DP-BJVC for younger children. Firstly, the conduits used for young children were greater in z-score than that for older patients (**Figure 1B**). Secondly, DP-BJVC showed an increase in diameter with age, that is, conduit dilatation probably resulted from calcification resistance as non-glutaraldehyde treated (24). We found that calcification in the failed DP-BJVC was mild and could be easily handled. The degree of dilatation is further refined by the flexible Dacron restraining device. All the 3 conduits developed aneurysmal dilatation and valvular regurgitation were implanted before 2013 without such device.

The PG across the DP-BJVC increased over time although only reaching statistical significance in the first year. This may be attributable to fairly fast somatic growth in young children. Additionally, the short-term anticoagulant therapy postoperatively might be helpful to reduce the subclinical conduit thrombosis (18). BJVC-related distal anastomotic stenosis has been reported as one of the main reasons for conduit failure. There were eight (9.4%) patients with distal anastomotic stenosis (PG ranged ≥50 mmHg) during the entire follow-up of our study, which trended to be less than that using glutaraldehyde-treated BJVC, with reported incidence range 13.5 to 22.0% (3, 7, 18). This finding may be as a result of better biocompatibility with lower inherent immunogenicity (16, 28). In contrast, the glutaraldehyde-treatment has been reported as a contributor to the formation of neo-intimal peeling at the distal anastomosis (18, 29).

Late infective endocarditis is a particular concern for BJVC (25). In a systematic review involving 840 patients from 55 studies using Contegra conduits, the pooled incidences of endocarditis was 7.1% during follow-up period ranging 9 to106 months (30). Furthermore, the infection usually occurred late after BJVC implantation, and its risk increased with time (31). In our cohort, only two (2.4%) patients developed with infective endocarditis during follow-up. This may be attributable to the favorable

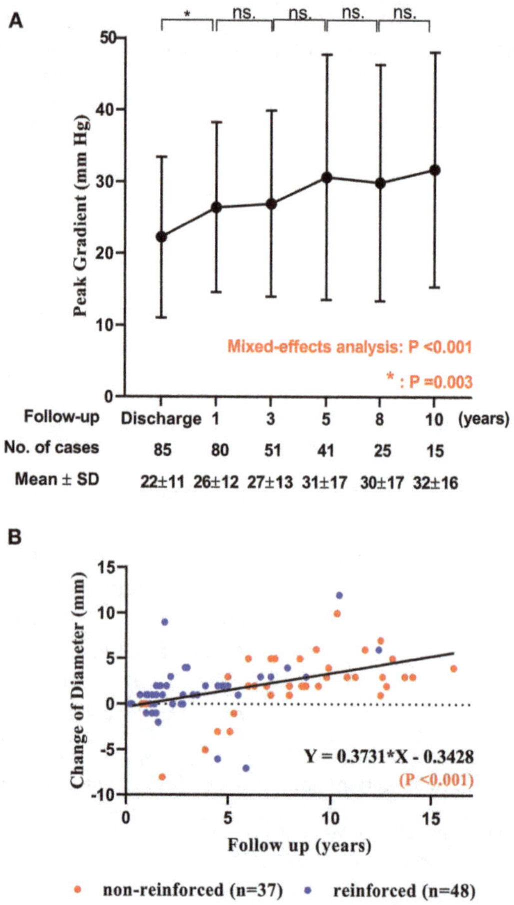

FIGURE 3 | The change of peak gradient and diameter of DP-BJVC. **(A)** Peak pressure gradient across the conduit measured by echocardiography before discharge and at 1, 3, 5, 8 and 10 years after implantation are presented with mean and standard deviation (SD). The gradient significantly increased with time (*P* <0.001). The comparisons of adjacent time show that the increase mainly occurred in the first postoperative year (*P* =0.003), which become slightly thereafter (*P* >0.05). ns, no significance. **(B)** The change of DP-BJVC diameter measured by echocardiography at the annular level from implantation to the last follow-up significantly and positively linear correction with the follow-up years. Each dot represents one patient. The diameter change of reinforced conduits (red dots) have similar regression coefficient with the non-reinforced conduits (blue dots. *P* = 0.806). Four conduits (arrows) had a diameter decrease over 5 mm early after implantation, which were all caused by stenosis and had been replaced.

hemodynamics and the lack of thrombosis as the site for bacterial adhesion due to anticoagulation treatment (1, 32).

LIMITATIONS

Our study has a couple of limitations. First, this is a cohort study, rather than a randomized and control trial. There were no control group using other types of conduits. During the study period, DP-BJVC was the only available material for RVOT reconstruction in our center, except for cryopreserved homograft used in a few children and ePTFE valved conduit (14) used in adolescents and adults recently. Second, the indications for conduit reintervention remain controversial and have been broadened over the past decade, which has influenced our management. The incidence of conduit reintervention substantially increased in the past 5 years.

CONCLUSION

Our novel designed DP-BJVC performed satisfactory functionality and durability in midterm follow-up, particularly for those younger than or equal to 3 years old. It showed advantages in resistance to calcification and infection, as well as appropriate dilation with age. DP-BJVC is a promising alternative for RVOT reconstruction in children with CHD.

AUTHOR CONTRIBUTIONS

J-GH and Z-SW developed the conduit. Z-SW and JL make substantial contributions to conception and design. TQ contributed to data collection and draft the article. All authors contributed to the article and approved the submitted version.

SUPPLEMENTARY MATERIAL

Supplementary Figure 1 | Intraoperative photographs of failed DP-BJVC in two patients. **(A)** 10.4 years after implantation in Rastelli operation for pulmonary atresia, the lumen surface of the conduit was smooth without visible thrombosis and calcification. **(B)** 10.3 years after implantation for truncus arteriosus repair, the conduit was aneurysmal dilated with mild calcification. Residual valve tissue is displayed with tweezers.

Supplementary Figure 2 | Results of mixed-effects analysis and Sidak's multiple comparisons of peak gradient across the DP-BJVC during follow-ups. Peak gradient across the conduit significant increased during follow-up (*P* = 0.0019). The difference mainly occurred during the first year after implantation (t1 vs. t0, *P* = 0.0027), and no significant difference was found thereafter (Ps > 0.3). t0, before discharge (*n* = 85); t1, 1 year after implantation (*n* = 80); t2, 3 years after implantation (*n* = 51); t3, 5 years after implantation (*n* = 41); t4, 8 years after implantation (*n* = 25); t5, 10 years after implantation (*n* = 15).

Supplementary Figure 3 | Examples of imaging examinations of implanted DP-BJVC. **(A,B)** Echocardiography at 2 years after Rastelli operation for pulmonary atresia. The conduit valve leaflets (PV) are clearly visible in 2-dimensional in the long-axis view along the conduit. Pulse-wave Doppler signal at conduit level showed normal laminar flow. **(C,D)** Cardiac CT examination at 10 years after truncus arteriosus repair. The conduit (PA) was mildly dilated in the proximal end, with scattered calcification at the distal (white arrow). The size of the right ventricle was normal. **(E,F)** Cardiac CT examination at 11 years after Rastelli operation for pulmonary atresia. The conduit was well-shaped with scattered calcification. **(G,H)** Cardiac MRI at 12 years after Rastelli operation for corrected transposition of the great arteries, showing the normal-sized heart and unobstructed ventricular outflow tracts.

Supplementary Figure 4 | Severe aneurysmal dilatation of DP-BJVC in a 3.5 years old girl. The conduit was reinforced with a Dacron ring. However, the diameter dilated almost 170% (from 12 to 20 mm) after 23 months at the level of annulus, which was even larger at the proximal and distal level. Although the conduit is currently in a undesirable state due to the extremely heavy afterload, it indirectly reflect that the annulus restraining device does not strictly limit the diameter of the conduit.

Supplementary Figure 5 | The results of comparison of diameter change between reinforced and non-reinforced DP-BJVC. The change of diameter significantly and positively linear correlated with follow-up time both in non-reinforced and reinforced conduit, with regression coefficient (slopes) of 0.53 and 0.48 respectively. The differences between the slopes are not significant ($P = 0.806$).

REFERENCES

1. Herrmann JL, Brown JW. Seven decades of valved right ventricular outflow tract reconstruction: the most common heart procedure in children. *J Thorac Cardiovasc Surg.* (2020) 160:1284–8. doi: 10.1016/j.jtcvs.2020.04.137
2. Breymann T, Blanz U, Wojtalik MA, Daenen W, Hetzer R, Sarris G, et al. European Contegra multicentre study: 7-year results after 165 valved bovine jugular vein graft implantations. *Thorac Cardiovasc Surg.* (2009) 57:257–69 doi: 10.1055/s-0029-1185513
3. Dave H, Mueggler O, Comber M, Enodien B, Nikolaou G, Bauersfeld U, et al. Risk factor analysis of 170 single-institutional contegra implantations in pulmonary position. *Ann Thorac Surg.* (2011) 91:195–302; discussion 202–3. doi: 10.1016/j.athoracsur.2010.07.058
4. Patel PM, Tan C, Srivastava N, Herrmann JL, Rodefeld MD, Turrentine MW, et al. Bovine jugular vein conduit: a mid- to long-term institutional review. *World J Pediatr Congenit Heart Surg.* (2018) 9:489–95. doi: 10.1177/2150135118779356
5. Falchetti A, Demanet H, Dessy H, Melot C, Pierrakos C, Wauthy P. Contegra versus pulmonary homograft for right ventricular outflow tract reconstruction in newborns. *Cardiol Young.* (2019) 29:505–10. doi: 10.1017/S1047951119000143
6. Patel PM, Herrmann JL, Rodefeld MD, Turrentine MW, Brown JW. Bovine jugular vein conduit versus pulmonary homograft in the Ross operation. *Cardiol Young.* (2020) 30:323–7. doi: 10.1017/S1047951119003007
7. Brown JW, Ruzmetov M, Rodefeld MD, Eltayeb O, Yurdakok O, Turrentine MW. Contegra versus pulmonary homografts for right ventricular outflow tract reconstruction: a ten-year single-institution comparison. *World J Pediatr Congenit Heart Surg.* (2011) 2:541–9. doi: 10.1177/2150135111415711
8. Poynter JA, Eghtesady P, McCrindle BW, Walters HL 3rd, Kirshbom PM, Blackstone EH, et al. Congenital heart surgeons: association of pulmonary conduit type and size with durability in infants and young children. *Ann Thorac Surg.* (2013) 96:1695–701; discussion 1701–2. doi: 10.1016/j.athoracsur.2013.05.074
9. Sandica E, Boethig D, Blanz U, Goerg R, Haas NA, Laser KT, et al. Bovine jugular veins versus homografts in the pulmonary position: an analysis across two centers and 711 patients-conventional comparisons and time status graphs as a new approach. *Thorac Cardiovasc Surg.* (2016) 64:25–35. doi: 10.1055/s-0035-1554962
10. Tod TJ, Dove JS. The association of bound aldehyde content with bioprosthetic tissue calcification. *J Mater Sci Mater Med.* (2016) 27:8. doi: 10.1007/s10856-015-5623-z
11. Manji RA, Zhu LF, Nijjar NK, Rayner DC, Korbutt GS, Churchill TA, et al. Glutaraldehyde-fixed bioprosthetic heart valve conduits calcify and fail from xenograft rejection. *Circulation.* (2006) 114:318–27. doi: 10.1161/CIRCULATIONAHA.105.549311
12. Naso F, Gandaglia A. Different approaches to heart valve decellularization: a comprehensive overview of the past 30 years. *Xenotransplantation.* (2017) 25:e12354. doi: 10.1111/xen.12354
13. Bibevski S, Ruzmetov M, Fortuna RS, Turrentine MW, Brown JW, Ohye RG. Performance of synergraft decellularized pulmonary allografts compared with standard cryopreserved allografts: results from multiinstitutional data. *Ann Thorac Surg.* (2017) 103:869–74. doi: 10.1016/j.athoracsur.2016.07.068
14. Miyazaki T, Yamagishi M, Maeda Y, Taniguchi S, Fujita S, Hongu H, et al. Long-term outcomes of expanded polytetrafluoroethylene conduits with bulging sinuses and a fan-shaped valve in right ventricular outflow tract reconstruction. *J Thorac Cardiovasc Surg.* (2018) 155:2567–76. doi: 10.1016/j.jtcvs.2017.12.137
15. Feng YG, Wu ZS, Hu JG, Hu TH, Zhang JC, Xu ZJ, et al. [Morphologic and physiochemical properties of bovine jugular conduit stabilized by dye-mediated poto-oxidation]. *Zhong Nan Da Xue Xue Bao Yi Xue Ban.* (2004) 29:429–31.
16. Lu WD, Zhang M, Wu ZS, Hu TH. Decellularized and photooxidatively crosslinked bovine jugular veins as potential tissue engineering scaffolds. *Interact Cardiovasc Thorac Surg.* (2009) 8:301–5. doi: 10.1510/icvts.2008.194076
17. Lu WD, Zhang M, Wu ZS, Hu TH, Xu ZJ, Liu W, et al. The performance of photooxidatively crosslinked acellular bovine jugular vein conduits in the reconstruction of connections between pulmonary arteries and right ventricles. *Biomaterials.* (2010) 31:2934–43. doi: 10.1016/j.biomaterials.2009.12.046
18. Boethig D, Schreiber C, Hazekamp M, Blanz U, Pretre R, Asfour B, et al. Risk factors for distal Contegra stenosis: results of a prospective European multicentre study. *Thorac Cardiovasc Surg.* (2012) 60:195–204. doi: 10.1055/s-0031-1298062
19. Zoghbi W, Enriquez-Sarano M, Foster E, Grayburn P, Kraft C, Levine R, et al. Recommendations for evaluation of the severity of native valvular regurgitation with two-dimensional and Doppler echocardiography. *J Am Soc Echocardiogr.* (2003) 16:777–802. doi: 10.1016/S0894-7317(03)00335-3
20. Prior N, Alphonso N, Arnold P, Peart I, Thorburn K, Venugopal P, et al. Bovine jugular vein valved conduit: up to 10 years follow-up. *J Thorac Cardiovasc Surg.* (2011) 141:983–7. doi: 10.1016/j.jtcvs.2010.08.037
21. Hawkins JA, Hillman ND, Lambert LM, Jones J, Di Russo GB, Profaizer T, et al. Immunogenicity of decellularized cryopreserved allografts in pediatric cardiac surgery: comparison with standard cryopreserved allografts. *J Thorac Cardiovasc Surg.* (2003) 126:247–52; discussion 252–3. doi: 10.1016/S0022-5223(03)00116-8
22. Moore MA, Phillips RE Jr, McIlroy BK, Walley VM, Hendry PJ. Evaluation of porcine valves prepared by dye-mediated photooxidation. *Ann Thorac Surg.* (1998) 66 (6 Suppl):S245–8. doi: 10.1016/S0003-4975(98)01118-7
23. Xu XH, Wu ZS, Yin BL, Hu JG, Yang YF. [Structural and hemodynamic study of right ventricular outflow tract reconstruction with valved bovine jugular vein conduit in the canine model by color Doppler echocardiography]. *Zhong Nan Da Xue Xue Bao Yi Xue Ban.* (2007) 32:599–603.
24. Lu WD, Wang AP, Wu ZS, Zhang M, Hu TH, Lei GY, et al. Calcification resistance for photooxidatively crosslinked acellular bovine jugular vein conduits in right-side heart implantation. *J Biomed Mater Res A.* (2012) 100:2644–53. doi: 10.1002/jbm.a.34203
25. Beckerman Z, De Leon LE, Zea-Vera R, Mery CM, Fraser CD. Jr. High incidence of late infective endocarditis in bovine jugular vein valved conduits. *J Thorac Cardiovasc Surg.* (2018) 156:728–34. e2. doi: 10.1016/j.jtcvs.2018.03.156
26. Karamlou T, Blackstone EH, Hawkins JA, Jacobs ML, Kanter KR, Brown JW, et al. Pulmonary conduit working group for the members of the congenital heart surgeons: can pulmonary conduit dysfunction and failure be reduced in infants and children less than age 2 years at initial implantation? *J Thorac Cardiovasc Surg.* (2006) 132:829–38. doi: 10.1016/j.jtcvs.2006.06.034
27. Ugaki S, Rutledge J, Al Aklabi M, Ross DB, Adatia I, Rebeyka IM. An increased incidence of conduit endocarditis in patients receiving bovine jugular vein grafts compared to cryopreserved homograft for right ventricular outflow reconstruction. *Ann Thorac Surg.* (2015) 99:140–6. doi: 10.1016/j.athoracsur.2014.08.034
28. Wojtalik M, Mrowczynski W, Zeromski J, Bartkowski R. Does contegra xenograft implantation evoke cellular immunity in children? *Interact Cardiovasc Thorac Surg.* (2003) 2:273–8. doi: 10.1016/S1569-9293(03)00058-6
29. Meyns B, Van Garsse L, Boshoff D, Eyskens B, Mertens L, Gewillig M, et al. The Contegra conduit in the right ventricular outflow tract

induces supravalvular stenosis. *J Thorac Cardiovasc Surg.* (2004) 128:834–40. doi: 10.1016/j.jtcvs.2004.08.015

30. Sharma A, Cote AT, Hosking MCK, Harris KC. A systematic review of infective endocarditis in patients with bovine jugular vein valves compared with other valve types. *JACC Cardiovasc Interv.* (2017) 10:1449–58. doi: 10.1016/j.jcin.2017.04.025
31. Hascoet S, Mauri L, Claude C, Fournier E, Lourtet J, Riou JY, et al. Infective endocarditis risk after percutaneous pulmonary valve implantation with the melody and sapien valves. *JACC Cardiovasc Interv.* (2017) 10:510–7. doi: 10.1016/j.jcin.2016.12.012
32. Robichaud B, Hill G, Cohen S, Woods R, Earing M, Frommelt P, et al. Bioprosthetic pulmonary valve endocarditis: incidence, risk factors, clinical outcomes. *Congenit Heart Dis.* (2018) 13:734–9. doi: 10.1111/chd.12639

18

Technical Aspects and Considerations of Meso-Rex Bypass Following Liver Transplantation with Left Lateral Segment Grafts

Christina Dalzell[1], Paola A. Vargas[2], Kyle Soltys[2,3], Frank Di Paola[2], George Mazariegos[2,3] and Nicolas Goldaracena[2*]

[1] School of Medicine, University of Virginia, Charlottesville, VA, United States, [2] Division of Transplant Surgery, Department of Surgery, University of Virginia Health System, Charlottesville, VA, United States, [3] Department of Surgery, Hillman Center for Pediatric Transplantation, UPMC Children's Hospital of Pittsburgh, University of Pittsburgh School of Medicine, Pittsburgh, PA, United States

***Correspondence:**
Nicolas Goldaracena
n.goldaracena@virginia.edu

In pediatric patients with extrahepatic portal vein obstruction and complications of portal hypertension, but with normal liver function, a meso-Rex bypass (MRB) connecting the superior mesenteric vein to the intrahepatic left portal is the favored surgical management. Pediatric patients with a history of a partial liver transplant (LT), especially living donors, are at greater risk for portal vein complications. Hence, an adequate knowledge of this technique and its additional challenges in the post-LT patient setting is crucial. We provide an overview of the available literature on technical aspects for an MRB post-LT. Preoperative considerations are highlighted, along with intraoperative considerations and postoperative management. Special attention is given to the even-more-demanding aspect of performing an MRB post-liver transplantation with a left lateral segment. Surgical alternatives are also discussed. In addition, we report here a unique case in which this surgical technique was performed on a complex pediatric patient with a history of a living-donor LT with a left lateral segment graft over a decade ago.

Keywords: extrahepatic portal vein obstruction (EHPVO), living donor liver transplant (LDLT), left lateral segment graft, meso-Rex bypass, pediatric surgery

INTRODUCTION

The meso-Rex bypass (MRB), first described by de Ville de Goyet et al. involves using a vein conduit to direct flow from the superior mesenteric vein (SMV) to the left portal vein within the Rex recess in those patients with extrahepatic portal vein obstruction (EHPVO) but an otherwise normal intrinsic liver function (1, 2). It is a common approach to deal with the portal hypertension complications derived from a portal vein thrombosis (PVT) following liver transplantation in those pediatric patients with otherwise functioning liver grafts. It differs from the other mainstay of treatment, a portosystemic shunt (PSS), because blood flow is still directed from the splanchnic system through the non-cirrhotic liver, which may benefit pediatric patients who are still undergoing growth and development (1). This approach requires a profound knowledge of the extrahepatic and intrahepatic anatomy. In this regard, the Rex recess can be identified by its relationship to specific landmarks—it lies within the umbilical scissure between segments II, III, and IV and the anterior part of the recess ends in the umbilical ligament. Understanding this anatomy provides surgeons with the opportunity to have this technique in their arsenal ready to be used when needed (2).

In the non-transplant patient, the most common cause of EHPVO is umbilical vein catheterization in the neonatal period (3). Other causes include previous abdominal surgeries and infection (2, 3). It is less likely related to coagulation disorders than its counterpart in adult patients, and the cause of thrombus formation can also be idiopathic in some cases (2). The main indications for surgical management of EHPVO include complications of portal hypertension such as splenomegaly, severe thrombocytopenia, and variceal bleeding (1, 4).

The cases of EHPVO after liver transplantation (LT) have been previously described in the literature (5, 6). Vascular complications, including portal vein obstruction (PVO), have been found to be associated with living donor liver transplantation (LDLT), especially when performed for biliary atresia (7–10). Furthermore, the creation of an MRB in pediatric patients who have received a partial graft has also been described in the literature (6, 11–15). However, MRB creation after LDLT with a left lateral segment (LLS) is associated with unique challenge due to the loss of important landmarks (6). In this study, we aim to gather and present the technical aspects of MRB in the post-LT setting. In addition, we describe our experience with MRB in a 15-year-old girl with a history of LDLT with an LLS graft when she was 9 months old presenting with EHPVO and life-threatening complications of portal hypertension over a decade after LT.

Preoperative Considerations

Planning an MRB creation post-LT requires a multidisciplinary evaluation of the patient. An important facet of preoperative workup is to exclude the presence of intrinsic liver disease and confirm anatomy using both non-invasive and invasive imaging techniques (16). Liver biopsy is often required to rule out intrinsic liver disease as a cause of portal hypertension (2). Hypercoagulable states or disorders must also be excluded with coagulation labs including commonly inherited hypercoagulable disorders (2). Surveillance esophagogastroduodenoscopy (EGD) should be performed to manage varices preoperatively, especially after a recent bleed (2). Preoperative abdominal imaging is necessary to confirm the patency of the mesenteric vein and left portal vein. This can been achieved with either abdominal ultrasound (US) with Doppler or low-dose postcontrast portal venous phase computed tomography of the abdomen (16, 17). In some cases, MRI or MR venography can also be used to better visualize the SMV-portal vein confluence (16, 17). The patency of the internal jugular vein (IJV), if intended to be used as jump graft, should also be confirmed with US preoperatively. In cases where the anatomy remains difficult to visualize due to variants, post-transplant, or collateralization, transjugular wedged hepatic venous portography is also an important technique (16, 17). This technique is invasive and is performed by interventional radiology. After right internal jugular (IJ) access is obtained, a catheter is directed into the left hepatic vein and a balloon is used to "wedge" and prevent outflow. This allows for retrograde portal venography *via* the injection of contrast (17). Pressure measurements can also be obtained during this procedure, including right atrial, caval, wedged hepatic vein and free hepatic vein pressures.

Intraoperative Considerations

In terms of the operation, the patient is positioned supine with the head and neck slightly facing right in order to have access to the left IJ, which is usually the preferred side for vein grafting. The IJV is the preferred vascular autograft due to excellent long-term patency rates when compared to unrelated or prosthetic grafts (6). The surgery can be performed through a midline or subcostal laparotomy (2). The approach followed will defer slightly if the creation of the MRB is in a patient with no previous liver surgery vs. a post-transplant patient. Likewise, the approach use for a full graft liver will defer from the approach used for a partial liver given that the usual anatomical landmarks are lost in the latter, making this procedure more challenging in these circumstances. The typical steps followed when creating an MRB in a patient with no previous abdominal surgeries include dividing the round ligament and falciform ligament to gain access to the umbilical scissure and identifying the Rex recess (2). Once the umbilical scissure is dissected, the intrahepatic left portal vein is identified and dissected. For this, it is crucial to resect the liver parenchyma bridging the scissure. This will not only allow exposure and access to the intrahepatic left portal vein but will also avoid the compression of the bypass and ensure a good patency of the graft postoperatively. The intrahepatic left portal vein is dissected for a length of approximately 3 cm on its ventral and lateral aspects, and all small branches taking off the Rex recess into segments 2, 3, and 4 of the liver are dissected and encircled with vessel loops in order to be safely occluded when the anastomosis is pursued. Next, a mesocolic window is created to expose the SMV. The left IJV, the preferred autologous vein graft for the MRB, is procured. The anastomoses are created using 7-0 absorbable Prolene sutures (2). The first anastomosis is typically performed to the Rex recess. A small Satinsky clamp is placed in the Rex recess, and the central portion of the intrahepatic left portal vein is anastomosed end to side to the vein autograft in a running fashion. The clamp is released to ensure that the bypass fills with blood from a patent intrahepatic system. Later, the distal end of the jump graft vein is positioned across the mesocolon and anastomosed to the SMV in an end-to-side fashion (2, 18).

The main difference when performing this procedure in a transplanted patient with a left lateral partial graft is that the anatomical references and landmarks that allow us to easily identify and locate the rex Recess are basically lost. Therefore, preoperative imaging and workup play a key role as a route map. Also, once the hilar structures are identified, one should stay above the biliary plate and understand that the Rex will be in close proximity to the cut edge of the liver that, due to hypertrophy, has rotated to the right upper quadrant.

Postoperative Management

Postsurgical imaging includes Doppler US to confirm bypass patency and measure flow (17). This is typically performed at postoperative days 1 and 3 and then at monthly intervals until 6 months post-bypass creation (17). Later, US are adequate only if clinically demanded due to new signs of portal hypertension (17, 19). CT and MRI can be used to supplement in cases with complex anatomy or if there is a concern for bypass patency (19). Anticoagulation remains a hallmark of treatment after bypass creation (2). In a study by Bhat et al. focused on evaluating the postoperative anticoagulation factors associated with bypass thrombosis, warfarin use was more common in pediatric patients with thrombosed bypass versus open bypass [63% versus 20%; OR 6.5 (95% CI 1.3–315) $p = 0.022$] (20). Thus, heparin is typically used in the immediate post-transplant period until the patient can be discharged on an oral regimen (20). Aspirin and dipyridamole have been reported in the literature, with patients typically discharged on a 3–6-month regimen (2, 6). In our experience, once the patient can tolerate orally, we start them on 81 mg of aspirin daily to maintain for life as the only antithrombotic treatment/prophylaxis.

MESO-REX POST-LT

Meso-Rex Post-LT With Whole Liver Grafts

The creation of an MRB following LT comes with unique challenges. MRB creation after a whole deceased donor liver transplantation (DDLT) has been documented in a few case reports and case series (5, 11, 21–23). In an early series by de Ville de Goyet et al. five pediatric patients who underwent LT with a whole graft and developed PVT underwent a successful MRB creation (11). In a case report by Han et al. an adult DDLT recipient underwent MRB creation for portal vein cavernous malformation complicated by hypersplenism and elevated hepatic enzymes (21). A fresh iliac deceased-donor venous allograft was used to connect the left portal vein to the splenic vein. At 6-month follow-up, the bypass remained patent (21). In another case report by Bachman-Braun et al. a pediatric patient with a history of WLT after failed Kasai for biliary atresia developed complications of prehepatic portal hypertension due to PVT (5). She underwent MRB creation with a deceased donor iliac vein. At 6 months after surgery, the patient again developed symptoms of portal hypertension and required surgical revision (5). A large collateral vein was identified and used as an autologous vein conduit to revise the previous bypass (5). In a cohort study by Krebs-Schmitt et al., 14 pediatric patients developed PVT after WLT and underwent MRB creation (22). In this post-LT population, 8 bypass using an autologous jugular vein graft remained patent (22). Two patients who had an autologous jugular vein graft required revision and all 4 patients who had a cryopreserved iliac vein homograft required revision (22). Thus, MRB creation is an effective treatment for EHPVO in both adult and pediatric patients with a history of WLT (**Figure 1A**).

Meso-Rex Post-LT With Partial Grafts

Portal vein obstruction is especially common after pediatric LDLT transplantation performed for biliary atresia (10, 24). It is also more common in partial grafts than whole grafts; hence, there are more reports of MRB creation in this patient population (24, 25). A review published in 2012 by de Ville de Goyet et al. includes the instances of MRB creation in reduced or LLS grafts (6). The first case was performed by de Ville de Goyet et al. for a pediatric patient with biliary atresia who received a reduced-size graft (26). From 1992 to 2012, there are reports of 28 pediatric patients undergoing MRB creation with a history of biliary atresia and partial liver transplantation, including reduced-size grafts (segments unspecified) and LLS grafts (6, 11–15, 26). This includes 12 patients who had received an LLS graft from a living-related donor (12, 13, 15). Out of the LDLT patients, 11/12 had long-term survival (12, 13, 15). One patient passed away due to pulmonary sepsis on postoperative day 50 (15). One bypass revision was also required in a patient who received an unrelated donor vascular autograft (12). When WLT transplant recipients were also included for a total of 51 cases of MRB creation after LT, the overall patient survival was 96% with a 100% long-term patency rate with the use of the IJV for the bypass (6).

CASE PRESENTATION

Our patient was a 15-year-old girl with a history of a living-related donor liver transplant with an LLS graft at 9 months old for biliary atresia following a failed Kasai procedure. Her postoperative transplant course was complicated by persistent thrombocytopenia and hypersplenism. She underwent partial splenic artery embolization in 2013 for increasing splenomegaly and thrombocytopenia, consistent with splenic sequestration. In 2014, she had an evidence of PVT with cavernous transformation on imaging and presented with a gastrointestinal (GI) bleeding consistent with esophageal varices and portal hypertensive gastropathy on endoscopy. Since that initial episode in 2014, she underwent repeat surveillance EGD with banding but had no further episodes of bleeding. Her screening endoscopy result in early 2021 showed continued portal hypertensive gastropathy. The computed tomography scan of her abdomen and pelvis 4 months prior to MRB creation showed splenomegaly, measuring 15.6 cm craniocaudal. Preoperative lab results included a platelet count of 81.000. Due to her risk of GI bleeding due to continued portal hypertension, a decision was made to proceed with MRB creation (**Figure 1B**).

As part of her preoperative evaluation, the patient underwent portal venogram and transjugular liver biopsy, which showed no signs of intrinsic liver disease. Other aspects of preoperative evaluation included echocardiography and an US of bilateral IJVs and subclavian veins.

The patient was taken to the operating room for MRB creation (**Figure 2**). A bilateral subcostal incision was made. The LLS graft was hypertrophied and was mobilized and dissected off the right abdominal wall. The hilar structures were identified (**Figure 2A**), and a very small bridge of liver parenchyma connecting segment 3 and the small portion of segment 4 was found. This area was

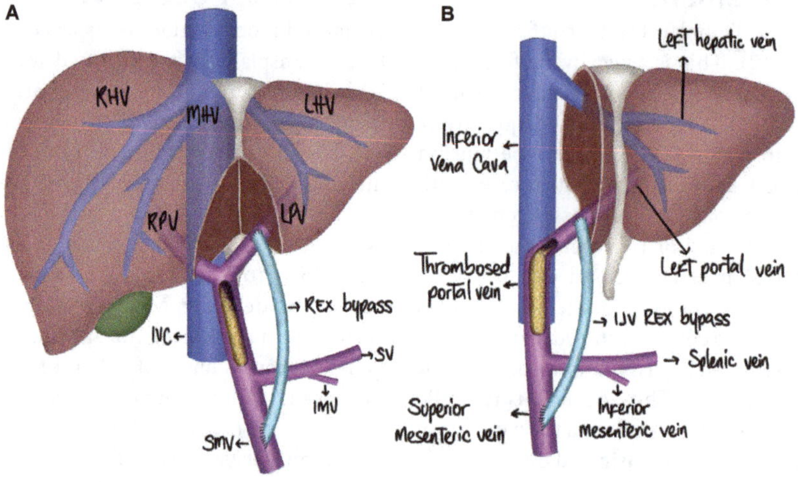

FIGURE 1 | Schematic representation of an MRB creation. **(A)** Meso-Rex post-LT with whole liver grafts. **(B)** Meso-Rex post-LT with partial grafts (LLS). IJV, internal jugular vein; IMV, inferior mesenteric vein; IVC, inferior vena cava; LHV, left hepatic vein; LPV, left portal vein; MHV, middle hepatic vein; RHV, right hepatic vein; RPV, right portal vein; SMV, superior mesenteric vein; SV, splenic vein.

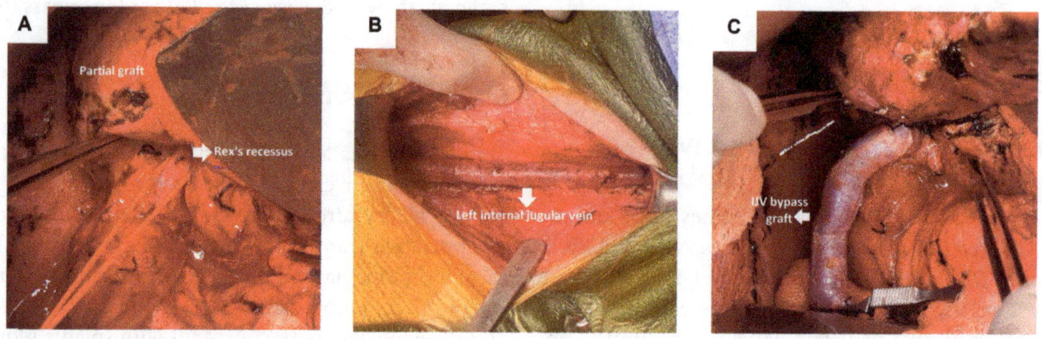

FIGURE 2 | Important steps during an MRB creation. **(A)** Identification of the hilar structures. **(B)** Exposure of the left IJV. **(C)** Anastomosis of the left portal vein and proximal end of the left IJV.

carefully dissected to identify the left portal vein (Rex recess). The portal plate and vein were subsequently exposed, and individual branches draining into the portal vein were isolated and protected with vessel loops. Next, the SMV was identified at the root of the mesentery.

The SMV was dissected and exposed distal to the lesser arcuate branches and proximal to the middle colic vein. Next, an incision was made along the anterior border of the left sternocleidomastoid muscle to expose the left IJV. The vein was taken as proximal as possible, down to its takeoff from the subclavian vein (**Figure 2B**).

The following step consisted of the creation of the meso-Rex bypass anastomosis. The portal plate was opened with scissors, and good back bleeding was noted prior to starting the anastomosis. The anastomosis of the left portal vein and proximal end of the left IJV was constructed in a running end-to-side fashion with 7-0 Prolene (**Figure 2C**). Portal venography was performed and confirmed good flow into the liver from the bypass graft (**Figure 3**). The graft was tunneled through a hole in the mesentery to the prepared area of the SMV. The SMV was opened, and a running end-to-side anastomosis was completed with 7-0 Prolene. The patient tolerated the procedure well, with no immediate postoperative complication and minimal blood loss.

She remained in the hospital for 1 week and was transitioned from a heparin drip (5 units/kg/h) to aspirin 81 mg daily when tolerating the PO intake. On POD #0, 1, and 3, US showed a patent bypass with appropriate flow. By the second postoperative week, her platelet count had increased to 228.000. On a follow-up US 2 months after MRB creation, her spleen size had decreased to 12.9 cm. At more than 8 months after the procedure, the patient's postoperative course has been uneventful. She remains on aspirin 81 mg daily.

DISCUSSION

The creation of a MRB in the post-LT is a challenging procedure. Despite its complexity, with a proper interdisciplinary management and comprehensive patient assessment, excellent postoperative outcomes and survival rates can be achieved. We presented the case of MRB creation in a female patient

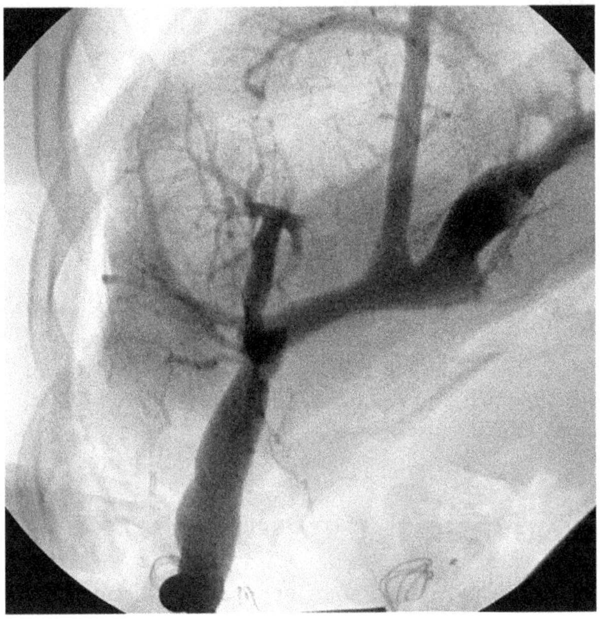

FIGURE 3 | Portal venography via the anastomosed graft with evidence of good flow into the liver.

who underwent LDLT 14 years prior with an LLS graft from a living-related donor. MRB creation was pursued due to the complications of portal hypertension related to EHPVO. Her postoperative course has remained unremarkable. In contrast to previous case studies, this is the first reported case in which this surgical technique was performed on an LLS graft from a living donor over a decade after the original transplant.

Biliary atresia is the most common indication for pediatric LT (9). An increase in the incidence of PVT following LT in patients with biliary atresia has been well established in the literature (7, 9, 27). Portal vein hypoplasia is a classic anatomic feature in patients with biliary atresia, which increases the challenge of anastomotic construction and thus the risk for post-transplant PVT (2, 5, 6). PVT is limited to the extrahepatic portal vein in children and can occur acutely after surgery in 5–10% of cases, or years later, often manifesting with signs of portal hypertension (6). A study by Ou et al. focused on evaluating pre-and post-transplant ultrasonographic findings in patients with biliary atresia who underwent LDLT to predict PVO (7). On multivariate analysis, the only pretransplant independent risk factor associated with post-transplant portal vein occlusion was the small main portal vein size <4 mm (p = 0.008). This is consistent with another study by de Ville de Goyet et al. showing that the portal vein size <5 mm is associated with portal vein complications on multivariate analysis after LDLT (11).

There are small case series and case reports on MRB creation after pediatric liver transplantation (6). A few cases describe this procedure in an LLS graft after LDLT. In a series by Gibelli et al. two patients with biliary atresia underwent LDLT and developed PVT on postoperative day 1. They subsequently underwent bypass creation on the same day (15). In a case report by Rivera et al., MRB creation was performed in a 13-month-old baby during the living-related donor transplant operation due to intraoperative PVT (13). In another case report by Caruso et al. a female child with biliary atresia underwent LDLT with surgical ligation of the splenic artery at 8 months. She had an episode of GI bleeding at age 5, with an evidence of complete PVT on imaging (28). The patient subsequently underwent MRB creation. However, the bypass thrombosed 4 months later and she had to undergo splenorenal shunt creation (28).

Meso-Rex bypass creation is especially difficult in patients with a partial graft. As evidenced by the case reports above, it is an uncommon procedure. The anatomic criteria, including a patent SMV and Rex recess with thrombus limited to the extrahepatic portal vein, must be met (6). This was confirmed on preoperative portal venography in our patient. Preoperative liver biopsy is also required to exclude cirrhosis before creating an MRB that will bring back blood to the transplanted liver. Bypass creation in an LLS graft is especially difficult because of the loss of landmarks in identifying the Rex recess and due to the route the bypass must take (6). In our patient, over a decade after a failed Kasai procedure and subsequent transplant, the graft was shifted to the right upper quadrant. IJV autograft is preferred, especially in the post-transplant setting, and has been associated with the best patency and overall outcomes, whereas the use of an unrelated donor vein or prosthetic material has been associated with a higher incidence of bypass thrombosis (6, 22).

Meso-Rex bypass creation differs from the other surgical option, a PSS, because it still allows blood flow through the liver. Studies have compared outcomes after the two techniques, with conflicting results (1, 29). In a retrospective study by Lautz et al., a cessation of variceal bleeding occurred in 96% of patients who underwent meso-Rex bypass versus 100% in PSS (29). However, there was a significant improvement in the platelet count, international normalized ratio, and serum ammonia level in the meso-Rex bypass group (29). In a systematic review by Zielsdorf et al., MRB creation was associated with a higher rate of bypass thrombosis (14.1% versus 5.8%; p = 0.021) and reoperation for thrombosis or stenosis (11.8% versus 4.1%; p = 0.019) versus PSS (1). Importantly, the neurological benefits of restoring portal blood flow to the liver have been established with meso-Rex bypass creation (30). In this study, neurocognitive testing was performed before and 1 year after surgery (30). Both PSS and MRB groups demonstrated similar fluid cognitive ability at initial evaluation; however, only the MRB group showed significant improvement 1 year after the surgery (30). In another study, patients who underwent MRB showed a significant improvement in their height and weight postoperatively (31). The negative association of EHPVO with growth has a multifactorial etiology, including a decrease in nutrient flow to the liver, malabsorption from portal hypertensive gastropathy, and early satiety from splenomegaly (4). These cognitive and growth benefits have led many surgeons to favor MRB over PSS creation in pediatric patients with non-cirrhotic livers.

Portal vein angioplasty with or without stent placement has also been described as an option for portal vein complications in pediatric LDLT (32). In a retrospective study of 75 pediatric patients who underwent LDLT, there were 6 late-onset PV complications. The initial treatment of portal vein stenosis in 4 patients was PTA with stent placement (n = 1) and PTA with balloon dilation (n = 3). In the remaining 2 patients, the portal vein was unable to be cannulated due to complete obstruction (n = 1) and restenosis with total thrombosis after the previous PTA with stent placement (n = 1), so they underwent a successful MRB creation (32). Hence, although PTA may be a first-line option in patients with stenotic portal veins, MRB creation is preferred in late-onset portal vein complications due to complete obstruction.

CONCLUSION

In summary, MRB creation in patients following LT is a challenging procedure that requires careful preoperative planning with an adequate, multidisciplinary approach and close follow-up. We demonstrated that patients with a long-term history of LDLT, presenting with advanced complications of portal hypertension, could benefit from MRB with an autologous IJV graft. Despite being a technically challenging procedure, we demonstrated an uncomplicated postoperative course with an adequate patient recovery. A MRB creation for chronic PVT with symptomatic portal hypertension is safe and feasible and remains the favored option for pediatric patients, even years after transplant with partial grafts.

AUTHOR CONTRIBUTIONS

NG, PV, and CD participated in conception and design of the manuscript, and writing and drafting of the manuscript. KS, FD, and GM participated in critical revision of the manuscript for important intellectual content. All authors approved the final version of the manuscript.

ACKNOWLEDGMENTS

We acknowledge Andres Ramos for providing assistance with the illustrations in the manuscript.

REFERENCES

1. Zielsdorf S, Narayanan L, Kantymyr S, Barbetta A, Kwon Y, Etesami K, et al. Surgical shunts for extrahepatic portal vein obstruction in pediatric patients: a systematic review. *HPB.* (2021) 23:656–65. doi: 10.1016/j.hpb.2020.11.1149
2. di Francesco F, Grimaldi C, de Ville de Goyet J. Meso-Rex bypass–a procedure to cure prehepatic portal hypertension: the insight and the inside. *J Am Coll Surg.* (2014) 218:e23–36. doi: 10.1016/j.jamcollsurg.2013.10.024
3. Bertocchini A, Falappa P, Grimaldi C, Bolla G, Monti L, de Ville de Goyet J. Intrahepatic portal venous systems in children with noncirrhotic prehepatic portal hypertension: anatomy and clinical relevance. *J Pediatr Surg.* (2014) 49:1268–75. doi: 10.1016/j.jpedsurg.2013.10.029
4. Khanna R, Sarin SK. Noncirrhotic Portal Hypertension: current and Emerging Perspectives. *Clin Liver Dis.* (2019) 23:781–807. doi: 10.1016/j.cld.2019.07.006
5. Blachman-Braun R, Lopez-Verdugo F, Alonso D, Book L, Feola GP, Rodriguez-Davalos MI. Revision of meso-Rex bypass utilizing a collateral vein in a patient with portal steal phenomenon after liver transplant: a case report. *Int J Surg Case Rep.* (2019) 60:230–3. doi: 10.1016/j.ijscr.2019.05.051
6. de Ville de Goyet J, Lo Zupone C, Grimaldi C, D'Ambrosio G, Candusso M, Torre G, et al. Meso-Rex bypass as an alternative technique for portal vein reconstruction at or after liver transplantation in children: review and perspectives. *Pediatr Transplant.* (2013) 17:19–26. doi: 10.1111/j.1399-3046.2012.01784.x
7. Ou HY, Concejero AM, Huang TL, Chen TY, Tsang LL, Chen CL, et al. Portal vein thrombosis in biliary atresia patients after living donor liver transplantation. *Surgery.* (2011) 149:40–7. doi: 10.1016/j.surg.2010.04.018
8. Ueda M, Oike F, Kasahara M, Ogura Y, Ogawa K, Haga H, et al. Portal vein complications in pediatric living donor liver transplantation using left-side grafts. *Am J Transplant.* (2008) 8:2097–105. doi: 10.1111/j.1600-6143.2008.02360.x
9. Neto JS, Fonseca EA, Feier FH, Pugliese R, Candido HL, Benavides MR, et al. Analysis of factors associated with portal vein thrombosis in pediatric living donor liver transplant recipients. *Liver Transpl.* (2014) 20:1157–67. doi: 10.1002/lt.23934
10. Moon JI, Jung GO, Choi GS, Kim JM, Shin M, Kim EY, et al. Risk factors for portal vein complications after pediatric living donor liver transplantation with left-sided grafts. *Transplant Proc.* (2010) 42:871–5. doi: 10.1016/j.transproceed.2010.02.059
11. de Ville de Goyet J, Gibbs P, Clapuyt P, Reding R, Sokal EM, Otte JB. Original extrahilar approach for hepatic portal revascularization and relief of extrahepatic portal hypertension related to later portal vein thrombosis after pediatric liver transplantation. Long term results. *Transplantation.* (1996) 62:71–5. doi: 10.1097/00007890-199607150-00015
12. Stenger AM, Broering DC, Gundlach M, Bloechle C, Ganschow R, Helmke K, et al. Extrahilar mesenterico-left portal shunt for portal vein thrombosis after liver transplantation. *Transplant Proc.* (2001) 33:1739–41. doi: 10.1016/s0041-1345(00)02663-4
13. Rivera J, Fusaro F, de Magnée C, Clapuyt P, Reding R. Meso-Rex shunt for immediate portal revascularization in pediatric liver transplantation: first report. *Pediatr Transplant.* (2012) 16:E235–7. doi: 10.1111/j.1399-3046.2011.01576.x
14. Vannevel G, Clapuyt P, Reding R, Menten R. Spontaneous meso-portal shunt following orthotopic liver transplantation in a child. *Pediatr Radiol.* (2010) 40:S92–4. doi: 10.1007/s00247-010-1758-8
15. Gibelli NE, Tannuri AC, Tannuri U, Santos MM, Pinho-Apezzato ML, Maksoud-Filho JG, et al. Rex shunt for acute portal vein thrombosis after pediatric liver transplantation in children with biliary atresia. *Transplant Proc.* (2011) 43:194–5. doi: 10.1016/j.transproceed.2010.11.011
16. Cárdenas AM, Epelman M, Darge K, Rand EB, Anupindi SA. Pre- and postoperative imaging of the Rex shunt in children: what radiologists should know. *AJR Am J Roentgenol.* (2012) 198:1032–7. doi: 10.2214/AJR.11.7963
17. Carollo V, Marrone G, Cortis K, Mamone G, Caruso S, Milazzo M, et al. Multimodality imaging of the Meso-Rex bypass. *Abdom Radiol.* (2019) 44:1379–94. doi: 10.1007/s00261-018-1836-1
18. Superina R, Shneider B, Emre S, Sarin S, de Ville de Goyet J. Surgical guidelines for the management of extra-hepatic portal vein obstruction. *Pediatr Transplant.* (2006) 10:908–13. doi: 10.1111/j.1399-3046.2006.00598.x
19. Chaves IJ, Rigsby CK, Schoeneman SE, Kim ST, Superina RA, Ben-Ami T. Pre- and postoperative imaging and interventions for the meso-Rex bypass in children and young adults. *Pediatr Radiol.* (2012) 42:220–72. doi: 10.1007/s00247-011-2283-0
20. Bhat R, Lautz TB, Superina RA, Liem R. Perioperative strategies and thrombophilia in children with extrahepatic portal vein obstruction undergoing the meso-Rex bypass. *J Gastrointest Surg.* (2013) 17:949–55. doi: 10.1007/s11605-013-2155-z
21. Han D, Tang R, Wang L, Li A, Huang X, Shen S, et al. Case report of a modified Meso-Rex bypass as a treatment technique for late-onset portal vein cavernous transformation with portal hypertension after adult deceased-donor liver transplantation. *Medicine.* (2017) 96:e7208. doi: 10.1097/MD.0000000000007208

22. Krebs-Schmitt D, Briem-Richter A, Grabhorn E, Burdelski M, Helmke K, Broering DC, et al. Effectiveness of Rex shunt in children with portal hypertension following liver transplantation or with primary portal hypertension. *Pediatr Transplant.* (2009) 13:540–4. doi: 10.1111/j.1399-3046.2008.01109.x
23. Gibelli NE, Tannuri U, de Pinho-Apezzato ML, Tannuri AC, Maksoud-Filho JG, Velhote MC, et al. "Rex shunt" for the treatment of portal vein thrombosis after pediatric liver transplantation: a case report. *Transplant Proc.* (2009) 41:955–6. doi: 10.1016/j.transproceed.2009.01.055
24. Alfares BA, Bokkers RPH, Verkade HJ, Dierckx RAJO, Gupte G, Franchi-Abella S, et al. Portal vein obstruction after pediatric liver transplantation: a systematic review of current treatment strategies. *Transplant Rev.* (2021) 35:100630. doi: 10.1016/j.trre.2021.100630
25. Alvarez F. Portal vein complications after pediatric liver transplantation. *Curr Gastroenterol Rep.* (2012) 14:270–4. doi: 10.1007/s11894-012-0257-5
26. de Ville de Goyet J, Clapuyt P, Otte JB. Extrahilar mesenterico-left portal shunt to relieve extrahepatic portal hypertension after partial liver transplant. *Transplantation.* (1992) 53:231–2.
27. Takahashi Y, Nishimoto Y, Matsuura T, Hayashida M, Tajiri T, Soejima Y, et al. Surgical complications after living donor liver transplantation in patients with biliary atresia: a relatively high incidence of portal vein complications. *Pediatr Surg Int.* (2009) 25:745–51. doi: 10.1007/s00383-009-2430-y
28. Caruso S, Miraglia R, Carollo V, Maruzzelli L, Luca A. Multidetector CT-guided endovascular treatment of a splenic artery aneurysm in a child with split-liver transplant and surgically ligated splenic artery origin. *Pediatr Radiol.* (2012) 42:1134–7. doi: 10.1007/s00247-012-2355-9
29. Lautz TB, Keys LA, Melvin JC, Ito J, Superina RA. Advantages of the meso-Rex bypass compared with portosystemic shunts in the management of extrahepatic portal vein obstruction in children. *J Am Coll Surg.* (2013) 216:83–9. doi: 10.1016/j.jamcollsurg.2012.09.013
30. Mack CL, Zelko FA, Lokar J, Superina R, Alonso EM, Blei AT, et al. Surgically restoring portal blood flow to the liver in children with primary extrahepatic portal vein thrombosis improves fluid neurocognitive ability. *Pediatrics.* (2006) 117:e405–12. doi: 10.1542/peds.2005-1177
31. Menon P, Rao KL, Bhattacharya A, Thapa BR, Chowdhary SK, Mahajan JK, et al. Extrahepatic portal hypertension: quality of life and somatic growth after surgery. *Eur J Pediatr Surg.* (2005) 15:82–7. doi: 10.1055/s-2004-830341
32. Cho YP, Kim KM, Ha TY, Ko GY, Hwang JY, Park H, et al. Management of late-onset portal vein complications in pediatric living-donor liver transplantation. *Pediatr Transplant.* (2014) 18:64–71. doi: 10.1111/petr.12204

19

Cerebral Oxygenation and Activity During Surgical Repair of Neonates with Congenital Diaphragmatic Hernia

Sophie A. Costerus[1†], Dries Hendrikx[2†], Joen IJsselmuiden[1], Katrin Zahn[3], Alba Perez-Ortiz[4], Sabine Van Huffel[2], Robert B. Flint[5,6], Alexander Caicedo[2], René Wijnen[1], Lucas Wessel[3], Jurgen C. de Graaff[7], Dick Tibboel[1] and Gunnar Naulaers[8,9]*

[1] Department of Paediatric Surgery, Erasmus Medical Center - Sophia Children's Hospital, Rotterdam, Netherlands, [2] ESAT-STADIUS Division, Department of Electrical Engineering, KU Leuven, Leuven, Belgium, [3] Department of Paediatric Surgery, University Hospital Mannheim, Mannheim, Germany, [4] Neonatal Intensive Care Unit, University Hospital Mannheim, Mannheim, Germany, [5] Division of Neonatology, Department of Paediatrics, Erasmus Medical Center - Sophia Children's Hospital, Rotterdam, Netherlands, [6] Department of Pharmacy, Erasmus Medical Center, Rotterdam, Netherlands, [7] Department of Anaesthesiology, Erasmus Medical Center, Rotterdam, Netherlands, [8] Department of Development and Regeneration, KU Leuven, Leuven, Belgium, [9] Neonatal Intensive Care Unit, University Hospitals Leuven, Leuven, Belgium

***Correspondence:**
Sophie A. Costerus
s.costerus@erasmusmc.nl

Background and aim: Neonatal brain monitoring is increasingly used due to reports of brain injury perioperatively. Little is known about the effect of sedatives (midazolam) and anesthetics (sevoflurane) on cerebral oxygenation ($rScO_2$) and cerebral activity. This study aims to determine these effects in the perioperative period.

Methods: This is an observational, prospective study in two tertiary pediatric surgical centers. All neonates with a congenital diaphragmatic hernia received perioperative cerebral oxygenation and activity measurements. Patients were stratified based on intraoperatively administrated medication: the sevoflurane group (continuous sevoflurane, bolus fentanyl, bolus rocuronium) and the midazolam group (continuous midazolam, continuous fentanyl, and continuous vecuronium).

Results: Intraoperatively, $rScO_2$ was higher in the sevoflurane compared to the midazolam group (84%, IQR 77–95 vs. 65%, IQR 59–76, $p = <0.001$), fractional tissue oxygen extraction was lower (14%, IQR 5–21 vs. 31%, IQR 29–40, $p = <0.001$), the duration of hypoxia was shorter (2%, IQR 0.4–9.6 vs. 38.6%, IQR 4.9–70, $p = 0.023$), and cerebral activity decreased more: slow delta: 2.16 vs. 4.35 μV^2 ($p = 0.0049$), fast delta: 0.73 vs. 1.37 μV^2 ($p = <0.001$). In the first 30 min of the surgical procedure, a 3-fold increase in fast delta (10.48–31.22 μV^2) and a 5-fold increase in gamma (1.42–7.58 μV^2) were observed in the midazolam group.

Conclusion: Sevoflurane-based anesthesia resulted in increased cerebral oxygenation and decreased cerebral activity, suggesting adequate anesthesia. Midazolam-based anesthesia in neonates with a more severe CDH led to alarmingly low $rScO_2$ values, below hypoxia threshold, and increased values of EEG power during the first 30 min of surgery. This might indicate conscious experience of pain. Integrating population-pharmacokinetic models and multimodal neuromonitoring are needed for personalized pharmacotherapy in these vulnerable patients.

Keywords: neonates, surgery, midazolam, sevoflurane, cerebral activity, cerebral oxygenation

INTRODUCTION

Clinicians are increasingly monitoring the neonatal brain during high-risk neonatal surgery, due to the increased number of neonates who develop brain injury perioperatively, and subsequently impaired neurodevelopmental outcome (1–4).

Multimodal brain monitoring is needed to monitor the interplay between cerebral oxygenation and activity (5). Near-infrared spectroscopy (NIRS) presents a continuous, non-invasive measurement of regional cerebral oxygen saturation ($rScO_2$), with reference values between 55 and 85% for awake neonates (6). Baseline $rScO_2$ can vary as a result of sensor placement (7, 8), sensor type (9, 10), and the measurement device (11, 12). Furthermore, it is possible to analyse cerebral oxygen consumption by using the fractional tissue oxygen extraction (FTOE) (13). Intraoperative use of NIRS has been explored, but no coherent results have been reported in non-cardiac neonatal surgery (5) and NIRS-guided treatment guidelines are only available in pediatric cardiac surgery (14).

The activity of the neonatal brain is quantified using electroencephalography (EEG), which measures the overall electrical activity of the cortical pyramidal neurons (15). Consequently, EEG has a great sensitivity of showing changes in neural functioning (16). The power of the EEG is computed in different frequency bands. Delta oscillations (δ: 0.5–4 Hz) dominate the neonatal EEG and regulate basic homeostatic need (17), which can be divided into slow delta (δ_1: 0.5–2 Hz) or fast delta (δ_2: 2–4 Hz). Noxious-evoked EEG activity can be studied by analyzing gamma oscillations (γ: 32–100 Hz) over the contralateral somatosensory cortex and by analyzing the fast delta band (δ_2) (18). Strong increased gamma γ oscillations and increased energy in the fast delta δ_2 band was shown to reflect nociceptive pain in neonates following heel lance (18).

To date, little is known about the effect of anesthetic approaches on cerebral oxygenation (5, 19). In this prospective center comparison study, neonates with a congenital diaphragmatic hernia (CDH), treated according to a standardized international guideline (20) received two different anesthetic approaches intraoperatively: midazolam with analgesia and muscle relaxation vs. an sevoflurane with analgesia and muscle relaxation. We hypothesize that cerebral oxygenation is affected to a lesser extent by the administration a sedative-agent (midazolam), compared to the administration of anesthetic-agent (sevoflurane), assuming that the cerebral activity is less affected by a sedative-agent compared to an anesthetic-agent. The aim of this study was to determine the effects of midazolam vs. sevoflurane on cerebral oxygenation and cerebral activity in the perioperative period.

MATERIALS AND METHODS

This is an observational, prospective center comparison study on perioperative neuromonitoring in neonates with a CDH. All patients underwent surgery in a tertiary pediatric referral center: the Sophia Children's Hospital (Rotterdam, the Netherlands), or the Mannheim University Hospital (Mannheim, Germany), which treat ~20 and 60 neonates a year, respectively. Local institutional review board approval (Erasmus MC, Rotterdam, The Netherlands, MEC-2017-145, and Universitätsmedizin Mannheim, Mannheim, Germany 2018-578N-MA) and written informed consent of parents or legal guardians were obtained.

Patients

This study focused on neonates with a CDH, a major non-cardiac anomaly, that requires surgical repair within the 1st days of life. CDH neonates were eligible for inclusion if surgical repair was scheduled between July 2018 and April 2020 within the first 28 days of life, regardless of the type of surgery (open or thoracoscopic surgery), or the need for extracorporeal membrane oxygenation (ECMO) therapy until 24 h before surgery, for which both centers used the same entry criteria (20). Neonates were excluded if they had major cardiac or chromosomal anomalies, syndromes associated with altered cerebral perfusion, or syndromes associated with major neurodevelopmental impairment. In addition, neonates on ECMO during the start of the procedure were also excluded. Patients were treated according to the CDH-EURO consortium guidelines (20).

Perioperative Management

The neonates enrolled in this study were stratified in two groups. In Rotterdam, surgery was performed in the operating room (OR) and anesthesia was sevoflurane based (end expired concentration between 1 and 2%), with bolus fentanyl (induction 1-5 ug kg^{-1}) and rocuronium (0.5–1.0 mg kg^{-1}) performed by a pediatric anaesthesiologist. Patients operated at the OR underwent thoracoscopic surgery if they were hemodynamically stable and if the liver was not herniated. In Mannheim, surgery was performed at the neonatal intensive care unit (NICU), and anesthesia was based on continuous midazolam (70–100 ug kg^{-1} h^{-1}), fentanyl (2-5 ug kg^{-1} h^{-1}), vecuronium (0.10–0.30 mg kg^{-1}), and bolus fentanyl (2–10 ug kg^{-1}), performed by a neonatologist/ECMO specialist according to center specific routine for many years. Performing surgery in the NICU was partly based on the cardiorespiratory instability of the patient. Repeated administration of analgesia was based on clinical evaluation.

Data Collection

Patient demographics were collected according to the international consensus about standardized reporting for CDH (21). Measurements were performed in a continuous fashion, started at least 6 h before surgery and continued up to 24 h after surgery. Perioperative management, such as the administration of medication and the analysis of arterial blood gasses, was recorded in the patient data management system (HiX, Chipsoft BV, Amsterdam, the Netherlands).

Heart rate (HR), intra-arterial mean arterial blood pressure (MABP) and peripheral arterial oxygen saturation (SpO_2) were measured at 1 Hz (Primus, Draeger, Luebeck, Germany). $rScO_2$ was measured at a sampling rate of 1 Hz using NIRS (neonatal sensor, INVOS 5100C, Covidien, Boulder, Colorado, United States) with a hypoxic threshold of 63% for this device-sensor combination (10, 11). EEG was recorded using a 4-channel EEG at 256 Hz (Rotterdam: BrainRT, OSG, Rumst, Belgium, Mannheim: Braintrend, Fritz Stephan GMBH, Gackenbach, Germany). The power of the EEG was computed in the slow delta (δ_1: 0.5–2 Hz), fast delta (δ_2: 2–4 Hz), and gamma (γ: 32–100 Hz) frequency bands. Clinicians were blinded for EEG, but not for $rScO_2$.

In Rotterdam, the Shell+ RT software Suite of the BrainRT was reprogrammed for real-time data extraction. In Mannheim, AnStat software (Carepoint, Ede, the Netherlands) was used for real-time data extraction. Both software extracted data in the same manner. The vasoactive-inotropic score (VIS) reflects the need and grade of vasoactive/inotropic pharmaceutical intervention and was calculated to quantify necessity of cardiovascular support (22).

Data Processing and Statistical Analysis

The signal processing pipeline started with three pre-processing steps. First, artifacts were detected and removed. For EEG, segments were excluded from the analysis if the absolute amplitude exceeded 500 μV, which is the maximum voltage that could be detected by the monitor. For the other signals, segments outside of the physiological range, segments containing motion artifacts were removed. Second, the spectral power in the EEG was computed using the continuous wavelet transform and ridge extraction (23). Three frequency bands of interest were defined: slow delta δ_1 (0.5–2 Hz), fast delta δ_2 (2–4 Hz), and gamma γ (30–100 Hz) frequency bands. Third, FTOE was computed from $rScO_2$ and SpO_2 values as FTOE = (SpO_2 - $rScO_2$)/SpO_2. Since $rScO_2$ mainly reflects the oxygenation of the venous return from the brain, FTOE defines the amount of oxygen extracted in the brain.

After these processing steps, signal parameters were extracted in four data windows: the *preoperative* window (Pr: 6–3 h before the start of surgery), the *intraoperative* window (In: entire surgical procedure), and two *postoperative* windows (Po3: 3–6 h and Po15: 15–18 h after the end of surgery). These data windows were used to balance the data and to remove transitional effects, such as artifacts of transport, artifacts of care, the effect of intraoperative administered medication.

T-test was used for the comparison of the patient demographics. Generalized least-squares models were used for the statistical analysis of the primary endpoint, since they showed to be the best fit for the data as indicated by the Akaike information criterion (24). *Post-hoc* comparisons were based on analysis of marginal means, implemented with Tukey's correction for multiple comparisons. All statistical computations were carried out in R, with significance defined as $\alpha < 0.05$ (25).

Correlations

Three correlations were studied to determine their effect on our results. Firstly, the correlation between vasoactive and inotropic medication on $rScO_2$ and FTOE was studied to clarify possible effects of cerebral vasoconstriction. Secondly, the correlation between the dosage of anesthesia and cerebral oxygenation and activity was studied to clarify dosage related changes in $rScO_2$ and EEG-power values. Thirdly, the correlation between cerebral oxygenation and activity was investigated to study whether the assumption of reduced cerebral activity resulting in increased $rScO_2$ holds true in this study.

Endpoints

The primary endpoint of this study was measurement of the differential effect of sevoflurane vs. midazolam on cerebral oxygenation perioperatively. The secondary endpoint of this study was measurement of the differential effect of sevoflurane vs. midazolam on cerebral activity and the vital parameters perioperatively.

The primary endpoint of this study was measurement of the differential effect of sevoflurane vs. midazolam on cerebral oxygenation perioperatively. The secondary endpoint of this study was measurement of the differential effect of sevoflurane vs. midazolam on cerebral activity and the vital parameters perioperatively.

RESULTS

Demographics

Informed consent was obtained in 49 CDH neonates. Five patients were excluded following the absence of multiple signals due to data transfer and/or storage problems, six patients were excluded due to the need of extracorporeal membrane oxygenation (ECMO) treatment and one patient was excluded due to cardiopulmonary resuscitation intra-operatively. Therefore, 37 neonates could be analyzed: 20 neonates in the sevoflurane group (all patients from Rotterdam and received surgery in the OR), 17 neonates in the midazolam group (all patients from Mannheim and received surgery in the NICU) (**Appendix 1**). In the midazolam group, five neonates received VA-ECMO treatment until 1 day before surgery. Both groups were comparable (**Table 1**), except for a lower amount of herniated livers (25 vs. 71%, $p = 0.005$), a lower VIS preoperatively (0, IQR 0–5 vs. 17, IQR 10–25, $p = <0.001$), a lower postnatal age on the day of surgery (3 days, IQR 2–4 vs. 6 days, IQR 3–12, $p = 0.008$), more thoracoscopic surgery

(40 vs. 23%, $p = 0.026$), and shorter surgery (95 min, IQR 70–125 vs. 182 min, IQR 114–203, $p = <0.001$) in the sevoflurane group compared to the midazolam group. Eight patients who underwent thoracoscopic surgery were converted to an open approach because of the need for a patch.

Anesthesia

Preoperatively, in the sevoflurane group, five neonates were not sedated while on mechanical ventilation, two neonates received continuous administration of morphine, seven neonates received continuous administration of midazolam, and six neonates received continuous administration of both midazolam and morphine (**Appendix 2**). In the midazolam group, all neonates received continuous midazolam, supplemented with continuous administration of fentanyl (**Appendix 2**) and were intubated multiple days before surgery. The patients in the sevoflurane group that were intubated and sedated before start of surgery received comparable dosages of midazolam (47 ug kg^{-1} h^{-1}, IQR 0–92 and 40 ug kg^{-1} h^{-1}, IQR 30–50, $p = 0.735$, respectively, **Table 1**) compared to the midazolam group.

Intraoperatively, the end expired sevoflurane concentration was 1.5% (IQR 1.1–1.9). Time between the start of administration of sevoflurane and start of the surgical procedure was 66 min (IQR 45–76.6). In six neonates, the preoperative continuous midazolam administration was continued intraoperatively and in two neonates the preoperative continuous morphine administration was continued intraoperatively during sevoflurane anesthesia (**Appendix 2**). Three neonates received a bolus of propofol (2.9, 3.7, and 7.3 mg kg^{-1} for endotracheal intubation). In the midazolam group, the midazolam dosage was 100 ug kg^{-1} h^{-1} (IQR 68–100). The time between the administration of midazolam and the start of the surgical procedure was 21 min (IQR 1–30). The midazolam dosage in the sevoflurane group of those in whom the midazolam was continued from PICU ($n = 6$) was significantly lower (47 ug kg^{-1} h^{-1}, IQR 0–67, $p = 0.003$) compared to the midazolam group (100 ug kg^{-1} h^{-1}, IQR 68–100) (**Table 1**). The fentanyl bolus dosage during the induction of anesthesia was lower in the sevoflurane group compared to the midazolam group (2 ug kg^{-1}, IQR 2–3 vs. 5 ug kg^{-1}, IQR 4–7 vs. $p = <0.001$), although the cumulative fentanyl bolus dosages that were administrated intraoperatively did not differ (10 ug kg^{-1}, IQR 7–17 vs. 6 ug kg^{-1}, IQR 4–12, $p = 0.119$). Yet, the midazolam group received additional continuous administration of fentanyl (4 ug kg^{-1} h^{-1}, IQR 3–5), whereas the sevoflurane group did not.

Postoperatively, the midazolam dosages did not differ significantly between the sevoflurane (39 ug kg^{-1} h^{-1}, IQR 26–99) and the midazolam group (48 ug kg^{-1} h^{-1}, IQR 20–50) (**Table 1** and **Appendix 2**).

Vital Parameters

Preoperatively, HR was significantly lower in the sevoflurane group (137 bpm, IQR 126–141) compared to the midazolam group (142 bpm, IQR 138–152) (**Figure 1A**, **Appendix 3**). MABP did not differ, although the VIS was significantly lower in the sevoflurane group (0, IQR 0–5) than in the midazolam group (17, IQR 10–25). Intraoperatively, HR and MABP significantly dropped in sevoflurane group (HR: 138 bpm, IQR 132–156 and MABP: 44 mmHg, IQR42–48) compared to the midazolam group (HR: 162 bpm, IQR 153–171 and 55 mmHg, IQR 50–60). Intraoperatively, the VIS score was again significantly lower in the sevoflurane group (9, IQR 5–17) than in the midazolam group (17, IQR 12–35).

Three until 6 h postoperatively, HR remained significantly lower in the sevoflurane group (127 bpm, IQR 120–135) compared to the midazolam group (141 bpm, IQR 139–148). VIS was still significantly lower in the sevoflurane group (2, IQR 0–11) compared to the midazolam group (17, IQR 10–28).

Fifteen until 18 h postoperatively, HR remained significantly lower in the sevoflurane group (131 bpm, IQR 127–135) compared to the midazolam group (144 bpm, IQR 137–153). SpO_2 and $PaCO_2$ did not differ between the group perioperatively.

Cerebral Oxygenation

Preoperatively, $rScO_2$, FTOE and duration of cerebral hypoxia did not differ significantly between the groups (**Figure 1**).

Intraoperatively, the $rScO_2$ values were significantly higher in the sevoflurane group (84%, IQR 77–95) compared to the midazolam group (65%, IQR 59–76, $p < 0.001$). The opposite was true for FTOE, which was lower in the sevoflurane group (14%, IQR 5–21) compared to the midazolam group (31%, IQR 29–40, $p < 0.001$). The duration of hypoxia was significantly shorter in the sevoflurane group (2%, IQR 0.4–9.6) compared to the midazolam group (38.6%, IQR 4.9–70, $p = 0.023$).

Three until 6 h and 15 until 18 h postoperatively, $rScO_2$, FTOE, and the duration of cerebral hypoxia did not differ between the groups.

Cerebral Activity

Preoperatively, power in the EEG slow delta δ_1 and gamma γ frequency bands was significantly higher in the sevoflurane group (7.9 μV^2, IQR 5.5–8.6; 0.19 μV^2, IQR 0.16–0.28) compared to the midazolam group (4.1 μV^2, IQR 3.4–6.2, $p = 0.009$ vs. 0.12 μV^2, IQR 0.09–0.14, $p = 0.0017$), but not for the fast delta δ_2 frequency (2.0 μV^2, IQR 1.5–2.3 vs. 1.7 μV^2, IQR 1.4–2.5) (**Figure 1**).

Intraoperatively, slow delta δ_1, fast delta δ_2 and gamma γ power decreased in the sevoflurane group and remained decreased during the entire intraoperative period. In the midazolam group a 3-fold increase of fast delta δ_2 power was observed in the first 30 min of the surgical procedure, which decreased later on. A comparable increase was observed for the gamma γ frequency, which was characterized by a 5-fold increase (**Figure 2**). The intraoperative median values of slow delta δ_1*and* fast delta δ_2 power decreased significantly in the sevoflurane group (2.2 μV^2, IQR 1.9–3.0, 0.73 μV^2, IQR 0.59–0.91) compared to the midazolam group (4.4 μV^2, IQR 3.1–6.0, $p = 0.0002$, 1.6 μV^2, IQR 1.0–1.7, $p = <0.001$), but not for gamma γ power (0.09 μV^2, IQR 0.08–0.10, 0.10 μV^2, IQR 0.08–0.11).

Higher maximal sevoflurane concentration (end expired concentration) was not associated with lower cerebral activity (**Figure 3**). Higher maximum dosages of midazolam were associated with lower cerebral activity ($p = 0.023$) (**Figure 3**).

TABLE 1 | Patient demographics of the sevoflurane and the midazolam group.

	Sevoflurane group	Midazolam group	*p*-value
N	20	17	
Male	55% (11)	59% (10)	0.821
Gestational age (wk)	38+1 (36+5 – 38+5)	37+6 (34+5 – 38+1)	0.111
Birth weight (kg)	3.0 (2.7–3.3)	2.8 (1.9–3.1)	0.070
Apgar 5 min	8 (8,9)	8 (7-8)	0.478
o/e LHR	50 (41–58)	40 (33-54)	0.337
Preoperative mechanical ventilation (%)	85% (17)	100%	0.101
Preoperative VA-ECMO	0%	29% (5)	0.022
Intraoperative VA-ECMO	0%	0%	1.00
Left sided defect (%)	85% (17)	65% (11)	0.977
Liver-up	25% (5)	71% (12)	0.005
Age at surgery (d)	3 (2–4)	6 (3-12)	0.008
Thoracoscopy/laparotomy	40/60% (8/12)	23/77% (4/13)	0.026
Conversion	100% (8)	0%	0.002
Duration of surgery (min)	95 (70–125)	182 (114–203)	0.000
Defect size (*n*)	6A, 8B, 5C, 1D	1A, 9B, 6C,1D	0.185
Patch (%)	60% (12)	88% (15)	0.056
VIS-score preoperative	0 (0–5)$	17 (10–25)$	0.000
VIS-score intraoperative	9 (5-25)$	17 (12–35)$	0.010
VIS-score postoperative (ug/kg)	2 (0–11)$	17 (10–28)$	0.001
Rocuronium bolus dosage intraoperative (mg/kg)	0.8 (0.6–1.0)	-	
Vecoronium bolus dosage during induction (mg/kg)	-	0.2 (0.15–0.21)	
Vecoronium perfusor dosage intraoperative (mg/kg/h)	-	0.09 (0.05–0.10)	
Fentanyl bolus dosages during induction (ug/kg)	2.3 (1.7–2.9)	5 (4–7)	0.000
Cumulative fentanyl bolus dosages intraoperative (ug/kg/h)	6.2 (4.1–11.5)	10 (7–28)	0.119
Fentanyl perfusor dosages intraoperative (ug/kg/h)	-	4 (3–5)	
Sevoflurane concentration [end expired concentration (%)]	1.5 (1.1–1.9)*	-	-
Midazolam perfusor dosage preoperative (ug/kg/h)	47 (0–92)	40 (30–50)	0.735
Midazolam perfusor dosage intraoperative (ug/kg/h)	47 (0–67)	100 (68–100)	0.003
Midazolam perfusor dosage postoperative (ug/kg/h)	39 (26–99)	50 (20–50)	0.647
Midazolam bolus intraoperative (%)	5% (1)	59% (10)	0.000

$*Data presented as median (IQR) or (range).*

**Range of the mean values.*

The neonates who received a bolus of propofol had EEG delta frequency power (2.15–2.16 μV^2) comparable to the other neonates in the sevoflurane group. Three until 6 h postoperatively, the EEG slow delta δ_1, fast delta δ_2, and gamma γ frequencies increased again in the sevoflurane group (5.0 μV^2, IQR 4.2–6.0, 1.4 μV^2, IQR 1.2–1.7, 0.11 μV^2, IQR 0.10–0.13), decreased in the midazolam group (2.9 μV^2, IQR 2.4–4.8, 1.36 μV^2, IQR 0.95–1.93, 0.11 μV^2, IQR 0.08–0.13) compared to the intraoperative period.

Fifteen until 18 h postoperatively, the EEG slow delta δ_1, fast delta δ_2, and gamma γ frequencies increased further in the sevoflurane group (6.7 μV^2, IQR 5.6–7.6, 1.7 μV^2, IQR 1.5–2.4, 0.14 μV^2, IQR 0.10–0.17), increased in the midazolam group (3.1 μV^2, IQR 2.4–4.8, 1.31 μV^2, IQR 0.98–2.23, 0.13 μV^2, IQR 0.08–0.17) compared to the intraoperative period.

Correlations

Preoperative, no correlation between $rScO_2$ or FTOE and cerebral activity was observed (**Figure 4**).

Intraoperatively, a significantly ($p = 0.01$) positive correlation between $rScO_2$ and cerebral activity in the midazolam group was found (**Figure 4**). In contrast, there was no correlation between FTOE and cerebral activity. Higher maximum dosages of midazolam resulted in a significant decrease in $rScO_2$ and slow delta EEG power (**Figure 3**). The same trend was observed for maximum sevoflurane concentration, although not significant. In the sevoflurane group, $rScO_2$ was negatively correlated with VIS ($R^2 = 0.23$, $p = 0.04$) and positively correlated with FTOE ($R^2 = 0.21$, $p = 0.04$). These correlations were not found in the midazolam group.

Postoperatively, $rScO_2$ was negatively correlated with VIS ($R^2 = 0.35$, $p = 0.01$) and FTOE positively correlated with VIS (R^2

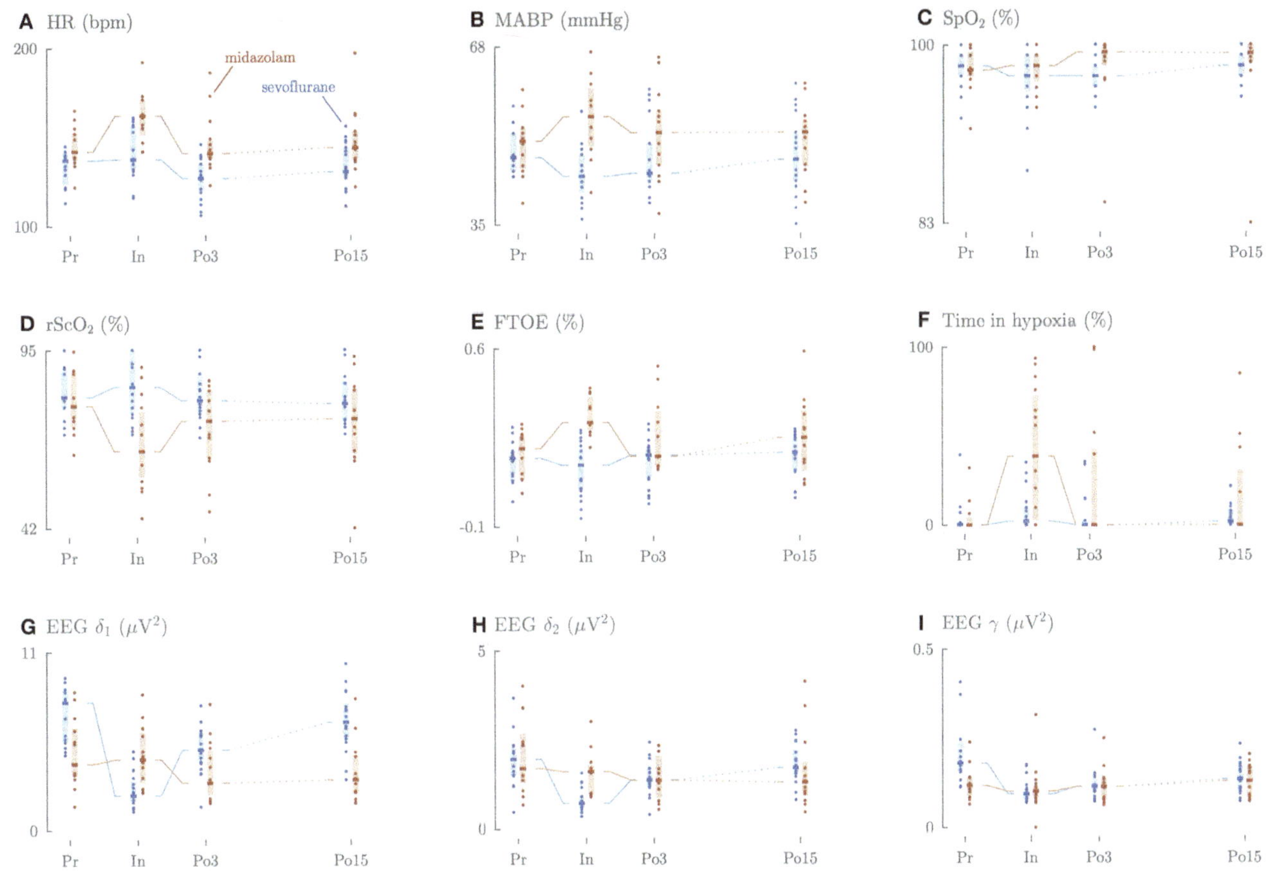

FIGURE 1 | Longitudinal overview of the perioperative changes in HR **(A)**, MABP **(B)**, SpO_2 **(C)**, rSO_2 **(D)**, FTOE **(E)**, time in hypoxia **(F)**, slow delta **(G)**, fast delta **(H)**, gamma **(I)** power.

$= 0.32$, $p = 0.001$) in the sevoflurane group, and not in the midazolam group.

DISCUSSION

In our study surgery during sevoflurane-based anesthesia resulted in stable cerebral oxygenation, decreased oxygen consumption and decreased cerebral activity. The EEG power did not indicate pain stimuli awareness. Surgery during midazolam-based anesthesia resulted in low $rScO_2$, increased cerebral oxygen consumption and increased cerebral activity throughout the first 30 min of the surgical procedure. The increased EEG power of the fast delta and the gamma band indicated conscious pain perception.

Intraoperatively, $rScO_2$ values were observed to be significantly higher in the sevoflurane group compared to the midazolam group, which reached alarmingly low $rScO_2$ values (**Figure 1**). In the sevoflurane group, we observed a stable $rScO_2$ and a decreased FTOE, despite a reduction in MABP (**Figure 1**), which is in line with a study in children between 0 and 2 years (26). In the midazolam group, a decrease in $rScO_2$ and an increase in FTOE were observed, despite an increase in MABP and HR (**Figure 1**). Vascular resistance and subsequently cerebral perfusion are affected by the partial pressure of carbon dioxide ($PaCO_2$) and by vasoactive and inotropic medication (27, 28). In this study, both groups had comparable $PaCO_2$ levels, which were stable and within clinical range. In the sevoflurane group, increased VIS was associated with lower $rScO_2$ values and higher FTOE intra- and postoperatively, which might reflect increased vascular resistance. Yet, the hemodynamic support, mostly with norepinephrine, was the highest in the midazolam group (**Table 1**), without affecting $rScO_2$ or FTOE. A recent study signals that norepinephrine elevates MABP, while reducing cerebral perfusion in adults (29). This is in line with our result in the sevoflurane group.

A recent study showed that higher sevoflurane doses significantly correlated with more suppressed background patterns (30). This correlation was not observed in our study, but this could be due to the relatively small range in sevoflurane concentrations that were administered (**Figure 3**). Overall, EEG power didn't decrease during midazolam-based anesthesia, but increased midazolam dose was found to be associated with a decrease in brain activity. The median time between bolus administration or increased perfusor dosages of midazolam and the start of surgical procedure was 21 min. During the first 30 min of surgery, a 3-fold increase in δ_2 power and a 6-fold

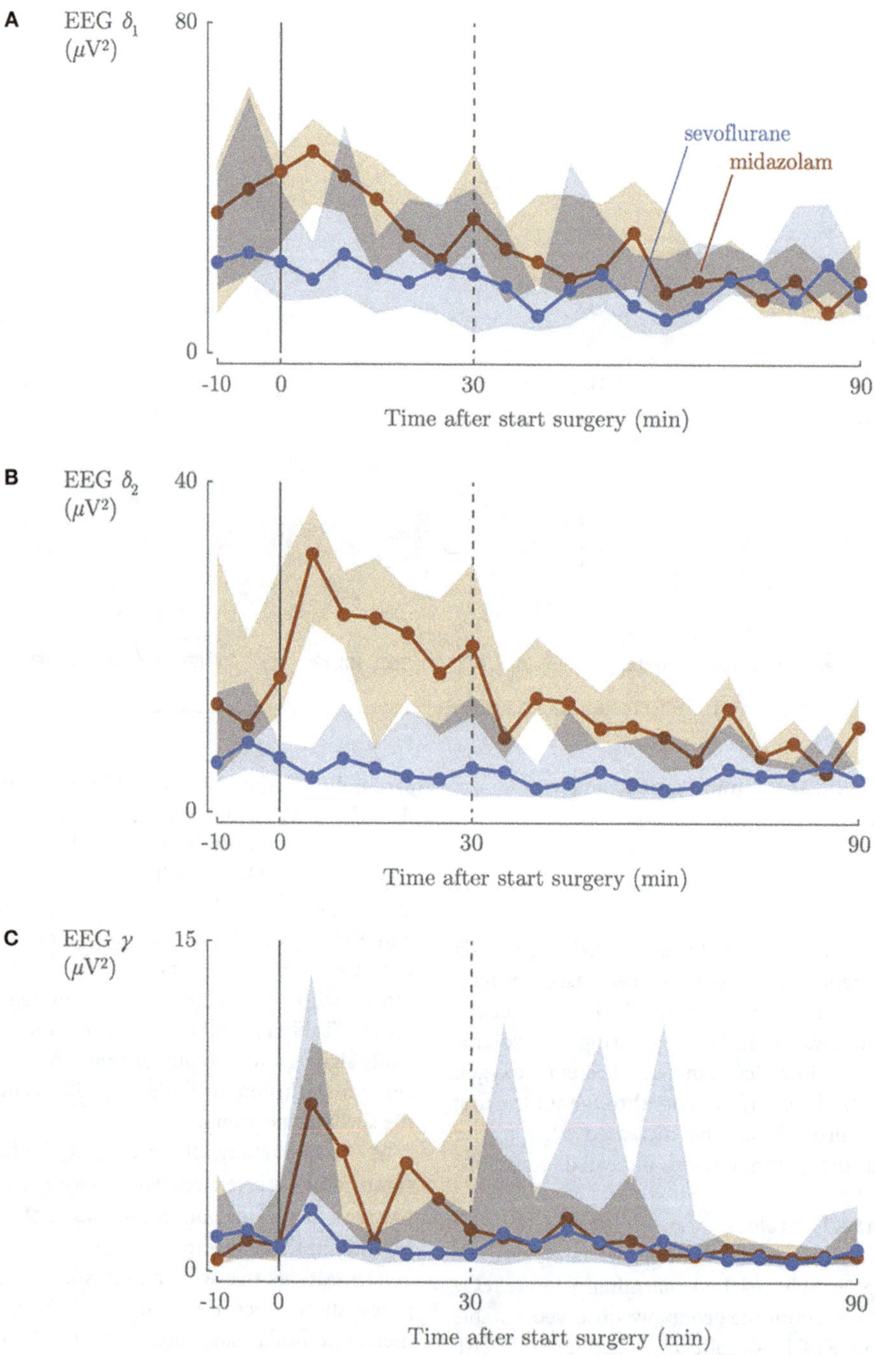

FIGURE 2 | Intraoperative cerebral activity; slow delta **(A)**, fast delta **(B)**, gamma **(C)** power. Blue, sevoflurane group; red, midazolam group; 0, start surgical procedure.

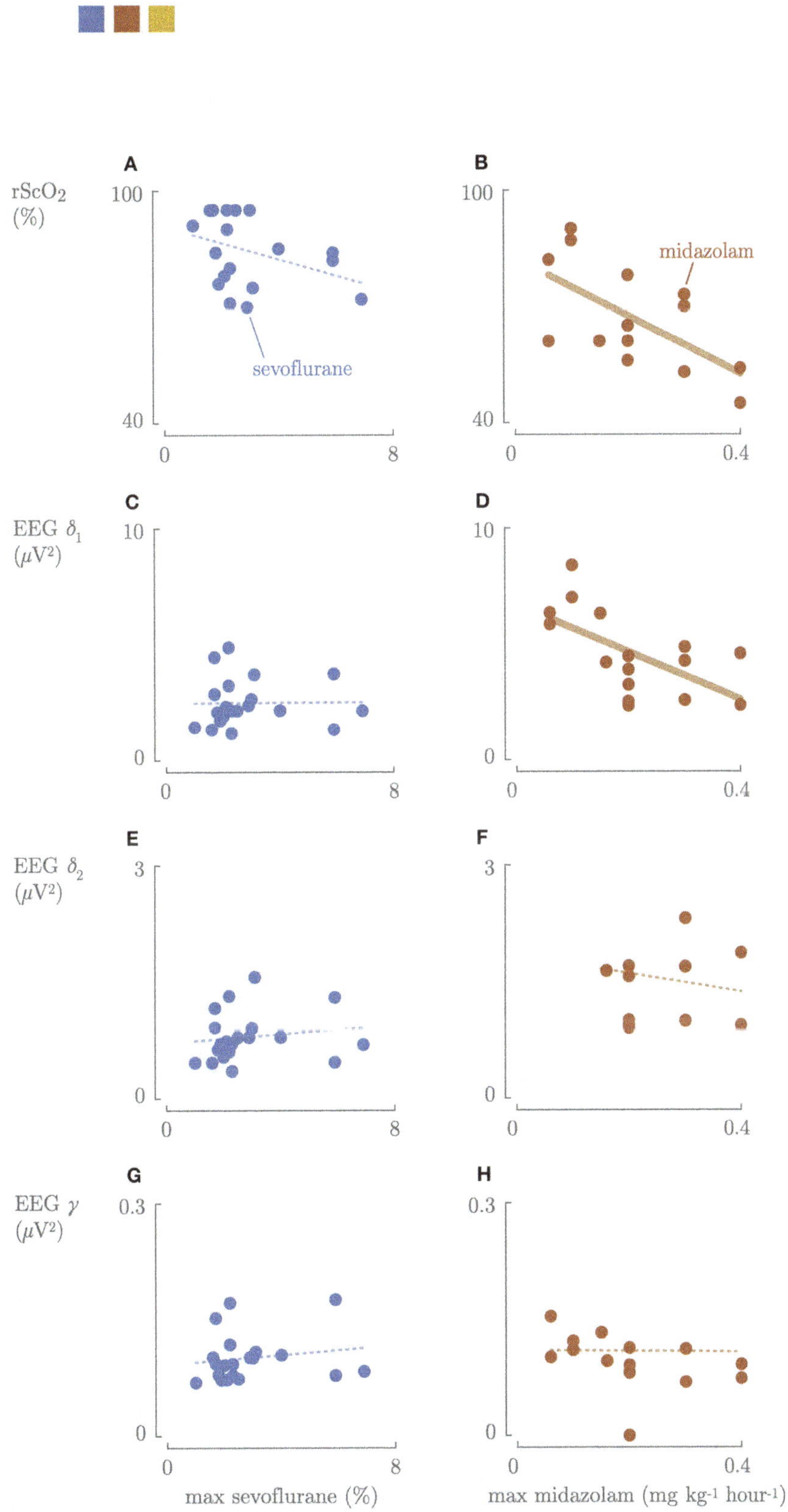

FIGURE 3 | Correlation between the maximum sevoflurane concentration or maximum dosages of midazolam cerebral oxygenation **(A,B)** and cerebral activity: slow delta **(C,D)**, fast delta **(E,F)**, gamma **(G,H)** power. Blue, sevoflurane group; red, midazolam group; fat line, significant correlation.

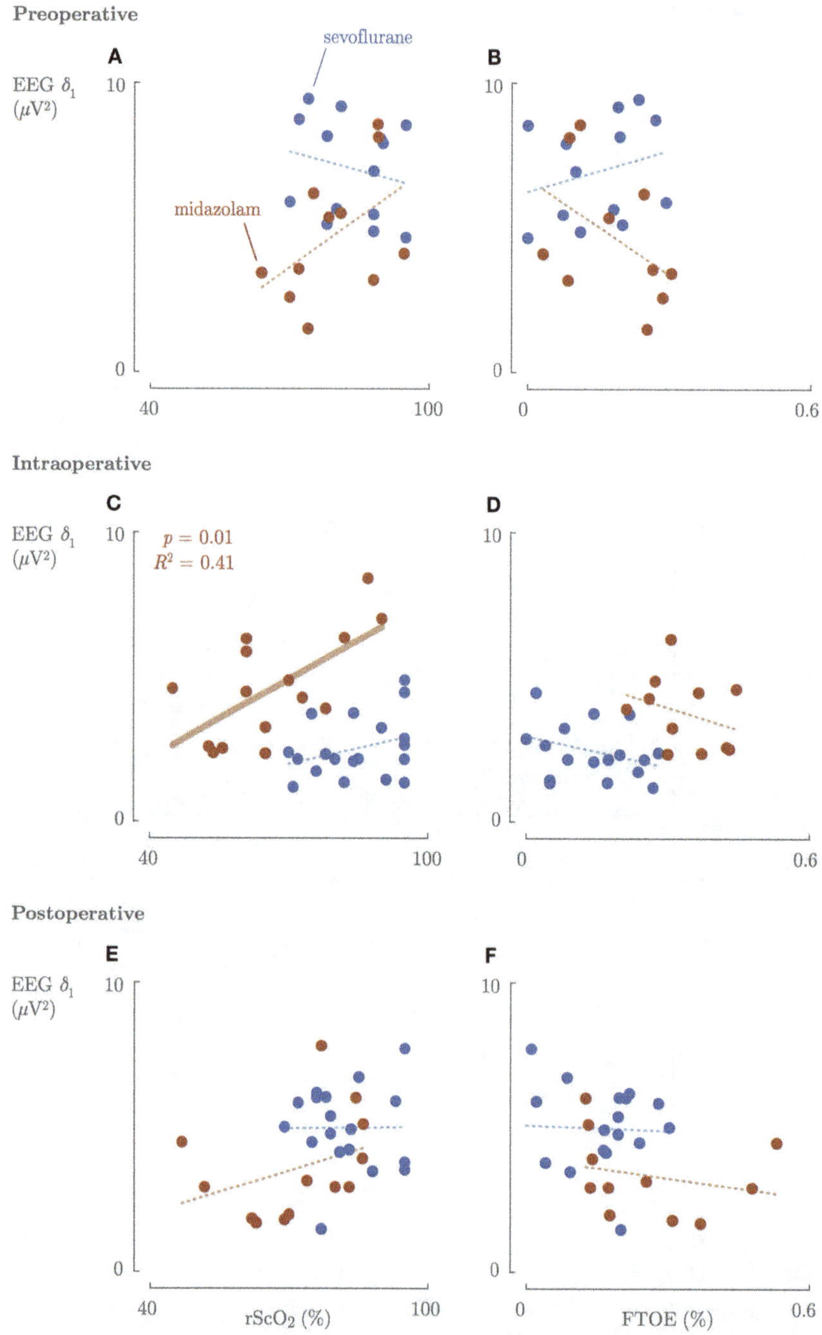

FIGURE 4 | Correlation between the cerebral activity and cerebral oxygenation and oxygen consumption preoperative **(A,B)**, intraoperative **(C,D)**, and postoperative **(E,F)**. Blue, sevoflurane group; red, midazolam group; fat line, significant correlation.

increase in gamma γ power were observed, suggesting that nociceptive stimuli were registered by the brain (**Figure 2**) (18). After 30 min, the power in the different EEG bands stabilized to lower values. This might indicate that the increase in midazolam dose requires (at least) 21 plus 30 min to reach a new steady state concentration, and/or that surgery started too soon after administering midazolam and analgesia, since cerebral activity decreased after 30 min. A loading dose helps to induce the effect quicker, although this was given in 59% of the neonates in the midazolam group.

Patients in the midazolam group received midazolam preoperatively for multiple days and had a median midazolam dosage of 0.1 mg $kg^{-1}h^{-1}$ intraoperatively. This is substantially higher than the dosing advice of 0.06 mg $kg^{-1}h^{-1}$ for sedation with midazolam in neonates with a gestational age above 32 weeks (31), although this dosing advice was already questioned by our research group (32). The elimination half-life of midazolam is ∼6 h in the 1st week of life in full-term neonates (33), although severity of disease and inflammation may also affect the elimination of midazolam in critically ill neonates (34). A recent Cochrane review concluded that midazolam was an effective sedative in neonates (35), although transient cerebral hypoperfusion was observed after a bolus of midazolam, as well as significant higher rates of adverse neurological events in neonates treated with midazolam compared to morphine (36, 37). In this study, neonates in the midazolam group all received continuous administration of fentanyl. Single use of fentanyl dosages of 50–100 ug kg^{-1} is a commonly used anesthetic approach during congenital cardiac surgery or if the neonate has limited hemodynamic reserve (38). A randomized trial in 1987 already proved the additional value of fentanyl in the stress response of neonates intraoperatively (39). Another study compared the effect of fentanyl with fentanyl plus midazolam on stress response during neonatal cardiac surgery, and concluded that intraoperative administration of fentanyl plus midazolam did not reduce stress response compared fentanyl (38). This suggests that high doses of fentanyl might be a better anesthetic approach than midazolam with lower dosages of fentanyl.

The strengths of this study are that both centers have long-lasting experience treating high-risk CDH patients and have acted as "founding fathers" for well-established international guidelines. In addition, neither the treatment modalities, nor the composition of the treatment teams changed during the study period. Both centers used validated pain assessment instruments (Comfort-B) as pharmacodynamic endpoint to evaluate and treat pain.

This study has two main limitations. First, exposure to medication was compared based on administered dosages instead of plasma concentrations, following the strict rules on blood sampling in neonates. Second, this is a center comparison study and not a randomized controlled trial. In this study, the neonates in the midazolam group were more critically ill. The neonates in the midazolam group were operated in the NICU, partly because of the preference of the clinicians and partly because of cardiorespiratory instability of the patient. In this group, the defect of the diaphragm was more severe (more patient with a herniated liver) and the neonates in this group needed more hemodynamic support preoperatively (higher VIS). Intraoperatively, however, the hemodynamic support did not differ between the midazolam and the sevoflurane group. In addition, we found a negative correlation between $rScO_2$ and VIS and a positive correlation between $rScO_2$ and FTOE in the sevoflurane group and not in the midazolam group. Furthermore, more critically ill patients may have a longer elimination time of midazolam.

CONCLUSION

This comparison of two approaches for CDH surgery showed that sevoflurane-based anesthesia resulted in increased cerebral oxygenation and decreased cerebral activity, suggesting adequate anesthesia. Midazolam-based anesthesia in neonates with a more severe CDH (more liver-up and higher VIS) led to alarmingly low $rScO_2$ values, below hypoxia threshold, and increased values of EEG power during the first 30 min of surgery. This might indicate conscious experience of pain.

These results stimulate the integration of population-pharmacokinetic models in combination with multimodal neuromonitoring to reach evidence-based perioperative pharmacotherapy in these vulnerable patients.

AUTHOR CONTRIBUTIONS

SC and DH: substantial contributions to the conception or design of the work, the acquisition, analysis, interpretation of data for the work, drafting the work, final approval of the version to be published, and agreed to be accountable for all aspects of the work in ensuring that questions related to the accuracy or integrity of any part of the work are appropriately investigated and resolved. JI, KZ, AP-O, SV, RF, AC, RW, LW, JG, DT, and GN: substantial contributions to the conception and design of the work, analysis, interpretation of data for the work, revising it critically for important intellectual content, final approval of the version to be published, and agreed to be accountable for all aspects of the work in ensuring that questions related to the accuracy or integrity of any part of the work are appropriately investigated and resolved. All authors contributed to the article and approved the submitted version.

FUNDING

Research supported by Bijzonder Onderzoeksfonds KU Leuven (BOF): C24/15/036. The effect of perinatal stress on the later outcome in preterm babies, EU: H2020 MSCA-ITN-2018: Integrating Functional Assessment measures for Neonatal Safeguard (INFANS), funded by the European Commission under Grant Agreement #813483. This research received funding from the Flemish Government (AI Research Program). SV and DH are affiliated to Leuven. AI—KU Leuven Institute for AI, B-3000, Leuven, Belgium. DH was a SB Ph.D. fellow at Fonds voor Wetenschappelijk Onderzoek (FWO), Vlaanderen, supported by the Flemish government.

ACKNOWLEDGMENTS

This project was performed by three centers of ERNICA (European Reference Network of Inherited and Congenital Anomalies). We would like to thank Dr. Leo van Wolfswinkel (MD, department of pediatric anaesthesiology, University Medical Center Utrecht, The Netherlands) for providing the Anstat software which made the data collection in Mannheim possible.

REFERENCES

1. Madderom MJ, Toussaint L, van der Cammen-van Zijp MH, Gischler SJ, Wijnen RM, Tibboel D, et al. Congenital diaphragmatic hernia with(out) ECMO: impaired development at 8 years. *Arch Dis Child Fetal Neonatal Ed.* (2013) 98:F316–22. doi: 10.1136/archdischild-2012-303020
2. Stolwijk LJ, Lemmers PM, Harmsen M, Groenendaal F, de Vries LS, van der Zee DC, et al. Neurodevelopmental outcomes after neonatal surgery for major noncardiac anomalies. *Pediatrics.* (2016) 137:e20151728. doi: 10.1542/peds.2015-1728
3. Leeuwen L, Schiller RM, Rietman AB, Van Rosmalen J, Wildschut ED, Houmes RJM, et al. Risk factors of impaired neuropsychologic outcome in school-Aged survivors of neonatal critical illness. *Crit Care Med.* (2018) 46:401–10. doi: 10.1097/CCM.0000000000002869
4. Stolwijk LJ, Keunen K, de Vries LS, Groenendaal F, van der Zee DC, van Herwaarden MYA, et al. Neonatal surgery for noncardiac congenital anomalies: neonates at risk of brain injury. *J Pediatr.* (2017) 182:335–41.e1. doi: 10.1016/j.jpeds.2016.11.080
5. Costerus S, van Hoorn C, Hendrikx D, Kortenbout J, Hunfeld M, Vlot J, et al. Towards integrative neuromonitoring of the surgical newborn: a systematic review. *Eur J Anaesthesiol.* (2020) 37:701–12. doi: 10.1097/EJA.0000000000001218
6. Dix LML, van Bel F, Lemmers PMA. Monitoring cerebral oxygenation in neonates: an update. *Front Pediatr.* (2017) 5:46. doi: 10.3389/fped.2017.00046
7. Sorensen LC, Leung TS, Greisen G. Comparison of cerebral oxygen saturation in premature infants by near-infrared spatially resolved spectroscopy: observations on probe-dependent bias. *J Biomed Opt.* (2008) 13:064013. doi: 10.1117/1.3013454
8. Kishi K, Kawaguchi M, Yoshitani K, Nagahata T, Furuya H. Influence of patient variables and sensor location on regional cerebral oxygen saturation measured by INVOS 4100 near-infrared spectrophotometers. *J Neurosurg Anesthesiol.* (2003) 15:302–6. doi: 10.1097/00008506-200310000-00002
9. Kleiser S, Ostojic D, Nasseri N, Isler H, Bucher HU, Bassler D, et al. *In vivo* precision assessment of a near-infrared spectroscopy-based tissue oximeter (OxyPrem v13) in neonates considering systemic hemodynamic fluctuations. *J Biomed Opt.* (2018) 23:1–10. doi: 10.1117/1.JBO.23.6.067003
10. Kleiser S, Ostojic D, Andresen B, Nasseri N, Isler H, Scholkmann F, et al. Comparison of tissue oximeters on a liquid phantom with adjustable optical properties: an extension. *Biomed Opt Express.* (2018) 9:86–101. doi: 10.1364/BOE.9.000086
11. Kleiser S, Nasseri N, Andresen B, Greisen G, Wolf M. Comparison of tissue oximeters on a liquid phantom with adjustable optical properties. *Biomed Opt Express.* (2016) 7:2973–92. doi: 10.1364/BOE.7.002973
12. Alderliesten T, Dix L, Baerts W, Caicedo A, van Huffel S, Naulaers G, et al. Reference values of regional cerebral oxygen saturation during the first 3 days of life in preterm neonates. *Pediatr Res.* (2016) 79:55–64. doi: 10.1038/pr.2015.186
13. Naulaers G, Meyns B, Miserez M, Leunens V, Van Huffel S, Casaer P, et al. Use of tissue oxygenation index and fractional tissue oxygen extraction as non-invasive parameters for cerebral oxygenation: a validation study in piglets. *Neonatology.* (2007) 92:120–6. doi: 10.1159/000101063
14. Aly SA, Zurakowski D, Glass P, Skurow-Todd K, Jonas RA, Donofrio MT. Cerebral tissue oxygenation index and lactate at 24 hours postoperative predict survival and neurodevelopmental outcome after neonatal cardiac surgery. *Congenit Hear Dis.* (2017) 12:188–95. doi: 10.1111/chd.12426
15. Britton JW, Frey LC, Hopp JL, Korb P, Koubeissi MZ, Lievens WE, et al. *Electroencephalography (EEG): An Introductory Text and Atlas of Normal and Abnormal Findings in Adults, Children, and Infants.* Chicago, IL: American Epilepsy Society (2016).
16. Bruns N, Blumenthal S, Meyer I, Klose-Verschuur S, Felderhoff-Müser U, Müller H. Application of an amplitude-integrated EEG monitor (cerebral function monitor) to neonates. *J Vis Exp.* (2017) 6:55985. doi: 10.3791/55985
17. Knyazev GG. EEG delta oscillations as a correlate of basic homeostatic and motivational processes. *Neurosci Biobehav Rev.* (2012) 10:2. doi: 10.1016/j.neubiorev.2011.10.002
18. Fabrizi L, Verriotis M, Williams G, Lee A, Meek J, Olhede S, et al. Encoding of mechanical nociception differs in the adult and infant brain. *Sci Rep.* (2016) 6:28642. doi: 10.1038/srep28642
19. Cornelissen L, Kim SE, Lee JM, Brown EN, Purdon PL, Berde CB. Electroencephalographic markers of brain development during sevoflurane anaesthesia in children up to 3 years old. *Br J Anaesth.* (2018) 120:1274–86. doi: 10.1016/j.bja.2018.01.037
20. Snoek KG, Reiss IK, Greenough A, Capolupo I, Urlesberger B, Wessel L, et al. Standardized postnatal management of infants with congenital diaphragmatic Hernia in Europe: the CDH EURO consortium consensus - 2015 update. *Neonatology.* (2016) 110:66–74. doi: 10.1159/000444210
21. Lally KP, Lasky RE, Lally PA, Bagolan P, Davis CF, Frenckner BP, et al. Standardized reporting for congenital diaphragmatic hernia - an international consensus. *J Pediatr Surg.* (2013) 48:2408–15. doi: 10.1016/j.jpedsurg.2013.08.014
22. Gaies MG, Gurney JG, Yen AH, Napoli ML, Gajarski RJ, Ohye RG, et al. Vasoactive-inotropic score as a predictor of morbidity and mortality in infants after cardiopulmonary bypass. *Pediatr Crit Care Med.* (2010) 11:234–2348. doi: 10.1097/PCC.0b013e3181b806fc
23. Iatsenko D, McClintock PVE, Stefanovska A. Extraction of instantaneous frequencies from ridges in time-frequency representations of signals. *Signal Processing.* (2016) 1:24. doi: 10.1016/j.sigpro.2016.01.024
24. Akaike H. Akaike's information criterion. In: *International Encyclopedia of Statistical Science*, (eds) Lovric M. (Berlin, Heidelberg: Springer). doi: 10.1007/978-3-642-04898-2_110
25. R Core Team. A language and environment for statistical computing. *R Found Stat Comput.* (2018).
26. Rhondali O, Juhel S, Mathews S, Cellier Q, Desgranges FP, Mahr A, et al. Impact of sevoflurane anesthesia on brain oxygenation in children younger than 2 years. *Paediatr Anaesth.* (2014) 24:734–40. doi: 10.1111/pan.12397
27. McCann ME, Schouten ANJ. Beyond survival; influences of blood pressure, cerebral perfusion and anesthesia on neurodevelopment. *Paediatr Anaesth.* (2014) 24:68–73. doi: 10.1111/pan.12310
28. Greisen G. Autoregulation of cerebral blood flow in newborn babies. *Early Hum Dev.* (2005) 81:423–8. doi: 10.1016/j.earlhumdev.2005.03.005
29. Thorup L, Koch KU, Upton RN, Østergaard L, Rasmussen M. Effects of vasopressors on cerebral circulation and oxygenation: a narrative review of pharmacodynamics in health and traumatic brain injury. *J Neurosurg Anesthesiol.* (2020) 32:18–28. doi: 10.1097/ANA.0000000000000596
30. Stolwijk LJ, Weeke LC, De Vries LS, Van Herwaarden MYA, Van Der Zee DC, Van Der Werff DBM, et al. Effect of general anesthesia on neonatal aEEG — a cohort study of patients with non-cardiac congenital anomalies. *PLoS ONE.* (2017) 12:183581. doi: 10.1371/journal.pone.0183581
31. www.geneesmiddeleninformatiebank.nl. *Midazolam 5 mg/ml-actualisatie-SPC-07-2018.* (2020). Available online at: https://www.geneesmiddeleninformatiebank.nl/smpc/h22596_smpc.pdf (accessed September 4, 2021).
32. Völler S, Flint RB, Beggah F, Reiss I, Andriessen P, Zimmermann LJI, et al. Recently registered midazolam doses for preterm neonates do not lead to equal exposure: a population pharmacokinetic model. *J Clin Pharmacol.* (2019) 59:1300–8. doi: 10.1002/jcph.1429
33. Burtin P, Jacqz-Aigrain E, Girard P, Lenclen R, Magny JF, Betremieux P, et al. Population pharmacokinetics of midazolam in neonates. *Clin Pharmacol Ther.* (1994) 56:615–25. doi: 10.1038/clpt.1994.186
34. Pacifici GM. Clinical pharmacology of midazolam in neonates and children: effect of disease—a review. *Int J Pediatr.* (2014) 2014:309342. doi: 10.1155/2014/309342
35. Ng E, Taddio A, Ohlsson A. Intravenous midazolam infusion for sedation of infants in the neonatal intensive care unit. *Cochrane Database Syst Rev.* (2017) 1:CD002052. doi: 10.1002/14651858.CD002052.pub3
36. Harte GJ, Gray PH, Lee TC, Steer PA, Charles BG. Haemodynamic responses and population pharmacokinetics of midazolam following administration to ventilated, preterm neonates. *J Paediatr Child Health.* (1997) 33:335–8. doi: 10.1111/j.1440-1754.1997.tb01611.x
37. van Straaten HLM, Rademaker CMA, de Vries LS. Comparison of the effect of midazolam or vecuronium on blood pressure and cerebral blood flow velocity in the premature newborn. *Dev Pharmacol Ther.* (1992) 19:191–5. doi: 10.1159/000457484

38. Gruber EM, Laussen PC, Casta A, Andrew Zimmerman A, Zurakowski D, Reid R, et al. Stress response in infants undergoing cardiac surgery: a randomized study of fentanyl bolus, fentanyl infusion, and fentanyl-midazolam infusion. *Anesth Analg.* (2001) 92:882–90. doi: 10.1097/00000539-200104000-00016
39. Anand KJS, Sippell WG, Aynsley-Green A. Randomised trial of fentanyl anaesthesia in preterm babies undergoing surgery: effects on the stress response. *Lancet.* (1987) 1:62–6. doi: 10.1016/S0140-6736(87)91907-6

20

Transumbilical Single-Site Laparoscopic Intraperitoneal Closure of the Internal Inguinal Ring for Pediatric Inguinal Hernia

Yi Ji [1†], Yanan Li [1†], Xuepeng Zhang [1], Tong Qiu [1], Siyuan Chen [2] and Zhicheng Xu [1]*

[1] Department of Pediatric Surgery, West China Hospital of Sichuan University, Chengdu, China, [2] Pediatric Intensive Care Unit, Department of Critical Care Medicine, West China Hospital of Sichuan University, Chengdu, China

***Correspondence:**
Zhicheng Xu
xzcxewk@163.com

Background: A new novel technique for pediatric inguinal hernia (PIH) repair, namely, transumbilical single-site laparoscopic intraperitoneal closure (TUSLIC) of the internal inguinal ring (IIR) with a single instrument, was introduced. The short-term follow-up of TUSLIC for PIH was compared with that of transabdominal multiple-site laparoscopic extraperitoneal closure (TAMLEC) for PIH.

Methods: Descriptive variables, perioperative clinical features, and short-term outcomes were retrospectively analyzed and compared between the patients who underwent TUSLIC and those who underwent TAMLEC.

Results: In total, 289 patients were enrolled in this study. Of these, 190 patients received TUSLIC, and 99 patients received TAMLEC. The descriptive variables (including sex, age, weight, and preoperative diagnosis of patients) were comparable between the two groups (P-values were 0.12, 0.71, 0.69, and 0.23, respectively). The mean operative times for unilateral hernia repair and bilateral hernia repairs in TAMLEC group were significantly less than those in TUSLIC group ($P < 0.01$). The values of surgical site infection, umbilical bleeding, testicular atrophy, iatrogenic ascent of the testis, and secondary hydrocele were not significantly different between the two groups. There were no suture granulomas, and recurrence occurred in TUSLIC group, though at a significantly lower rate than in TAMLEC group ($P < 0.05$).

Conclusions: TUSLIC is a feasible, safe, and reliable minimally invasive method for PIH. Compared with TAMLEC, TUSLIC has the advantages of minimized complications and a low recurrence rate.

Keywords: pediatric inguinal hernia, transumbilical laparoscopic herniorrhaphy, internal inguinal ring, follow-up, outcomes

INTRODUCTION

The laparoscopic pediatric herniorrhaphy (LPH) operation was first described by Montupet in 1993 using a purse-string suture technique, in which the internal inguinal ring (IIR) was closed with nonabsorbable threads (1, 2). The method of laparoscopic percutaneous extraperitoneal closure of IIR, as introduced by Takehara, is one of the simplest and most reliable operations for pediatric inguinal hernia (PIH) (3). Conventional laparoscopic suturing procedures required three ports. These procedures are technically challenging and were not easily performed even by experienced pediatric surgeons (4).

The procedure of transabdominal multiple-site laparoscopic extraperitoneal closure (TAMLEC) of IIR has been developed for PIH repairs. However, extraperitoneal hernia sac ligation and knot burial subcutaneously in the management of TAMLEC have resulted in some complications, such as stitch sinus, infection, granuloma, and puckering of the skin. In addition, recurrent PIHs may occur due to loose sutures, which slowly cut through muscle tissue, especially in obese children with thick abdominal walls (5, 6). Recently, the percutaneous internal ring suturing (PIRS) requiring only a single umbilical port is used for pediatric inguinal hernia repair (3, 7–10). PIRS is technically easy with a short learning curve (11, 12). PIRS has satisfactory cosmesis and the advantage of identifying the patency of the contralateral processus vaginalis. However, it has been reported that PIRS had relatively higher rates of postoperative complications and recurrence (13). In the present study, we have established a new approach for PIH repair: transumbilical single-site laparoscopic intraperitoneal closure (TUSLIC) of IIR with a single instrument. In this study, we will present this new novel procedure of TUSLIC and analyze our initial experiences.

MATERIALS AND METHODS

Design and Study Population

This was a retrospective study of patients with PIH who underwent TUSLIC and TAMLEC between January 2020 and January 2021. Institutional review board approval for this retrospective case series was obtained at West China Hospital of Sichuan University. The inclusion criteria were as follows: patients age of 0–14 years and presence of clinically confirmed groin hernia (by ultrasonography examination); patients had received either TUSLIC or TAMLEC. The exclusion criteria were: patients with comorbidities, including Hirschsprung's disease (HD), abdominal tumors, and cryptorchidism. Patients' parents were given the option to choose the treatment (either TUSLIC or TAMLEC). The patients' parents or guardians gave written, informed consent.

Study Outcomes

Descriptive variables, perioperative clinical features, and short-term outcomes were analyzed and compared between the patients with TUSLIC and patients with TAMLEC. The primary outcome of this study was recurrence. Secondary outcomes included intraoperative and postoperative complications, conversions to open surgery, and operative time (ORT). We hypothesized that patients receiving TUSLIC might have less recurrence and postoperative complications than those receiving TAMLEC.

Abbreviations: PIH, pediatric inguinal hernia; TUSLIC, transumbilical single-site laparoscopic intraperitoneal closure; IIR, internal inguinal ring; TAMLEC, transabdominal multiple-site laparoscopic extraperitoneal closure; LPH, laparoscopic pediatric herniorrhaphy; HD, Hirschsprung's disease; PPV, potent processus vaginalis; ORT, operative time; SSI, surgical site infection; SD, standard deviation; 2-DGA, 2-dimensional gripping angle.

Surgical Technique

The Procedure of TAMLEC

In the TAMLEC procedure, the patient was placed in a supine position with a monitor at the patient's feet. The operator stood on the opposite side of the inguinal hernia, and the camera assistant stood on the other side. A 5 mm incision was made through the center of the umbilicus with the open Hasson technique (14) to establish the pneumoperitoneum at a pressure of 6–8 mmHg with a flow rate of 3–6 L/min. A 5 mm trocar and a 30° laparoscope were introduced into the peritoneal cavity. Then, a second 3 mm incision was made for direct insertion of a 3 mm grasper without a trocar at the intersection point between the anterior midline and the level of 2.0–4.0 cm distal to the umbilicus.

Laparoscopy was started by inspection of the pelvis and bilateral IIRs. A modified Kirschner wire with a single 2–0 non-absorbable thread was introduced vertically through a 2 mm eyelet at the surface projection of IIR to the preperitoneal space, in which the ilioinguinal nerve, as well as penetration of the peritoneum, were avoided. With the help of a 3 mm grasper traction on the peritoneum, the Kirschner wire easily traversed the epigastric vein and vas deferens in males beneath the peritoneum along the medial and inferior border of the IIR. The peritoneum was pierced medially by the wire, and the loop end of the thread was left intraperitoneally with the other end outside the abdomen when the wire was pulled out of body. Subsequently, the wire with another single 2–0 non-absorbable thread was inserted through the previous eyelet again, guided under the peritoneum of the superior and lateral border of the IIR, advanced over the spermatic cord vessels, and then pierced into the peritoneum where the loop end of the suture was left before. The end of the loop thread was placed through the loop at the tip of the Kirschner wire using a 3 mm grasper, after which the end of the double threads was pulled out by withdrawing the wire, the hernia sac was highly ligated extraperitoneally by tying both corresponding threads tightly, and the knots were buried subcutaneously.

If a contralateral potent processus vaginalis (PPV) was present, the TAMLEC procedure was repeated immediately without additional trocars and incisions. Finally, all the instruments were removed, the abdomen was desufflated, and the incisions (three in unilateral repair, four in bilateral repairs) over the abdominal wall were closed and covered with adhesive paper strips. In patients with hydrocele, the hydrocele was punctured from the scrotum.

The Procedure of TUSLIC

In the TUSLIC procedure, the patient was placed in a supine position with a monitor at the patient's feet. The surgeon stood on the head side of the patient. A 5 mm incision was made through the left rim of the umbilical ring with the open Hasson technique to establish pneumoperitoneum at a pressure of 6–8 mmHg with a flow rate of 3–6 L/min (**Figure 1**). A 5 mm trocar and a 30° laparoscope were introduced into the peritoneal cavity.

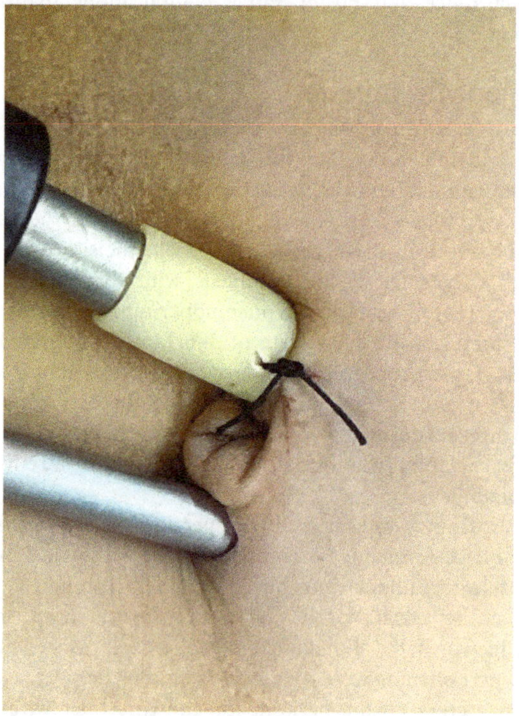

FIGURE 1 | A 5 mm trocar and a 30° laparoscope were introduced into the peritoneal cavity through the left rim of the umbilical ring with the open Hasson technique. Another 3.0 mm incision was made for placement of the 3 mm laparoscopic needle holder or scissors at the right rim of the umbilical ring without a trocar.

A

B

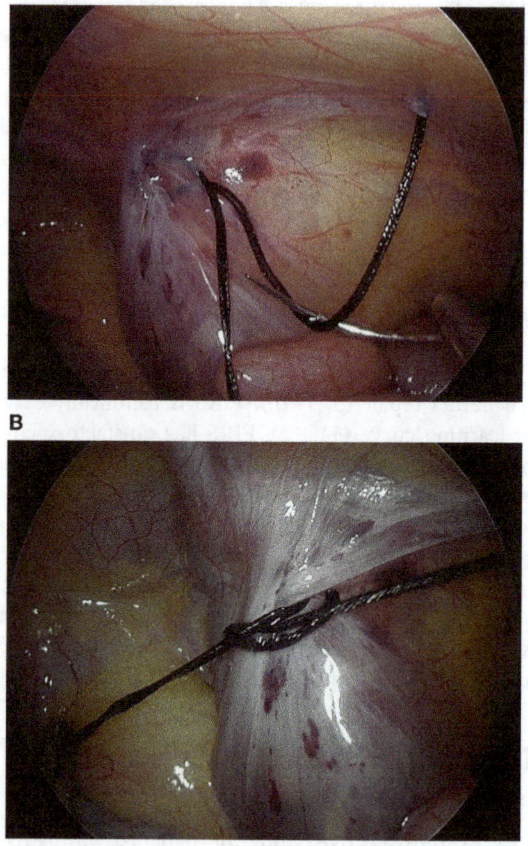

FIGURE 2 | The tip of the short end of the threads was grasped by a needle holder and rotated 360° either under or above the long limb of the thread, forming a loop that was passed through the first loop **(A)**. The loop was pushed in a downward and medial direction to the pelvic cavity, while the long end of the double threads outside the body was pulled upward **(B)**.

A second 3 mm incision was made for placement of the working instrument at the right rim of the umbilical ring without a trocar.

Laparoscopy was started by inspection of the pelvis and both IIRs. An 18-G vascular catheter was pierced into the preperitoneal space between the peritoneum and the structures of the vas deferens. The spermatic cord in males was expanded with 1–5 ml saline solution. The needle with double 2–0 braided polyester threads punctured the body surface from the outside at the right or left lower quadrant into the peritoneal cavity, 2 cm above and lateral to the IIR, leaving one end of the double threads outside the abdominal wall. Under direct vision, the needle was driven to pierce the peritoneum at 5 o'clock for the beginning point of suture, advanced carefully in front of the spermatic cord vessels and vas deferens, beneath the peritoneum along the inferior margin of IIR, and pulled out of the peritoneum at 7 o'clock. Then, the needle was manipulated headward and reinserted into the preperitoneal space at 7 o'clock, guided along the medial, superior, and lateral margins of the IIR, passed over the inferior epigastric vein, and then drawn from the previous peritoneum hole at 5 o'clock. If the opening of the IIR was large, more steps were carried out to ensure the uninterrupted circle seam surrounding the IIR.

Once the circular seam around the IIR was completely established without any skip areas, the long end of the double threads was held outside of the abdomen by the surgeon's left hand. The tip of the short end of the double threads was grasped and rotated 360 degrees either under or above the long limb of the

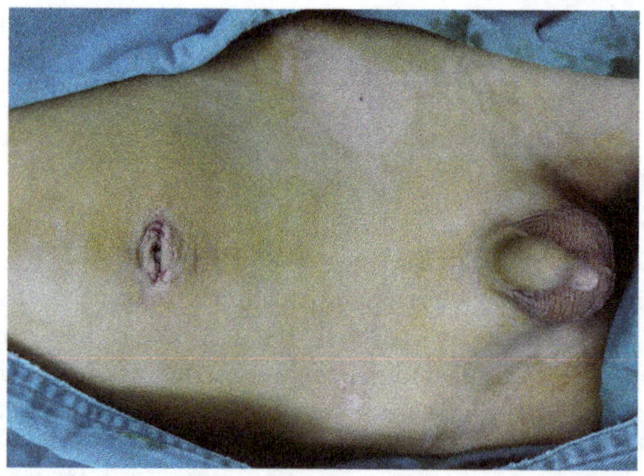

FIGURE 3 | The 5 and 3 mm incisions on the bilateral rims of the umbilical ring were closed. The puncture holes in the abdominal wall that were formed by the needle were left open without a dressing.

TABLE 1 | Data of the descriptive variables and perioperative features of the two groups.

Patients (*N*)	TUSLIC group (190)	TAMLEC group (99)	*P*
Sex (male/*N*)	0.88	0.82	0.12†
Age (months)			
Mean (SD)	30.5 ± 24.6	29.4 ± 21.8	0.71#
Median (IQR)	26.3 (19.2–35.6)	26.1 (18.4–33.9)	
Body weight (kg)			
Mean (SD)	16.7 ± 8.4	15.8 ± 13.1	0.69#
Median (IQR)	13.6 (11.5–17.0)	12.9 (11.2–16.6)	
Preoperative diagnosis			
Left	59	24	0.23†
Right	108	59	0.65†
Bilateral	23	16	0.34†
Unilateral:bilateral repairs	92:88	55:44	0.25†
ORT (unilateral) (min)	18.8 ± 4.8	12.2 ± 2.1	<0.01
ORT (bilateral) (min)	29.9 ± 5.6	21.5 ± 2.6	<0.01‡
Contralateral PPV (*N*)	65	28	0.31‡
Conversion (*N*)	0	0	1.0§

TUSLIC, transumbilical single-site laparoscopic intraperitoneal closure; TAMLEC, transabdominal multiple-site laparoscopic extraperitoneal closure; ORT, operative time; PPV, patent processus vaginalis; min, minutes; SD, standard deviation; IQR, interquartile range.

† *P-value was calculated using the chi-square test.*

P-value was calculated using the Mann–Whitney U-test.

‡ *P-value was calculated using an independent sample Student's t-test.*

§ *P-value was calculated with Fisher's exact test.*

TABLE 2 | Short-term follow-up data compared between the two groups.

Patients (*N*)	TUSLIC group (190)	TAMLEC group (99)	*P*
SSI (*N*)	2	0	0.31†
Umbilical bleeding	3	0	0.21†
Testicular atrophy (*N*)	0	0	N/A
Iatrogenic ascent of the testis	0	0	N/A
Secondary hydrocele (*N*)	0	1	0.17†
Suture granuloma (*N*)	0	4	0.01†
Recurrence (*N*)	0	3	0.04†
Follow-up (m)	9.8 ± 3.4	9.6 ± 3.2	0.81‡

TUSLIC, transumbilical single-site laparoscopic intraperitoneal closure; TAMLEC, transabdominal multiple-site laparoscopic extraperitoneal closure; SSI, surgical site infection; m, month; N/A, data not available.

† *P-value was calculated with Fisher's exact test.*

‡ *P-value was calculated using an independent sample Student's t-test.*

double threads, forming a loop (**Figure 2A**), which was passed through that loop and circulated twice around the long limb to make a surgeon's knot. The short end of the double threads was pushed in a downward and medial direction to the pelvic cavity, while the long end of the double threads was pulled upward (**Figure 2B**), which was repeated as above 2–3 times to form a locking knot. All threads were cut off, and a 5 mm long stump of the knot was left.

If a contralateral PPV was present, the TUSLIC procedure was performed simultaneously without additional trocars or incisions. Finally, all the instruments were removed, and the incisions at the bilateral rim of the umbilical ring were closed (**Figure 3**) and covered with adhesive paper strips. The puncture holes on the abdominal wall in the right or left lower quadrant were left open without dressing. In patients with hydrocele, the hydrocele was punctured from the scrotum.

Data Collection and Statistical Analysis

Patients were analyzed for their descriptive variables and perioperative clinical features (age at operation, sex, body weight, preoperative diagnosis, ORT, unilateral: bilateral repairs, contralateral PPV, and conversion) by reviewing their medical charts. The follow-up data, including the level of surgical site infection (SSI), umbilical bleeding, testicular atrophy, iatrogenic ascent of the testis, secondary hydrocele, suture granuloma, and recurrences, were collected at the last visit to our outpatient clinic according to the medical files.

Independent sample Student's t-tests (or Mann–Whitney U-test) and chi-squared tests (or Fisher's exact test) were used to compare continuous and categorical descriptive variables, respectively. The results are expressed as the mean with standard deviation (SD) or median with interquartile range. The software applied for statistical calculation was IBM SPSS 22.0 for Windows 10.0 (IBM Corp.). A P of <0.05 was considered statistically significant.

RESULTS

Data on Descriptive Variables and Perioperative Clinical Features

There were 299 patients with PIH under 14 years of age who underwent TUSLIC and TAMLEC between January 2020 and January 2021. Among them, 10 patients were excluded from the study because of combined comorbidities (four patients had HD, three patients had retroperitoneal lymphangioma, two patients had oval cystic teratoma, and one patient had cryptorchidism). The remaining 289 patients were enrolled in this study. Of them, 190 patients underwent TUSLIC, and 99 patients underwent TAMLEC. Among 190 patients in TUSLIC group, there were 168 males and 22 females with a mean age of 30.5 ± 24.6 months. Among 99 patients in TAMLEC group, there were 81 males and 18 females with a mean age of 29.4 ± 21.8 months. The descriptive variables, including sex, age, body weight, and preoperative diagnosis, between the two groups were comparable ($P > 0.05$; **Table 1**).

During the operation, all patients performed well in both groups. No patient needed to convert to conventional herniorrhaphy. The value of contralateral PPV was 34.2% in TUSLIC group, which was not significantly different from the 28.3% in TAMLEC group ($P = 0.31$). The ORTs for unilateral hernia repair and bilateral hernia repair in TAMLEC group were significantly lower than those in TUSLIC group ($P < 0.01$). No intraoperative complications occurred in the two groups.

Short-Term Follow-Up Results

The response rate for the telephone questionnaire and/or clinic interview was 94.8%, including 190 patients with TUSLIC (93.7%) and 99 patients with TAMLEC (97.0%). The data of 15 patients (TUSLIC 12, TAMLEC 3) were not collected. They had incorrect phone numbers, and no family member was contactable for the telephone or clinic interview.

The follow-up time was 9.8 ± 3.4 months in TUSLIC group and 9.6 ± 3.2 months in TAMLEC group ($P = 0.81$). Postoperative complications, including SSI, umbilical bleeding, testicular atrophy, iatrogenic ascent of the testis, and secondary hydrocele, were not significantly different between the two groups ($P > 0.05$; **Table 2**). Compared with TAMLEC group, there was no suture granuloma and recurrent PIH occurred in TUSLIC group ($P = 0.01$ and 0.04, respectively). In TAMLEC group, one obese patient and two patients with postoperative suture granuloma had inguinal hernias that recurred.

DISCUSSION

Transumbilical two-port laparoscopic intraperitoneal closure, which is a well-developed minimally invasive surgery for PIH, leaves almost invisible scars on the abdominal wall and avoids the disadvantages of extraperitoneal closure of IIR (15–18). However, it has not achieved wide acceptance because of its demanding techniques and difficult learning curve (19). In response to these challenges, the TUSLIC of IIR with a single instrument was established in January 2020, which is an improved transumbilical two-port laparoscopic intraperitoneal closure. In the present study, we provided evidence that TUSLIC is a safe and effective procedure for IIR in pediatric population. In addition, the results of our study revealed that TUSLIC had the advantages of minimized postoperative complications and a low recurrence rate comparing to those of TAMLEC. The peri- and postoperative complications, such as SSI, umbilical bleeding, testicular atrophy, iatrogenic ascent of the testis and secondary hydrocele after TUSLIC, were not significantly different from those after TAMLEC. However, the ORT during TUSLIC was significantly longer than that during TAMLEC due to the complex techniques in TUSLIC of IIR with the single instrument.

Recurrence rate is one of the most important outcome measures in PIH operation. It has been demonstrated that recurrence rates after open PIH repair and standard 3 port laparoscopic hernia repair ranged from 0.5 to 4% and 0.7 to 4.5%, respectively (8, 13, 20). In the present study, no cases of recurrence were recorded in patients receiving TUSLIC after a mean follow-up of 9.8 months.

Enlargement of the preperitoneal space with saline solution between the peritoneum along the inferior border of the IIR and the structures of the spermatic cord vessels and vas deferens is a prerequisite for successful TUSLIC. Moreover, normal saline for preperitoneal hydrodissection could predispose patients to the formation of preperitoneal local adhesions and fibrosis (21). It has been demonstrated that peritoneal trauma prior to repair could decrease the possibility of recurrence (3). Therefore, during passing of the threads, the saline liquid in the preperitoneal space may cause more tissue trauma, further promote the formation of healing around the IIR and reduce later recurrences.

Avoidance of damaging vas deferens and spermatic blood vessels is also a major concern during PIH operation. In TUSLIC, a volume of 1–5 ml of saline injection is needed for most patients. For children with a large opening of the hernia sac, a 5–10 ml or greater volume of saline injection could help unfold the redundant peritoneum along the inferior border of the IIR, which is convenient for seaming without a jumping zone and protects the spermatic cord vessels and vas deferens from damage. In the present study, no injury of epigastric or iliac blood vessels occurred in TUSLIC. These complications have been commonly reported in patients receiving PIRS (3, 10). Importantly, it has been revealed that more experienced pediatric surgeon had a lover incidence of these intraoperative complications (7, 12). However, questions still exist as whether TUSLIC, PIRS, or any other PIH repair technique may damage the spermatic cord. In this regard, testicular atrophy has been observed in patients who receiving open inguinal hernia repair. Remarkably, no case of testicular atrophy was recorded in a study of 188 patients receiving PIRS, with a median follow-up of 46 months (7).

During TUSLIC, it is important to note that when the working instrument repeatedly passes the incision at the right edge of the umbilicus, a false path into the peritoneal cavity may be formed, leading to more tissue trauma. This may have been responsible for the two cases of SSI and three cases of umbilical bleeding after TUSLIC. However, these complications were observed to decrease as we gained experience in TUSLIC. For small infants with a small abdominal space, the supine position is tilted 15° with the head down, the emptied bladder and the appropriately raised pneumoperitoneum, all of which can contribute a satisfactory working space. Similarly, it has been reported that complications significantly decreased after 10–25 or 30–35 patients in PIRS (7, 9).

Previous studies confirmed that there was a learning curve for intraoperative complications that reached the benchmarks after each pediatric surgeon performed at least 30-35 cases (11, 12).

The basic technique in TUSLIC is to control the needle tip direction with a single needle holder, which can be practiced by changing the 2-dimensional gripping angle (2-DGA) between the axis of the needle body and needle holder. The 2-DGA can be altered by adjusting the needle end when the needle tip is anchored by the sutured tissue or by rotating the needle body when the needle end is suspended by attached threads from the outside abdominal wall. However, the learning curve of TUSLIC may be long and steep, which requires much simulator training, even for a senior surgeon. Therefore, this may explain why the ORT in patients receiving TUSLIC was much longer than that of patients receiving TAMLEC or PIRS (20, 22–24).

Our study cohort included patients who aged 0–14 years. A subgroup of our patients were adolescents, with an age of 10–14 years. Form the pathophysiology of view, inguinal hernias in adolescent are more similar to that in children than in adults. We could not analyze clinical outcomes of the adolescent subgroup in our current study due to a relatively small sample size. However, no severe complications and recurrence were observed in our adolescent subgroup. In a recent study, the authors reported no postoperative complications and recurrences occurred in a group of 51 adolescents who receiving PIRS with an average follow-up of 44 months (25). These findings, together with our observation, further support that laparoscopic high ligation is a reliable procedure for inguinal hernia repair in adolescent patients.

It is important to consider the limitations of this study. First, this is a retrospective study conducted in a single institution and may not reflect all institutions. A multicenter randomized trial comparing the two treatment modalities is necessary. Second, the follow-up data for a small number of patients enrolled in this research were missing, which may have affected the final statistical results. Third, our study had a relative short follow-up period (mean about 9.5 months). This may be too short to draw some serious conclusions. A more convincing conclusion may require a longer follow-up in the future.

CONCLUSION

In conclusion, TUSLIC for PIH is a feasible, safe and reliable minimally invasive procedure for a well-trained surgeon. Compared with TAMLEC, TUSLIC has the advantages of a lower recurrence rate and fewer complications. The TUSLIC procedure for IIR with a single instrument may be considered an alternative option for PIH.

AUTHOR CONTRIBUTIONS

ZX designed the study. ZX and YJ collected data and managed its quality. ZX, YJ, YL, XZ, and TQ performed the statistical analysis and drafted the manuscript. SC and YJ contributed substantially to its revision. All authors read the manuscript carefully, approved the final version, and participated data interpretation.

FUNDING

This work was supported by the National Natural Science Foundation of China (grant numbers 81400862 and 81401606), the Key Project in the Science and Technology Program of Sichuan Province (grant number 2019YFS0322), the Science Foundation for The Excellent Youth Scholars of Sichuan University (grant number 2015SU04A15), and the 1·3·5 Project for Disciplines of Excellence Clinical Research Incubation Project, West China Hospital of Sichuan University (grant numbers 2019HXFH056, 2020HXFH048, and ZYJC21060).

REFERENCES

1. Zendejas B, Zarroug AE, Erben YM, Holley CT, Farley DR. Impact of childhood inguinal hernia repair in adulthood: 50 years of follow-up. *J Am Coll Surg.* (2010) 211:762–8. doi: 10.1016/j.jamcollsurg.2010.08.011
2. Montupet P, Esposito C. Laparoscopic treatment of congenital inguinal hernia in children. *J Pediatr Surg.* (1999) 34:420–3. doi: 10.1016/S0022-3468(99)90490-6
3. Takehara H, Yakabe S, Kameoka K. Laparoscopic percutaneous extraperitoneal closure for inguinal hernia in children: clinical outcome of 972 repairs done in 3 pediatric surgical institutions. *J Pediatr Surg.* (2006) 41:1999–2003. doi: 10.1016/j.jpedsurg.2006.08.032
4. Raveenthiran V, Agarwal P. Choice of repairing inguinal hernia in children: open versus laparoscopy. *Indian J Pediatr.* (2017) 84:555–63. doi: 10.1007/s12098-017-2354-9
5. Chang YT, Lee JY, Tsai CJ, Chiu WC, Chiou CS. Preliminary experience of one-trocar laparoscopic herniorrhaphy in infants and children. *J Laparoendosc Adv Surg Tech A.* (2011) 21:277–82. doi: 10.1089/lap.2010.0132
6. Ostlie DJ, Ponsky TA. Technical options of the laparoscopic pediatric inguinal hernia repair. *J Laparoendosc Adv Surg Tech A.* (2014) 24:194–8. doi: 10.1089/lap.2014.0081
7. Pogorelic Z, Cohadzic T, Jukic M, Nevescanin Biliskov A. Percutaneous internal ring suturing for the minimal invasive treatment of pediatric inguinal hernia: a 5-year single surgeon experience. *Surg Laparosc Endosc Percutan Tech.* (2021) 31:150–4. doi: 10.1097/SLE.0000000000000878
8. Pogorelic Z, Rikalo M, Jukic M, Katic J, Juric I, Furlan D, et al. Modified Marcy repair for indirect inguinal hernia in children: a 24-year single-center experience of 6826 pediatric patients. *Surg Today.* (2017) 47:108–13. doi: 10.1007/s00595-016-1352-2
9. Thomas DT, Gocmen KB, Tulgar S, Boga I. Percutaneous internal ring suturing is a safe and effective method for the minimal invasive treatment of pediatric inguinal hernia: experience with 250 cases. *J Pediatr Surg.* (2016) 51:1330–5. doi: 10.1016/j.jpedsurg.2015.11.024
10. Ergınel B, Akın M, Yildiz A, Karadağ CA, Sever N, Dokucu AI. Percutaneous internal ring suturing as a first choice laparoscopic inguinal hernia repair method in girls: a single-center study in 148 patients. *Pediatr Surg Int.* (2016) 32:697–700. doi: 10.1007/s00383-016-3903-4
11. Pogorelic Z, Huskic D, Cohadzic T, Jukic M, Susnjar T. Learning curve for laparoscopic repair of pediatric inguinal hernia using percutaneous internal ring suturing. *Children (Basel).* (2021) 8:294. doi: 10.3390/children8040294
12. Barroso C, Etlinger P, Alves AL, Osorio A, Carvalho JL, Lamas-Pinheiro R, et al. Learning curves for laparoscopic repair of inguinal hernia and communicating hydrocele in children. *Front Pediatr.* (2017) 5:207. doi: 10.3389/fped.2017.00207
13. Kilda A, Berzanskis M, Lukosiute-Urboniene A, Malcius D, Barauskas V. High recurrence rate of children's inguinal hernia after percutaneous internal ring suturing: a single-center study. *Hernia.* (2021) 25:797–801. doi: 10.1007/s10029-020-02316-1
14. Hasson HM. A modified instrument and method for laparoscopy. *Am J Obstetr Gynecol.* (1971) 110:886–7. doi: 10.1016/0002-9378(71)90593-X
15. Zhou X, Song D, Miao Q, Shan W. Transumbilical endoscopic surgery for completely enclosing inguinal hernias in children. *J Pediatr Surg.* (2011) 46:2417–20. doi: 10.1016/j.jpedsurg.2011.08.013
16. Zhou X, Peng L, Sha Y, Song D. Transumbilical endoscopic surgery for incarcerated inguinal hernias in infants and children. *J Pediatr Surg.* (2014) 49:214–7. doi: 10.1016/j.jpedsurg.2013.10.024
17. Jun Z, Juntao G, Shuli L, Li L. A comparative study on trans-umbilical single-port laparoscopic approach versus conventional repair for incarcerated inguinal hernia in children. *J Minim Access Surg.* (2016) 12:139–42. doi: 10.4103/0972-9941.169953
18. Xi HW, Duan WQ, Cui QQ, You ZH, Zhao Z, Zhang P. Transumbilical single-site laparoscopic inguinal hernia inversion and ligation in girls. *J Laparoendosc Adv Surg Tech A.* (2015) 25:522–5. doi: 10.1089/lap.2014.0383
19. Ismail M, Shalaby R. Single instrument intracorporeal knot tying during single port laparoscopic hernia repair in children: a new simplified technique. *J Pediatr Surg.* (2014) 49:1044–8. doi: 10.1016/j.jpedsurg.2014.02.082

20. Kara YA, Yagiz B, Balci O, Karaman A, Ozguner IF, Karaman I. Comparison of open repair and laparoscopic percutaneous internal ring suturing method in repairing inguinal hernia in children. *Cureus.* (2021) 13:e14262. doi: 10.7759/cureus.14262
21. Połubinska A, Breborowicz A, Staniszewski R, Oreopoulos DG. Normal saline induces oxidative stress in peritoneal mesothelial cells. *J Pediatr Surg.* (2008) 43:1821–6. doi: 10.1016/j.jpedsurg.2008.02.010
22. Wolak PK, Strzelecka A, Piotrowska A, Dabrowska K, Wolak PP, Piotrowska I, et al. The operative time for unilateral inguinal hernia repair in children performed with Percutaneous Internal Ring Suturing (PIRS) or open approach method. *J Clin Med.* (2021) 10:1293. doi: 10.3390/jcm10061293
23. Rao R, Smith M, Markel TA, Gray BW, Landman MP. Modified percutaneous internal ring suturing with peritoneal injury in children: matched comparison to open hernia repair. *Surg Endosc.* (2021) 35:854–9. doi: 10.1007/s00464-020-07457-z
24. Ergun E, Yagiz B, Kara YA, Abay AN, Balci O, Eryilmaz S, et al. Comparison of laparoscopic percutaneous internal ring suturing method and open inguinal hernia repair in children under 3 months of age. *Turk J Surg.* (2021) 37:215–21. doi: 10.47717/turkjsurg.2021.5157
25. Pogorelic Z, Batinovic T, Jukic M, Susnjar T. Percutaneous internal ring suturing is a safe and effective method for inguinal hernia repair in young adolescents. *J Laparoendosc Adv Surg Tech A.* (2022). doi: 10.1089/lap.2021.0393. [Epub ahead of print].

21

Successful Outcome After Intralesional Curettage for Spindle Cell Hemangioma of Fibula in an Infant

Tao Han[1†], Rufa Wang[2†] and Xiaoguang Zhou[3]*

[1] Department of Burns and Plastic Surgery, Children's Hospital of Nanjing Medical University, Nanjing, China, [2] Department of Orthopedic Surgery, Children's Hospital of Nanjing Medical University, Nanjing, China, [3] Neonatal Medical Center, Children's Hospital of Nanjing Medical University, Nanjing, China

***Correspondence:**
Xiaoguang Zhou
zxgnch@sina.com

Spindle cell hemangioma (SCH), a non-neoplastic reactive vascular lesion, rarely locates in bones. We herein report a successful case of intralesional curettage for an infant with SCH of fibula. An 11-month-old boy was admitted to our center with a painless mass in the right proximal calf. Preoperative digital radiograph demonstrated a massive vascular lesion with an irregular bone destruction of proximal fibula. The lesion was removed via the intralesional curettage approach and pathologically diagnosed as SCH. The patient gained bone structure recovery of right proximal fibula. Two years after the surgery, he experienced no local recurrence. For the management of SCH of fibula with partial bone destruction, we suggest early-stage intralesional curettage as its safety and effectiveness.

Keywords: spindle cell hemangioma, intralesional curettage, outcome, vascular lesions, fibula

INTRODUCTION

Spindle cell hemangioma (SCH), characterized by cavernous blood vessels and spindle cell proliferation, has recently been considered as a non-neoplastic reactive vascular lesion (1, 2). SCH often occurs at early age with high risk of recurrence after surgery due to its uncertain border with surrounding tissue. It commonly arises in the dermal or subcutaneous tissue of the distal extremities (3, 4). Reports on SCH cases involving bone are rare, most of which focus on histopathological description, but lack sufficient clinical and follow-up data (5, 6). Herein, we present a case of SCH in proximal fibula that was managed successfully by intralesional curettage and, moreover, discuss its clinical characteristics and long-term surgical outcome.

CASE REPORT

An 11-month-old boy patient presented to our center with a 2-month history of painless mass in the right proximal calf. The mass had been noted to be slowly enlarging in 3 weeks after presentation. No significant symptom was found in this patient. Initial workup performed included radiograph, three-dimensional CT (3d CT) reconstruction, and MRI. Radiographs of the right tibia and fibula indicated an irregular bone destruction of proximal fibula (**Figures 1A,B**), and the lytic bone destruction was confirmed by 3d CT reconstruction (**Figures 1C,D**). MRI revealed a massive vascular tumor with surrounding soft tissue hyperplasia and involvement of the proximal fibular epiphyseal plate (**Figures 1E,F**).

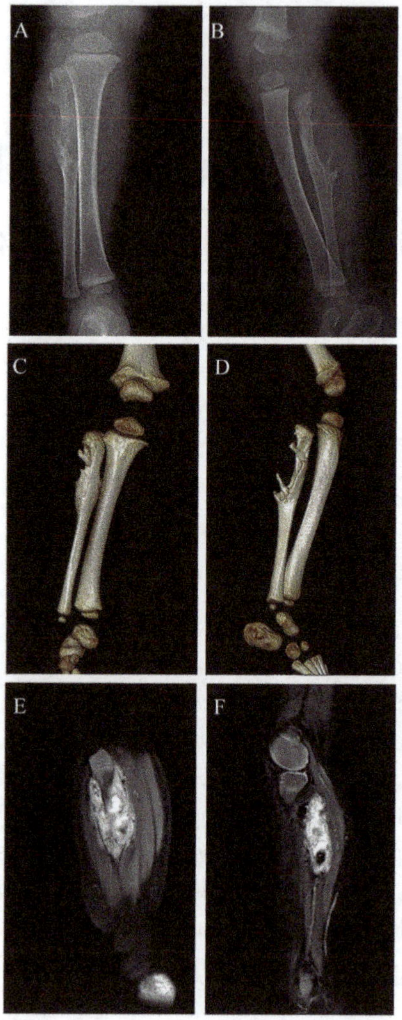

FIGURE 1 | Digital radiograph preoperatively: **(A,B)** Radiographs of the right tibia and fibula showing an irregular bone destruction of proximal fibula; **(C,D)** 3d CT reconstruction demonstrating lytic bone destruction of right proximal fibula; **(E,F)** MRI revealing a massive vascular tumor with surrounding soft tissue hyperplasia and involvement of the proximal fibular epiphyseal plate.

Considering partial bony structure of proximal fibula was normal, intralesional curettage was performed on the right proximal fibula under general anesthesia. After lesion exposure, a 4.02 × 0.0-cm-sized vascular mass was identified with extension to proximal fibular. Gross examination showed a reddish spongious solid mass, containing topical hemorrhage, partial thrombosis, and irregular bone destruction (**Figure 2A**). With protection of common peroneal nerve and peripheral vessels, complete curettage of lesion was performed to normal periosteum of fibular (**Figures 2B,C**). Histologically, the lesion was characterized by the fissure-like vessel lumens lined with flattened endothelial cells among the spindle cells (**Figure 3A**). The spindle-shaped cells arranged in fascicular pattern in solid area, with similar cell morphology and no atypia (**Figures 3B,C**). Immunohistochemically, the endothelial cells lining the vessel spaces stained positive for CD31, CD34, and ERG (**Figures 3D–F**). Therefore, with standard of international society for study of vascular anomalies (ISSVA) classification (7), the diagnosis of spindle cell hemangioma was made in this patient according to the clinical and histopathologic manifestations. On postoperative follow-up, this patient was asymptomatic without any evidence of recurrence. Two years after this surgery, he returned to hospital for outpatient review. Radiographs showed the reformation of the cortex of the proximal fibula (**Figures 4A,B**), and both uniform bone mineral density and continuous cortical of right proximal fibula were confirmed by 3d CT reconstruction (**Figures 4C,D**). Besides, MRI demonstrated remarkable regression of lesion without any signs of tumor growth through the fibula (**Figures 4E,F**).

DISCUSSION

This case is rare in comparison with majority of reported SCH cases and merits discussion on following points: location of lesion, selection of surgical intervention, histopathologic characteristics, and long-term postoperative follow-up. SCH is a benign vascular lesion which generally locates in the subcutis at the distal extremities and presents as solitary and multifocal masses. It also can be associated with several clinical syndromes,

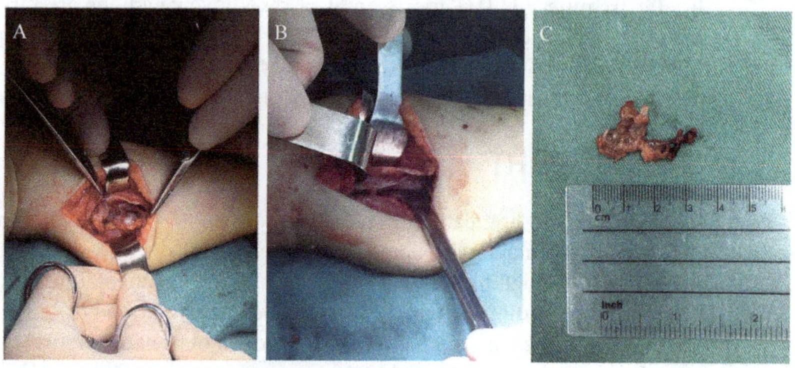

FIGURE 2 | The photograph during the surgery: **(A)** Intraoperative image of the surgical finding of a vascular mass attached to proximal fibula; **(B)** Complete curettage of lesion to normal fibular surface; **(C)** Macroscopic appearance of the excised lesion.

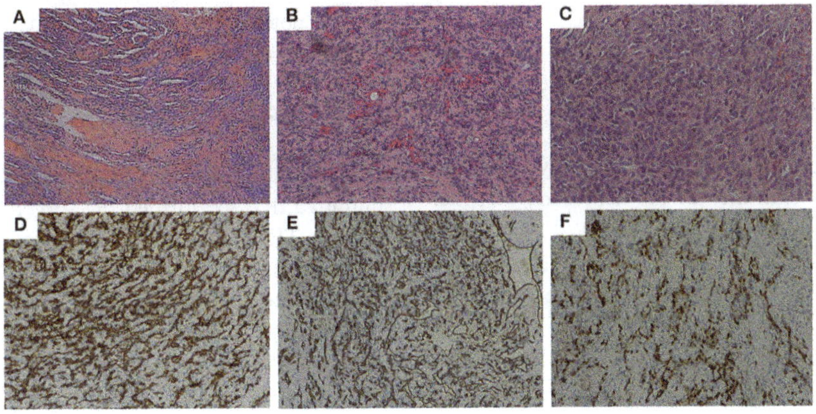

FIGURE 3 | Histopathological features: **(A)** (HE, ×40) the fissure-like vessel lumens lined with flattened endothelial cells among the spindle cells, **(B)** (HE, ×100), **(C)** (HE, ×200) the spindle shaped cells arranging in fascicular pattern in solid area. Immunohistochemical analysis revealing positive staining for **(D)** CD31 (×100), **(E)** CD34 (×100), and **(F)** ERG (×100) in the majority of spindle cells.

among which Maffucci syndrome is the most common (8, 9). In several uncommon cases, SCHs have been found in lips, nasal passage, temporal muscle, and even in lungs and spleen (2, 10–13). In comparison, the reported cases of SCH arising in bones are even more unusual so far (14–16). In our case, a solitary lesion of SCH involved the proximal fibula with surrounding soft tissue hyperplasia, while the superficial skin and tissues were normal.

To date, the main treatment choice for fibular tumor is segmental or subperiosteal resection, in case of local recurrence at surgical site (17–19). Wide excision for clear margin has always been first choice for SCHs, and repeated surgical resection is performed if a recurrence occurs (3, 20). However, given that preoperative digital radiograph indicated that the vascular mass on fibula was solitary, and part of both cortex and cancellous fibula were not involved, intralesional curettage was selected as the surgical intervention in this case for achieving the maximum retention of healthy bony structure. During the operation, complete curettage was performed to the normal fibular surface without residual lesion.

The histologic appearance in this case consisted of the fissure-like vessel lumens lined with flattened endothelial cells among the spindle cells, which arranged in fascicular pattern in solid area. CD31, CD34, and ERG, as vascular endothelial markers, were reported positive expression in various kinds of vascular tumors. In this case, immunohistochemical analysis revealed positive staining for CD31, CD34, and ERG in the majority of spindle cells, consistent with the diagnosis of SCH (21, 22). Metastasis of SCH is rare, although local recurrence may occur (20, 23). On the most recent imaging examination, 2 years after the initial surgery, our patient was still disease free and found to experience entire reformation of bone structure of the right proximal fibula. This indicates the safety and effectiveness of intralesional curettage for the management of this case.

In conclusion, for SCH of fibula with partial bone destruction, intralesional curettage renders a safe and efficient intervention at early stage. Meanwhile, our study was limited by lacking further evaluation for treatment approaches owing to small sample size.

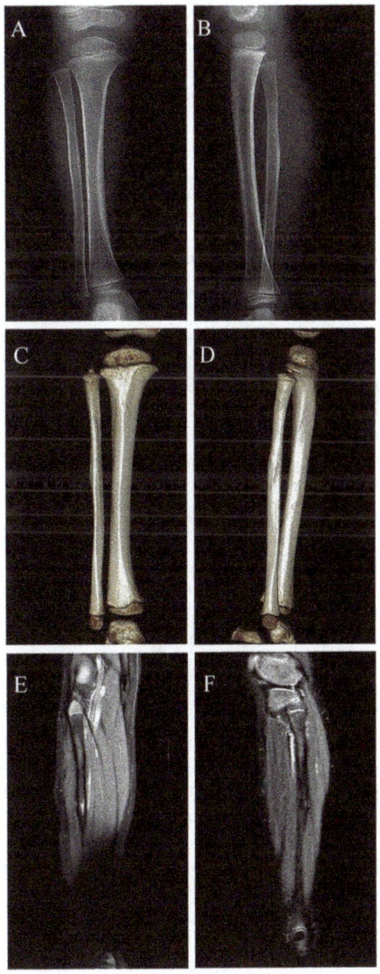

FIGURE 4 | Digital radiograph at 2 years postoperatively: **(A,B)** Radiographs showing reformation of the cortex of the proximal fibula; **(C,D)** 3d CT reconstruction demonstrating both uniform bone mineral density and continuous cortical of right proximal fibula; **(E,F)** MRI revealing remarkable regression of lesion without evidence of local recurrence.

Long-time and consistent follow-up could establish the efficacy of our management.

ETHICS STATEMENT

The studies involving human participants were reviewed and approved by the Ethics Committee of the Children's Hospital of Nanjing Medical University. Written informed consent to participate in this study was provided by the participants' legal guardian/next of kin. Written informed consent was obtained from the minor(s)' legal guardian/next of kin for the publication of any potentially identifiable images or data included in this article.

AUTHOR CONTRIBUTIONS

XZ revised the manuscript and approved the final manuscript as submitted. RW performed the surgery and conducted the data analyses. TH wrote sections of the article and edited the figures. TH and RW contribute to this work equally. All authors read and approved the final manuscript.

REFERENCES

1. Tosios KI, Gouveris I, Sklavounou A, Koutlas IG. Spindle cell hemangioma (hemangioendothelioma) of the head and neck: case report of an unusual (or underdiagnosed) tumor. *Oral Surg Oral Med Oral Pathol Oral Radiol Endod.* (2008) 105:216–21. doi: 10.1016/j.tripleo.2007.03.005
2. Gao BQ, Zhou DK, Qian XH, Zhang W, Ying LX, Wang WL. Spindle cell hemangioma of the spleen: A case report. *Medicine (Baltimore).* (2019) 98:e14555. doi: 10.1097/MD.0000000000014555
3. Liu H, Rao Y, Gu H, Yang X, Hu L, Sun Y, et al. Characteristic appearance of spindle cell hemangiomatosis, often misdiagnosed as venous malformation: A retrospective study of 11 cases. *J Dermatol.* (2020) 47:1424–31. doi: 10.1111/1346-8138.15571
4. Marusic Z, Billings SD. Histopathology of spindle cell vascular tumors. *Surg Pathol Clin.* (2017) 10:345–66. doi: 10.1016/j.path.2017.01.006
5. Maclean FM, Schatz J, McCarthy SW, Scolyer RA, Stalley P, Bonar SF. Epithelioid and spindle cell haemangioma of bone. *Skeletal Radiol.* (2007) 36:S50–7. doi: 10.1007/s00256-006-0135-z
6. Vijayan S, Naik M, Rao S, Hameed S. Spindle cell hemangioma of femur. *Clin Cancer Invest J.* (2015) 4:469–72. doi: 10.4103/2278-0513.148979
7. Miller DD, Gupta A. Histopathology of vascular anomalies: update based on the revised 2014 ISSVA classification. *Semin Cutan Med Surg.* (2016) 35:137–46. doi: 10.12788/j.sder.2016.053
8. Lekwuttikarn R, Chang J, Teng JMC. Successful treatment of spindle cell hemangiomas in a patient with Maffucci syndrome and review of literatures. *Dermatol Ther.* (2019) 32:e12919. doi: 10.1111/dth.12919
9. Gupta V, Mridha AR, Khaitan BK. Unsatisfactory response to sirolimus in Maffucci syndrome-associated spindle cell hemangiomas. *Dermatol Ther.* (2019) 32:e12851. doi: 10.1111/dth.12851
10. Murakami K, Yamamoto K, Sugiura T, Kirita T. Spindle cell hemangioma in the mucosa of the upper lip: a case report and review of the literature. *Case Rep Dent.* (2018) 2018:1370701. doi: 10.1155/2018/1370701
11. Tastemel Ozturk T, Suslu AE, Kavuncuoglu A, Gumeler E, Kosemehmetoglu K, Yalcin B. Spindle cell hemangioma of nasal passage and ethmoidal sinus in a 4-month old infant. *Arch Argent Pediatr.* (2021) 119:e36–40. doi: 10.5546/aap.2021.eng.e36
12. Minagawa T, Yamao T, Shioya R. Spindle cell hemangioendothelioma of the temporal muscle resected with zygomatic osteotomy: a case report of an unusual intramuscular lesion mimicking sarcoma. *Case Rep Surg.* (2011) 2011:481654. doi: 10.1155/2011/481654
13. Duqing X, Zhaohong W, Gefei W. Multiple spindle cell hemangiomas in both lungs: a rare case report and review of the literature. *J Cardiothorac Surg.* (2019) 14:86. doi: 10.1186/s13019-019-0906-y
14. Vaseenon T, Saengsin J, Pattamapaspong N, Settakorn J, Pruksakorn D. spindle cell hemangioma of the midfoot: a case report. *J Orthop Case Rep.* (2017) 7:75–9. doi: 10.13107/jocr.2250-0685.904
15. Hakozaki M, Tajino T, Watanabe K, Yamada H, Kikuchi S, Hojo H, et al. Intraosseous spindle cell hemangioma of the calcaneus: a case report and review of the literature. *Ann Diagn Pathol.* (2012) 16:369–73. doi: 10.1016/j.anndiagpath.2012.01.005
16. Tsukamoto S, Honoki K, Shimada K, Fujii H, Kido A, Takano M, et al. Periosteal spindle cell hemangioma of the fibula: a case report. *Skeletal Radiol.* (2013) 42:1165–8. doi: 10.1007/s00256-013-1603-x
17. Guo C, Zhang X, Gao F, Wang L, Sun T. Surgical management of proximal fibular tumors: risk factors for recurrence and complications. *J Int Med Res.* (2018) 46:1884–92. doi: 10.1177/0300060518762677
18. Mostafa MF. Subperiosteal resection of fibular aneurysmal bone cyst. *Eur J Orthop Surg Traumatol.* (2015) 25:443–50. doi: 10.1007/s00590-014-1527-8
19. Erler K, Demiralp B, Ozdemir MT, Basbozkurt M. Treatment of proximal fibular tumors with en bloc resection. *Knee.* (2004) 11:489–96. doi: 10.1016/j.knee.2003.10.005
20. Perkins P, Weiss SW. Spindle cell hemangioendothelioma. An analysis of 78 cases with reassessment of its pathogenesis and biologic behavior. *Am J Surg Pathol.* (1996) 20:1196–204. doi: 10.1097/00000478-199610000-00004
21. Sheehan M, Roumpf SO, Summerlin DJ, Billings SD. Spindle cell hemangioma: report of a case presenting in the oral cavity. *J Cutan Pathol.* (2007) 34:797–800. doi: 10.1111/j.1600-0560.2006.00708.x
22. Chavva S, Priya MH, Garlapati K, Reddy GS, Gannepalli A. Rare case of spindle cell haemangioma. *J Clin Diagn Res.* (2015) 9:ZD19–21. doi: 10.7860/JCDR/2015/11998.6080
23. Patel SV, Bass FD, Niemi WJ, Pressman MM. Spindle cell hemangioendothelioma: a case presentation and literature review of a rare lower extremity tumor. *J Foot Ankle Surg.* (1996) 35:309–11. doi: 10.1016/s1067-2516(96)80079-2

22

Outcomes and Prognostic Factors for Survival of Neonates with Necrotizing Enterocolitis

*Elena Sophia Elekta Dilean Siahaan, Wahyudhy Adriansyah, Andika Purba Sasmita, Aditya Rifqi Fauzi, Andi Dwihantoro and Gunadi**

Pediatric Surgery Division, Department of Surgery, Faculty of Medicine, Public Health and Nursing, Universitas Gadjah Mada/Dr. Sardjito Hospital, Yogyakarta, Indonesia

Correspondence:
Gunadi
drgunadi@ugm.ac.id

Background: Due to the survival of preterm neonates being continually improved, the modifiable prognostic factors of necrotizing enterocolitis (NEC) are essential to be investigated and considered in making a suitable treatment to decrease the prevalence and effect of NEC. Many prognostic factors have been associated with the survival of neonates with NEC; however, the studies show conflicting results. Moreover, the study from developing countries regarding NEC outcomes is minimal. Here, we aimed to determine the survival of neonates with NEC and associate it with the prognostic factors.

Methods: A retrospective study was conducted using medical records of neonates with NEC at our institution from January 2014 to December 2019.

Results: Fifty-two neonates with NEC were involved with the overall survival of 44.2%. Log-rank analysis showed that NEC staging and birth weight were significantly associated with the survival of neonates with NEC with a *p*-value of 0.010 and 0.002, respectively, while sex, APGAR score, platelet count, and type of treatment were not ($p = 0.068$, 0.752, 0.087, and 0.343, respectively). Multivariate analysis revealed that sex and NEC staging were strongly associated with the survival of neonates with NEC with a *p*-value of 0.018 [HR = 3.10 (95% CI = 1.21–7.93)] and 0.019 [HR = 0.44 (0.22–0.87)], respectively.

Conclusions: Our study shows that sex and NEC staging might affect the survival of neonates with NEC. It implies that NEC staging should be closely monitored and intervened as early as necessary to prevent further morbidity and mortality.

Keywords: developing country, necrotizing enterocolitis, prognostic factors, NEC staging, survival

INTRODUCTION

Necrotizing enterocolitis (NEC) is the leading cause of morbidity and mortality of neonates with intestinal disorders in the neonatal intensive care unit (NICU) (1). Its incidence is 1 per 1,000 live births, and more than 90% of cases are premature infants (2). Its incidence is increasing because of the increasing number of preterm birth and the advances in neonatal care (3, 4).

Due to the continually improving survival of preterm neonates, the modifiable prognostic factors of NEC are essential to be investigated and considered in making a suitable treatment to decrease the prevalence and effect of NEC (4). Many prognostic factors have been associated with the survival of neonates with NEC; however, the studies show conflicting results (1, 5, 6). Moreover, the study from developing countries regarding NEC outcomes is minimal (7, 8). Here, we aimed to determine the survival of neonates with NEC and associate it with the prognostic factors.

METHODS

Subjects and Necrotizing Enterocolitis Staging

A retrospective study was conducted using medical records of neonates with NEC at our institution from January 2014 to December 2019. We included 56 diagnosed with NEC, with the International Classification of Diagnosis (ICD) X code of P.77. According to modified Bell's staging, the diagnosis and staging of NEC were established, consisting of the severity of systemic, intestinal, radiographic, and laboratory findings (9). The exclusion criteria were incomplete medical records. We excluded four neonates due to incomplete medical records and investigated 52 neonates for final analysis.

The Ethical Committee of the Faculty of Medicine, Universitas Gadjah Mada/Dr. Sardjito Hospital, Indonesia, approved the study (KE/FK/0375/EC/2020).

Prognostic Factors

We evaluated the following prognostic factors for the survival of neonates with NEC: sex, birth weight, NEC staging, platelet count, APGAR score, and type of treatment. Birth weight was classified into extremely low birth weight (<1,000 g), very low birth weight (<1,500 g), low birth weight (<2,500 g), and normal (≥2,500 g) according to World Health Organization classification, while the platelet count was defined as thromb ocytosis (>350,000/mm^3), normal (≥150,000–350,000/mm^3), and thrombocytopenia (<150,000/mm^3) according to a previous study (6). The type of treatment is divided into conservative and surgical procedures, while the APGAR Score was classified as asphyxia (<8) and non-asphyxia (≥8).

Enteral Feeding

The decision to start enteral feeding was according to the following parameters: bowel sounds, no greenish gastric residual, and the volume of gastric residual was <1 ml/kg/day. Most of the enteral feeding was breastfeeding (94.2%) (**Table 1**).

Statistical Analysis

The survival of neonates with NEC was determined using a log-rank test, while the probabilities of the survival of the neonates were plotted using the Kaplan–Meier curve. The IBM SPSS Statistics version 16 (SPSS Chicago, IL, USA) was utilized to perform all statistical analyses.

Abbreviations: APGAR, appearance pulse grimace activity respiration; CI, confidence interval; HR, hazard ratio; NEC, necrotizing enterocolitis; NICU, neonatal intensive care unit.

TABLE 1 | Baseline characteristics of neonates with NEC in our institution.

Characteristics	*N* (%)
Sex	
Male	29 (55.8)
Female	23 (44.2)
Asphyxia (APGAR score)	
Yes (<8)	27 (51.9)
No (≥8)	25 (48.1)
Birth weight (g)	
Normal birth weight (≥2,500)	12 (23)
Low birth weight (<2,500)	20 (38.5)
Very low birth weight (<1,500)	17 (32.7)
Extremely low birth weight (<1,000)	3 (5.8)
Platelet count (/mm^3)	
Thrombocytosis (>350,000)	6 (11.5)
Normal (≥150,000–350,000)	20 (38.5)
Thrombocytopenia (<150,000)	26 (50)
NEC staging	
IA	18 (34.6)
IB	2 (3.9)
IIA	15 (28.9)
IIB	0
IIIA	7 (13.4)
IIIB	10 (19.2)
Type of treatment	
Conservative	39 (75)
Operative	13 (25)
Feeding	
Breastfeeding	49 (94.2)
Formula	3 (5.8)
Sepsis	
Yes	48 (92.3)
No	4 (7.7)
Mechanical ventilation	
PCAC	4 (7.7)
PCMV	15 (28.8)
SIMV	2 (3.8)
NIMV	4 (7.7)
CPAP	10 (19.2)
Survival	
Survived	23 (44.2)
- Male	14 (60.9)
- Female	9 (39.1)
Died	29 (55.8)
- Male	14 (48.3)
- Female	15 (51.7)

NEC, necrotizing enterocolitis.

RESULTS

Baseline Characteristics

We involved 52 neonates with NEC with overall survival of 44.2%. Most of them were male (55.8%), with asphyxia (51.9%), low birth weight or less (77%), thrombocytopenia (50%), sepsis (92.3%), and breastfeeding (94.2%) (**Table 1**).

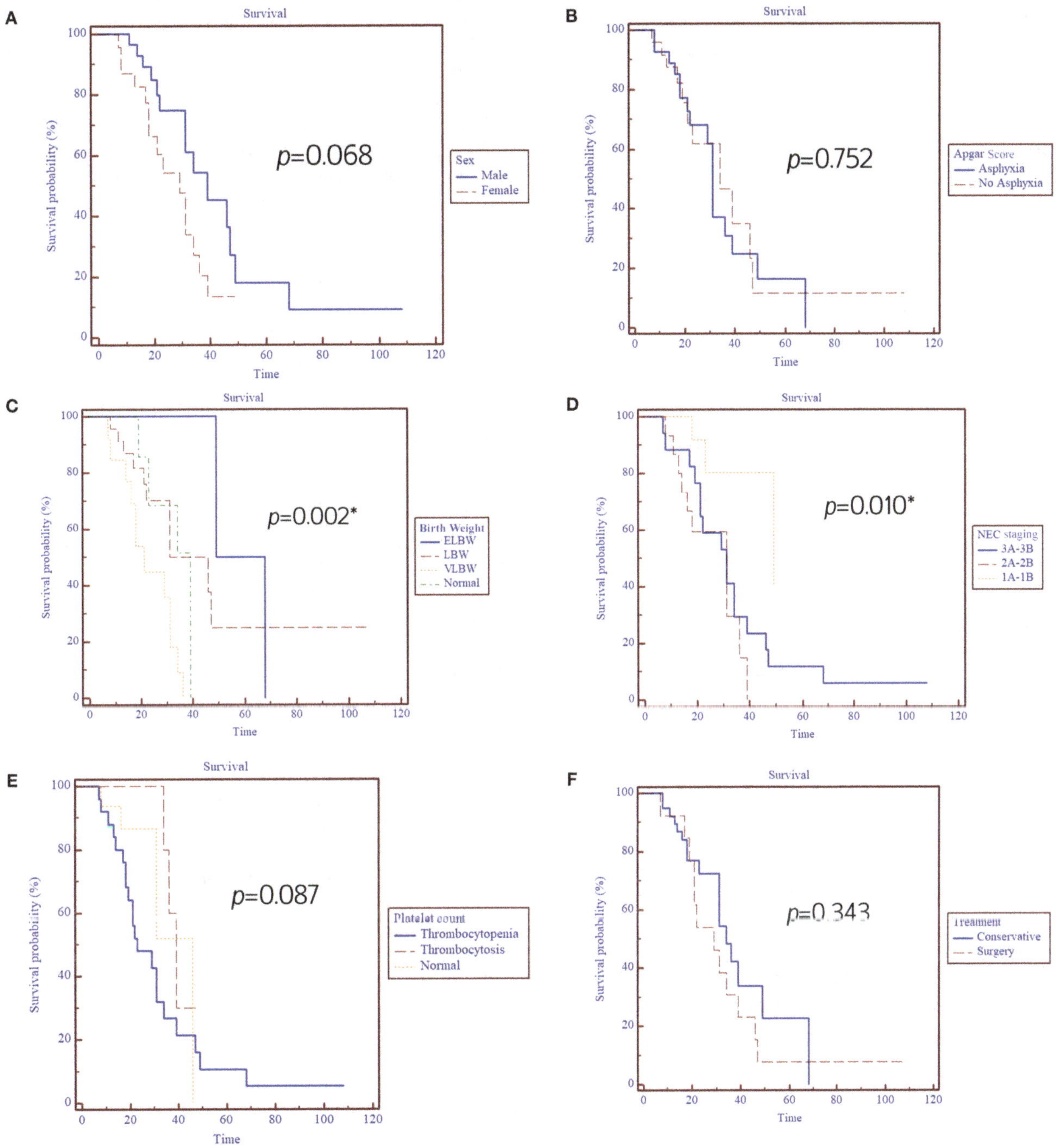

FIGURE 1 | Kaplan–Meier analysis for the association between prognostic factors: **(A)** Sex, **(B)** APGAR score, **(C)** Birth weight, **(D)** NEC staging, **(E)** Platelet count, **(F)** Treatment, and NEC patients' survival. *, significant $p < 0.05$.

Association Between Prognostic Factors and Survival of Neonates With Necrotizing Enterocolitis

Log-rank analysis showed that NEC staging and birth weight were significantly associated with the survival of neonates with NEC with *a* *p*-value of 0.010 and 0.002, respectively. At the same time, sex, APGAR score, platelet count, and type of treatment were not ($p = 0.068$, 0.752, 0.087, and 0.343, respectively) (**Figure 1**; **Table 2**).

TABLE 2 | Association between prognostic factors and survival of neonates with NEC in our institution.

Variables	HR (95% CI)	*p*-Value
Sex		
Female	1.89 (0.89–4.04)	0.068
Asphyxia		
APGAR score <8	1.12 (0.54–2.34)	0.752
Birth weight (Ref: normal birth weight)		
Low birth weight	0.87 (0.33–2.32)	0.002*
Very low birth weight	2.75 (0.83–9.13)	
Extremely low birth weight	0.45 (0.14–1.46)	
Platelet count (Ref: Normal)		
Thrombocytopenia	1.84 (0.75–4.53)	0.087
Thrombocytosis	0.62 (0.21–1.80)	
NEC staging (Ref: IA-IB)		
IIA–IIB	5.83 (2.07–16.40)	0.010*
IIIA–IIIB	3.89 (1.71–8.84)	
Type of treatment		
Surgery	1.41 (0.65–3.05)	0.343

**p* < 0.05; *CI, confidence interval; HR, hazard ratio; NEC, necrotizing enterocolitis; Ref, reference.*

TABLE 3 | Multivariate analysis of survival of neonates with NEC in our institution.

Variables	HR (95% CI)	*p*-value
Sex (female)	3.10 (1.21–7.93)	0.018*
Asphyxia	1.04 (0.36–2.98)	0.940
Birth weight	1.41 (0.82–2.41)	0.211
Platelet count	1.94 (0.93– 4.06)	0.079
NEC staging	0.44 (0.22–0.87)	0.019*
Type of treatment	1.84 (0.54–6.34)	0.332

**p* < 0.05; *CI, confidence interval; HR, hazard ratio; NEC, necrotizing enterocolitis.*

Multivariate Analysis of Prognostic Factors for Survival of Neonates With Necrotizing Enterocolitis

Multivariate analysis revealed that sex (female) and NEC staging were strongly associated with the survival of neonates with NEC with *a p*-value of 0.018 {hazard ratio [HR] = 3.10 [95% confidence interval (CI) = 1.21–7.93]} and 0.019 [HR = 0.44 [95% CI = 0.22–0.87)], respectively (**Table 3**).

DISCUSSION

Here, we show that the overall survival of our NEC neonates is 44.2%, which is similar to a previous study (10). One reason for the high mortality rate was withdrawal from critical care, while another reason was the unavailability of pediatric surgery services in some hospitals; thus, surgery was not possible (10). Our institution, as an academic referral hospital, has pediatric surgery services. However, our findings were not compatible with a previous report (10) since the type of treatment did not affect the outcome of NEC infants (**Table 3**).

We reveal that NEC staging is a strong prognostic factor for the survival of neonates with NEC. Our findings were compatible with a previous study that revealed that the NEC stage III in VLBW and LBW infants is an independent prognostic factor for the survival of neonates with NEC (7). Moreover, lower birth weight was significantly associated with NEC incidence and mortality (11, 12). Immaturity of the gastrointestinal tract, digestive function, circulation regulation, barrier function, and immune defense are essential factors in explaining NEC occurring in infants with LBW (13). We show new evidence to support this hypothesis by providing data from a population ethnically different from the previous report (7). The previous report showed that the prognostic factors for NEC had been expanded, including ethnicity (4). Moreover, due to the survival of preterm neonates being continually improved, it is suggested that clinicians and researchers should look for the prognostic factors for NEC, particularly the modifiable one, to be taken into consideration in making a suitable treatment to decrease the prevalence and effect of NEC (4).

Interestingly, female patients had a 3.1-fold higher risk of mortality than male patients. A previous study showed that male is a risk factor for mortality (11). These differences might be due to different ethnicities. Ethnicity has been considered as a prognostic factor for NEC (4). In addition, a previous study showed no association between sex and NEC (9). They suggested continuous assessment on the impact of sex on the severity of NEC since the male has tended to suffer from NEC (9).

Our study presented that thrombocytopenia almost reached a significant level affecting the mortality of NEC infants with the HR of ~2 ($p = 0.07$) (**Table 3**). Most neonates with advanced stages of NEC will have thrombocytopenia within 24–72 h of disease onset (14). Thrombocytopenia level is strongly correlated with the clinical staging of NEC, and a progressive decrease in thrombocyte level implies the development of intestinal gangrene (15). In addition, thrombocytopenia has been shown as a strong predictor of the mortality of neonates with NEC (16).

Treatment type is a significant prognostic factor in NEC patients (17). Infants with NEC who underwent surgery had higher morbidity and mortality than those who received conservative treatment (17, 18). However, our findings showed that type of treatment did not affect the mortality of NEC neonates. While Hull et al. (19) revealed that different surgical approaches affected the mortality of NEC neonates, none of the specific surgical approaches is suggested for NEC (19). It depends on several variables, including the birth weight, hemodynamic status, comorbidities, existing resources, intraoperative findings, and attending physician preference of the neonate (19).

Our study noted several limitations, including a small sample size and a single-center report, implying that a further multicenter study with larger sample size is necessary to clarify and confirm our findings. These weaknesses should be noted during the interpretation of our findings. Due to its retrospective design, we have difficulty evaluating the long-term complications of NEC, including neurodevelopmental impairment, poor growth, gastrointestinal sequels, such as strictures, adhesions, feeding difficulties, cholestasis, short bowel syndrome, and intestinal failure (20).

CONCLUSION

Our study shows that sex and NEC staging might affect the survival of neonates with NEC. It implies that NEC staging should be closely monitored and intervened as early as necessary to prevent further morbidity and mortality.

AUTHOR CONTRIBUTIONS

AD and G conceived the study. ESEDS, WA, APS, ARF, and G drafted the manuscript. ESEDS and G analyzed the data. AD and G facilitated all project-related tasks. All authors read and approved the final manuscript.

ACKNOWLEDGMENTS

We extend our thanks to Henggar Allest Pratama who provided excellent technical support and assistance during the study. We are also thankful to the English editing service staff at the Faculty of Medicine, Public Health and Nursing, Universitas Gadjah Mada, for checking the manuscript grammar. Some results for the manuscript are from ESEDS's thesis.

REFERENCES

1. Samuels N, van de Graaf RA, de Jonge RCJ, Reiss IK, Vermeulen MJ. Risk factors for necrotizing enterocolitis in neonates: a systematic review of prognostic studies. *BMC Pediatr.* (2017) 17:105. doi: 10.1186/s12887-017-0847-3
2. Stoll BJ, Hansen NI, Bell EF, Shankaran S, Laptook AR, Walsh MC, et al. Neonatal outcomes of extremely preterm infants from the NICHD neonatal research network. *Pediatrics.* (2010) 126:443–56. doi: 10.1542/peds.2009-2959
3. Sylvester KG, Liu GY, Albanese CT. Necrotizing enterocolitis. In: Coran AG, Caldamone A, Adzick NS, Krummel TM, Laberge JM, Shamberger R, editors. *Pediatric Surgery.* Philadelphia, PA: 7th ed. Elsevier Saunders (2012). p. 1187–207.
4. Alsaied A, Islam N, Thalib L. Global incidence of necrotizing enterocolitis: a systematic review and meta-analysis. *BMC Pediatr.* (2020) 20:344. doi: 10.1186/s12887-020-02231-5
5. Clark RH, Gordon P, Walker WM, Laughon M, Smith PB, Spitzer AR. Characteristics of patients who die of necrotizing enterocolitis. *J Perinatol.* (2012) 32:199–204. doi: 10.1038/jp.2011.65
6. Bracho-Blanchet E, Torrecilla-Navarrete ME, Zalles-Vidal C, Ibarra-Ríos D, Fernández-Portilla E, Dávila-Pérez R. Prognostic factors related to mortality in newborns with necrotising enterocolitis. *Cirugía y Cirujanos.* (2015) 83:286–91. doi: 10.1016/j.circen.2015.09.015
7. Bora R, Murthy NB. In resource limited areas complete enteral feed in stable very low birth weight infants (1000 1500 g) started within 24 h of life can improve nutritional outcome. *J Matern Fetal Neonatal Med.* (2017) 30:2572–7. doi: 10.1080/14767058.2016.1256992
8. Satardien M, Van Wyk L, Sidler D, Van Zyl JI. Outcomes of neonates requiring neonatal intensive care admission for necrotizing enterocolitis in a resource-restricted hospital in Cape Town, South Africa. *J Trop Pediatr.* (2021) 67:fmaa130. doi: 10.1093/tropej/fmaa130
9. Kim JH. Neonatal necrotizing enterocolitis: clinical features and diagnosis. In: UpToDate, Abrams SA, Kim MS, editors. *UpToDate.* Waltham, MA (2021) Available online at: https://www.uptodate.com/contents/search (accessed on March 31, 2021).
10. Qian T, Zhang R, Zhu L, Shi P, Yang J, Yang CY, et al. Necrotizing enterocolitis in low birth weight infants in China: Mortality risk factors expressed by birth weight categories. *Pediatr Neonatol.* (2017) 58:509–15. doi: 10.1016/j.pedneo.2016.10.004
11. Yeo SL. NICU update: state of the science of NEC. *J Perinat Neonatal Nurs.* (2006) 20:46–50. doi: 10.1097/00005237-200601000-00016
12. Stapleton TD, Kahn JM, Evans LE, Critchlow CW, Gardella CM. Risk factors for group B streptococcal genitourinary tract colonization in pregnant women. *Obstet Gynecol.* (2005) 106:1246–52. doi: 10.1097/01.AOG.0000187893.52488.4b
13. Lin HY, Chang JH, Chung MY, Lin HC. Prevention of necrotizing enterocolitis in preterm very low birth weight infants: is it feasible? *J Formos Med Assoc.* (2014) 113:490–7. doi: 10.1016/j.jfma.2013.03.010
14. Song R, Subbarao GC, Maheshwari A. Haematological abnormalities in neonatal necrotizing enterocolitis. *J Matern Fetal Neonatal Med.* (2012) 25(supple. 4):14–7. doi: 10.3109/14767058.2012.715005
15. Ververidis M, Kiely EM, Spitz L, Drake DP, Eaton S, Pierro A. The clinical significance of thrombocytopenia in neonates with necrotizing enterocolitis. *J Ped Surg.* (2001) 36:799–803. doi: 10.1053/jpsu.2001.22964
16. Kenton AB, Hegemier S, Smith EO, O'Donovan DJ, Brandt ML, Cass DL, et al. Platelet transfusions in infants with necrotizing enterocolitis do not lower mortality but may increase morbidity. *J Perinatol.* (2005) 25:173–7. doi: 10.1038/sj.jp.7211237
17. Hong CR, Han SM, Jaksic T. Surgical considerations for neonates with necrotizing enterocolitis. *Semin Fetal Neonatal Med.* (2018) 23:420 5. doi: 10.1016/j.siny.2018.08.007
18. Thyoka M, De Coppi P, Eaton S, Khoo K, Hall NJ, Curry J, et al. Advanced necrotizing enterocolitis part 1: mortality. *Eur J Ped Surg.* (2012) 22:008. doi: 10.1055/s-0032-1306263
19. Hull MA, Fisher JG, Gutierrez IM, Jones BA, Kang KH, Kenny M, et al. Mortality and management of surgical necrotizing enterocolitis in very low birth weight neonates: a prospective cohort study. *J Am Coll Surg.* (2014) 218:1148–55. doi: 10.1016/j.jamcollsurg.2013.11.015
20. Bazacliu C, Neu J. Necrotizing enterocolitis: long term complications. *Curr Pediatr Rev.* (2019) 15:115–24. doi: 10.2174/1573396315666190312093119

23

The Remission Effects of First Injection of Sclerotherapy for Pediatric Rectal Prolapse

Weimo Zhou[1†], *Yingzuo Shi*[2†], *Ming Zhang*[3] *and Li Li*[4*]

[1] Department of Pediatric Surgery, Guigang City People's Hospital, Eighth Affiliated Hospital of Guangxi Medical University, Guigang, China, [2] Department of Pediatric Surgery, Wuxi People's Hospital, Wuxi, China, [3] Clinical Laboratory, Zhucheng Maternal and Child Health Hospital, Zhucheng, China, [4] The Department of Pediatrics, Ganzhou People's Hospital, Ganzhou, China

***Correspondence:**
Li Li
lili0366@sina.com

Background: Pediatric rectal prolapse is a common issue in clinical practice. Among various managements, sclerotherapy is an important method to successfully treat pediatric rectal prolapse, especially for the first injection. The knowledge of the first injection of sclerotherapy can be revealed by a systemic review and meta-analysis of randomized clinical trials.

Methods: We performed a systematic search and a meta-analysis for the retrospective clinical studies of sclerotherapy in pediatric rectal prolapse. The comparison between remission and recurrence after the first injection of sclerotherapy was performed to find if the first injection of sclerotherapy can treat rectal prolapse completely. After a restricted selection, 17 studies involving 1,091 pediatric rectal prolapse subjects with sclerotherapy were enrolled in a variety of classifications of injection agents. The focused outcome was to check whether the first injection of sclerotherapy can achieve a remission status. The meta-analysis was performed by Review Manager 5.4.

Results: Among the subjects receiving sclerotherapy, the meta-analysis favors the remission status after receiving the first injection of sclerotherapy. The meta-analysis results showed significant remission tests for the overall effect and significant heterogeneities in odds ratio and the fixed-effects model. The significant therapeutic effects remained, however, even after testing in the relative risk and the random-effects model.

Conclusions: Despite significant heterogeneity and relatively low quality of evidence, the first injection of sclerotherapy may conceivably demonstrate therapeutic effects to help the patients of pediatric rectal prolapse achieve a remission status.

Keywords: pediatric, rectal prolapse, sclerotherapy, first injection, remission, meta-analysis

INTRODUCTION

Pediatric rectal prolapse is a significant issue in clinical practice. The weak pelvic musculature might predispose the children to such disease. In addition, the loose attachment of rectal mucosa to the muscularis will contribute to rectal prolapse (1). Most patients of pediatric rectal prolapse belong to the mucosal subtype, which is related to straining due to constipation during the toilet training process in children. Pediatric rectal prolapse in older children might be related to congenital neuromuscular abnormalities, autism or developmental delay, and anorectal malformations (2, 3).

The incidence rate of pediatric rectal prolapse was still not clear (4, 5). Spontaneous resolution would be around 60–90% in pediatric rectal prolapse. Compared to pediatric rectal prolapse, rectal prolapse in adults was rarely spontaneously resolving (2). Despite the high rate of spontaneous resolution, pediatric patients with rectal prolapse will suffer much if the condition will not spontaneously resolve. Therefore it is still necessary to receive the management if there is no spontaneous resolution. Before the ultimate choice of operation (6, 7), sclerotherapy would be an important procedure to relieve the pediatric prolapse (3, 5, 8–11). Therefore, it is important for us to understand the intermediate choice (sclerotherapy) between operation and conservative treatment. In this study, we planned to enroll the related articles of sclerotherapy in pediatric rectal prolapse. We wanted to confirm the remission effects of the first injection of sclerotherapy in pediatric rectal prolapse in the study design of systematic review and meta-analysis. We hypothesized that the first injection of sclerotherapy would favor remission rather than recurrence (no remission after the first injection of sclerotherapy and necessary subsequent injection of sclerotherapy).

METHODS

Literature Search and Selection Criteria

We used the following keywords: "rectal" or "rectum" or "prolapse" or "children" or "pediatric" or "sclerotherapy" and "rectal prolapse" to search and to collect the related articles in the PubMed, ScienceDirect, Embase, Web of Science, and Scopus databases. The articles were limited to those published or e-published online before December 2021.

The inclusion criteria of this study were as follows: (1) Sclerotherapy treatment for pediatric patients with rectal prolapse; (2) The studies with sclerotherapy outcome and related clinical profiles; (3) The studies with detailed data of sclerotherapy and pediatric rectal prolapse; (4) These studies were also published in English language in the journals of science citation index database; and (5) Retrospective or prospective study. The exclusion criteria were the following: (1) Some parts of detailed data were unavailable in the content of the articles (unavailable even after inquiring the corresponding authors about the data needed for this meta-analysis); (2) The authors did not respond or could not have access to the dataset, in which case the articles would be excluded as the category without detailed data; (3) The studies that do not belong to patients with rectal prolapse or sclerotherapy; and (4) Review articles.

Quality Assessment and Data Extraction

The study was conducted according to the preferred reporting items for systematic reviews and meta-analyses (PRISMA) guidelines (23). The risk of bias for each study was assessed by the random sequence generation, allocation concealment, blinding of participants and personnel, blinding of outcome assessment, incomplete outcome data, and selective reporting. We extracted the following data from the eligible articles. First, the success rate and patient number of the first injection of sclerotherapy in pediatric patients with rectal prolapse were gathered. Second, the remission rate and patient number under the first injection of sclerotherapy were collected. Third, the recurrence and patient number of the first injection of sclerotherapy in pediatric patients with rectal prolapse were gathered. Fourth, the probable side effects of sclerotherapy in pediatric patients with rectal prolapse was noted.

Data Extraction and Critical Appraisal

WZ reviewed the abstracts to screen the articles. WZ and YS performed the extraction of clinical outcome data from the text, tables, and figures of the enrolled articles independently. The enrolled articles had the clinical outcome data in the text, tables, figures, or supplementary material. Then, a collaborative review was performed to resolve any discrepancies. All authors participated to review the final results.

Meta-Analysis and Statistical Analysis

The odds ratio (OR) with 95% CI (a summary statistic) was obtained by the Mantel–Haenszel method for dichotomous variables. Chi-square tests were used to study heterogeneity between the enrolled studies. The derived I^2 statistic was used to estimate the statistical heterogeneity of studies included in the meta-analysis. The I^2 statistic was used to estimate the percentage of the total variation across studies due to heterogeneity rather than chance. The I^2 values of 25, 50, and 75% represented low, medium, and high heterogeneity, respectively. If the heterogeneity is high, the random-effects model will be used for the analysis and the fixed-effects model will be used for studies with low or moderate heterogeneity. Subgroup analyses were not possible due to the lack of patient-level data. All *P* values were two-sided. All statistical analyses were conducted with Review Manager Version 5.4 (The Cochrane Collaboration, London).

RESULTS

Description of Studies

The initial literature search through the dataset found 124 articles and the additional records from other sources were 14 articles. Then, 55 duplicates were removed and the residual 83 articles were screened according to the relevance of abstracts and titles. Of that, 40 articles were discarded after this step. Full-text contents of the remaining 43 articles were assessed for eligibility. Then, 27 articles were excluded due to review articles, not nurse-led studies, not randomized trials, and not perioperative setting. The qualitative analysis of these 16 articles was performed and no articles were excluded. Therefore, only 16 studies were included in this meta-analysis (1, 4, 5, 10–22). The flow diagram was

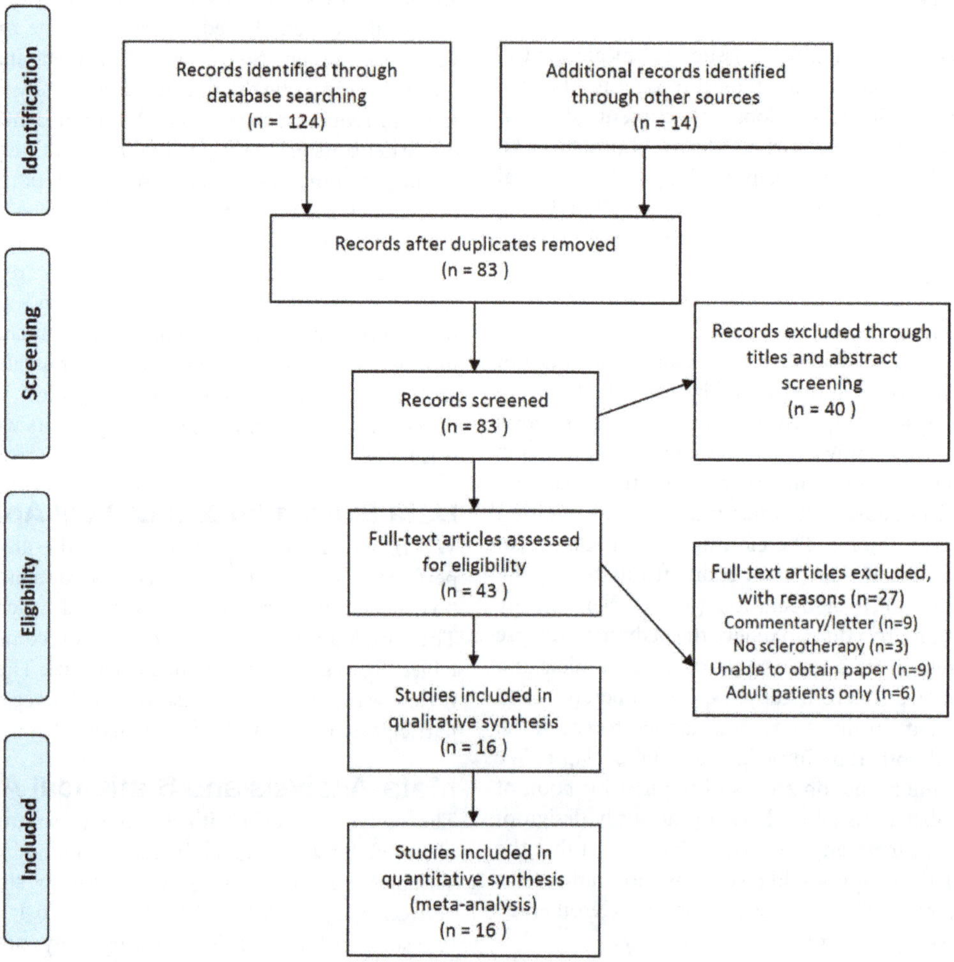

FIGURE 1 | The preferred reporting items for systematic reviews and meta-analyses (PRISMA) flow diagram of the current meta-analysis. The current meta-analysis followed the PRISMA guideline to identify the potentially relevant literature and to screen the identified literature using the abstract and title selection. The full text of screened literature was assessed to find the eligible studies and to include the suitable ones for the final meta-analysis.

presented according to the PRISMA guideline (**Figure 1**). The detailed characteristics of the 16 studies were also summarized in **Table 1**.

Odds of Remission for the First Injection of Sclerotherapy in Pediatric Rectal Prolapse

The I^2 was 95% CI, which revealed high heterogeneity. Therefore, the random-effects model was applied. The test for the overall effect was $Z = 5.07$ ($p < 0.00001$) and the meta-analysis results favored remission after the first injection of sclerotherapy in pediatric patients of rectal prolapse (**Figure 2**). However, the range of 95% CI of several studies included "1" (5, 15, 20). One study revealed the tendency to favor recurrence (13).

DISCUSSION

In the current meta-analysis, the results showed that the first injection of sclerotherapy might have a higher OR to help the pediatric patients with rectal prolapse achieve a remission status. However, the high heterogeneity and the 95% CI of several studies that included an OR of 1 might bias our findings. In a previously published review (24), they focused on the success rate of a single injection (77%), overall complication rate (14%), and the significant difference between different sclerosing agents (no significant differences). Based on their findings, our meta-analysis enrolled all kinds of sclerosing agents in the first injection of sclerotherapy, which should not have a bias from the different sclerosing agents. Our study also supported that there was a high OR of remission after the first injection of sclerotherapy on the pediatric rectal prolapse. Our results suggested that the first injection of sclerotherapy should play a crucial role in the treatment of pediatric patients with rectal prolapse.

In clinical practice, the management for pediatric rectal prolapse has yet to reach a consensus. There are over 100 surgical procedures in the field of rectal prolapse (25). The majority of infants and children can be spontaneously resolved without an aggressive management. Some patients can resolve after conservative management, such as medical treatment for constipation. However, a subgroup of patients might need

TABLE 1 | Summary of enrolled studies for sclerotherapy of pediatric rectal prolapse.

	Study design	Subjects	Injection agent	Remission vs. recurrence
Abes and Sarihan (12)	Retrospective	Rectal prolapse	Normal saline	15 vs. 1
Antao et al. (13)	Retrospective	Rectal prolapse (median age: 3.3 years (4 months–10 years)	Phenol	7 vs. 17
Bahador et al. (14)	Retrospective	Rectal prolapse (108 male, 45 female) (mean age: 2.2 years (9 months to 5 years).	96% ethyl alcohol	147 vs. 6
Batool et al. (15)	Retrospective	Prolonged rectal prolapse	Phenol in almond oil	29 vs. 21
Chan et al. (5)	Retrospective	Rectal prolapse	D50 water	9 vs. 5
Dolejs et al. (4)	Retrospective	Rectal prolapse	Phenol in peanut oil	35 vs. 16
Fahmy and Ezzelarab (16)	Retrospective	Rectal prolapse	Ethyl alcohol, phenol in almond oil, deflux	78 vs. 7
Freeman (1)	Retrospective	Rectal prolapse	Phenol in almond oil	18 vs. 0
Kay and Zachary (11)	Retrospective	Rectal prolapse (29 males, 22 females)	Normal saline	40 vs. 11
Malyshev and Gulin (17)	Retrospective	Rectal prolapse	Ethyl alcohol	339 vs. 14
Sahay et al. (18)	Retrospective	Rectal prolapse	Phenol	16 vs. 7
Sarmast et al. (19)	Retrospective	Rectal prolapse	Normal saline	48 vs. 2
Sasaki et al. (20)	Restrospective	Rectal prolapse 5 boys, 4 girls mean age: 6.5 years; (2.5–14 years)	Phenol in almond oil	6 vs. 3
Shah et al. (21)	Retrospective	Rectal prolapse median age: 2.5 years; (2–4.5 years)	Normal saline	12 vs. 5
Wyllie (10)	Retrospective	Rectal prolapse average age: 2.5 years	Phenol in almond oil	86 vs. 5
Zganjer et al. (22)	Retrospective	Rectal prolapse mean age: 6.2 years; (4–8 years)	Cow's milk	80 vs. 6

Study or Subgroup	remission Events	remission Total	recurrence Events	recurrence Total	Weight	Odds Ratio M-H, Random, 95% CI
Abes 2004	15	16	1	16	5.2%	225.00 [12.85, 3939.51]
Antao 2005	7	24	17	24	6.5%	0.17 [0.05, 0.59]
Bahador 2008	147	153	6	153	6.5%	600.25 [189.22, 1904.16]
Batool 2005	29	50	21	50	6.7%	1.91 [0.86, 4.22]
Chan 1998	9	14	5	14	6.3%	3.24 [0.69, 15.20]
Dolejs 2017	35	51	16	51	6.7%	4.79 [2.07, 11.05]
Fahmy 2004	78	85	7	85	6.6%	124.16 [41.59, 370.64]
Freeman 1984	18	18	0	18	4.2%	1369.00 [25.77, 72720.79]
Kay 1970	40	51	11	51	6.7%	13.22 [5.15, 33.90]
Malyshev 1973	339	353	14	353	6.7%	586.33 [275.32, 1248.66]
Sahay 2017	16	23	7	23	6.5%	5.22 [1.49, 18.35]
Sarmast 2015	48	50	2	50	6.0%	576.00 [77.92, 4257.71]
Sasaki 2004	6	9	3	9	6.0%	4.00 [0.56, 28.40]
Shah 2005	12	17	5	17	6.3%	5.76 [1.32, 25.19]
Wyllie 1979	86	91	5	91	6.5%	295.84 [82.66, 1058.85]
Zganjer 2008	80	86	6	86	6.5%	177.78 [55.00, 574.67]
Total (95% CI)		**1091**		**1091**	**100.0%**	**30.60 [8.16, 114.77]**
Total events	965		126			

Heterogeneity: Tau² = 6.60; Chi² = 283.96, df = 15 (P < 0.00001); I² = 95%

Test for overall effect: Z = 5.07 (P < 0.00001)

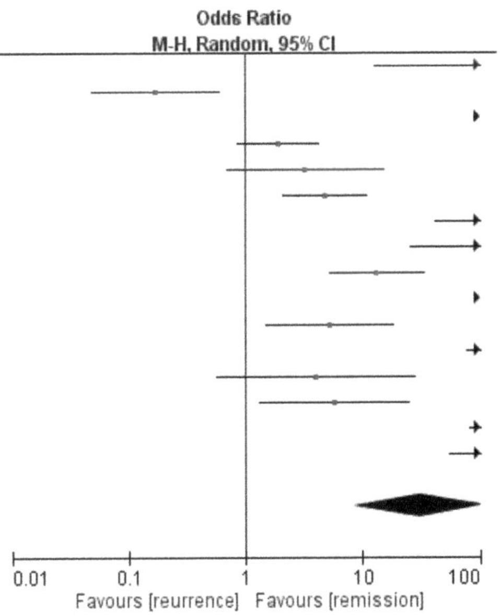

FIGURE 2 | The odds ratio of remission vs. recurrence for the first injection of sclerotherapy in the enrolled studies of pediatric rectal prolapse. The first injection of sclerotherapy showed a favorable result toward remission rather than recurrence. The heterogeneity was high and the result was statistically significant.

aggressive intervention due to persistent symptoms or the lack of spontaneous resolve (2). Therefore, when the clinicians make a clinical judgment, that is, whether they want to take a more aggressive management, sclerotherapy might be an intermediate choice between conservative treatment and surgery.

However, due to the high probability of spontaneous resolution (60–90%) of pediatric rectal prolapse (2), we can observe that it is difficult to enroll a high number of patients for the sclerotherapy, except the studies of Bahador et al. (14) and Malyshev et al. (17). Therefore, the meta-analysis results might be influenced by the two relatively big studies in patient numbers. In addition, the lack of standardization of sclerosing agents, the number, and the location of injections also contributed to the difficulty to standardize the treatment procedures of sclerotherapy. The proportion of patients who would experience a resolution of rectal prolapse with non-operative management remains unknown, even with a recent meta-analysis with such data (24). Another review article showed that the success rate of sclerotherapy in pediatric rectal prolapse was 79.5% (25), which was similar to the meta-analytic data of Hintz et al. (24). However, the review article just used a systematic review strategy to conclude the success rate of sclerotherapy. Therefore, we still need more data to confirm the remission effects of the first injection of sclerotherapy in pediatric rectal prolapse.

There were several limitations in the current study. First, the high heterogeneity and the relatively poor quality of data might bias our findings. Even if the random-effect model can adjust such bias, the influences for our study results were still significant. Second, the lack of demographic data for the "real subgroup" of sclerotherapy in most enrolled studies might limit our ability to analyze the subgroup differences. The lack of demographic data was because we focused on sclerotherapy for pediatric rectal prolapse. However, not all enrolled studies would provide the demographic data "purely" for "sclerotherapy for rectal prolapse," which is the reason for the lack of some demographic data in **Table 1**. Third, the lack of a detailed information on subgroups was also an obstacle in performing the subgroup analysis. Fourth, the different kinds of sclerosing agents were included in the current study, which might bias our interpretations. However, the meta-analysis of Hintz et al. suggested that there was no significant difference in the treatment effects between different sclerosing agents (24). Fifth, all the enrolled studies had a retrospective design, which would also influence our meta-analysis results. The references we searched also revealed that the published studies were all retrospective, probably due to the characteristics of the clinical practice of pediatric rectal prolapse, and it might be difficult to enroll such patients in a design of randomized clinical trials or double-blinded trials. Further studies of randomized trials might be warranted to confirm the treatment and remission effects of the first injection of sclerotherapy.

CONCLUSION

Despite significant heterogeneity and a relatively low quality of evidence, the first injection of sclerotherapy might demonstrate the therapeutic effects to help the patients of pediatric rectal prolapse achieve remission status. However, more randomized trials with more standardization of sclerotherapy procedures will be warranted in the future to confirm the remission effects of the first injection of sclerotherapy in pediatric rectal prolapse.

AUTHOR CONTRIBUTIONS

WZ reviewed the abstracts to screen the articles. WZ and YS performed the extraction of clinical outcome data from text, tables, and figures of the enrolled articles independently. MZ checked the manuscript and gave instructions. LL provided the idea of the study design and gave instructions. All authors contributed to the article and approved the submitted version.

REFERENCES

1. Freeman NV. Rectal prolapse in children. *J R Soc Med.* (1984) 77 Suppl 3:9–12.
2. Saadai P, Trappey AF, Langer JL. Surgical management of rectal prolapse in infants and children. *Eur J Pediatr Surg.* (2020) 30:401–5. doi: 10.1055/s-0040-1716725
3. Corman ML. Rectal prolapse in children. *Dis Colon Rectum.* (1985) 28:535–9. doi: 10.1007/BF02554107
4. Dolejs SC, Sheplock J, Vandewalle RJ, Landman MP, Rescorla FJ. Sclerotherapy for the management of rectal prolapse in children. *J Pediatr Surg.* (2017). doi: 10.1016/j.jpedsurg.2017.10.015
5. Chan WK, Kay SM, Laberge JM, Gallucci JG, Bensoussan AL, Yazbeck S. Injection sclerotherapy in the treatment of rectal prolapse in infants and children. *J Pediatr Surg.* (1998) 33:255–8. doi: 10.1016/S0022-3468(98)90441-9
6. Puri B. Rectal prolapse in children: laparoscopic suture rectopexy is a suitable alternative. *J Indian Assoc Pediatr Surg.* (2010) 15:47–9. doi: 10.4103/0971-9261.70634
7. Laituri CA, Garey CL, Fraser JD, Aguayo P, Ostlie DJ, St Peter SD, et al. 15-Year experience in the treatment of rectal prolapse in children. *J Pediatr Surg.* (2010) 45:1607–9. doi: 10.1016/j.jpedsurg.2010.01.012
8. Chew SS, Marshall L, Kalish L, Tham J, Grieve DA, Douglas PR, et al. Short-term and long-term results of combined sclerotherapy and rubber band ligation of hemorrhoids and mucosal prolapse. *Dis Colon Rectum.* (2003) 46:1232–7. doi: 10.1007/s10350-004-6720-0
9. Qvist N, Rasmussen L, Klaaborg KE, Hansen LP, Pedersen SA. Rectal prolapse in infancy: conservative versus operative treatment. *J Pediatr Surg.* (1986) 21:887–8. doi: 10.1016/S0022-3468(86)80015-X
10. Wyllie GG. The injection treatment of rectal prolapse. *J Pediatr Surg.* (1979) 14:62–4. doi: 10.1016/S0022-3468(79)80578-3
11. Kay NR, Zachary RB. The treatment of rectal prolapse in children with injections of 30 per cent saline solutions. *J Pediatr Surg.* (1970) 5:334–7. doi: 10.1016/0022-3468(70)90190-9
12. Abes M, Sarihan H. Injection sclerotherapy of rectal prolapse in children with 15 percent saline solution. *Eur J Pediatr Surg.* (2004) 14:100–2. doi: 10.1055/s-2004-815855
13. Antao B, Bradley V, Roberts JP, Shawis R. Management of rectal prolapse in children. *Dis Colon Rectum.* (2005) 48:1620–5. doi: 10.1007/s10350-005-0074-0
14. Bahador A, Foroutan HR, Hosseini SM, Davani SZ. Effect of submucosal alcohol injection on prolonged rectal prolapse in infants and children. *J Indian Assoc Pediatr Surg.* (2008) 13:11–3. doi: 10.4103/0971-9261.42566
15. Batool T, Akhtar J, Ahmed S. Management of idiopathic rectal prolapse in children. *J Coll Physicians Surg Pak.* (2005) 15:628–30.
16. Fahmy MA, Ezzelarab S. Outcome of submucosal injection of different sclerosing materials for rectal prolapse in children. *Pediatr Surg Int.* (2004) 20:353–6. doi: 10.1007/s00383-004-1197-4
17. Malyshev YI, Gulin VA. Our experience with the treatment of rectal prolapse in infants and children. *Am J Proctol.* (1973) 24:470–2.
18. Sahay R, Murthi G, Lindley R. Outcomes following sclerotherapy for mucosal rectal prolapse with oily phenol injection: single-centre review. *Pediatr Surg Int.* (2017) 33:363–5. doi: 10.1007/s00383-016-4035-6
19. Sarmast MH, Askarpour S, Peyvasteh M, Javaherizadeh H, Mooghehi-Nezhad M. Rectal prolapse in children: a study of 71 cases. *Przeglad gastroenterologiczny.* (2015) 10:105–7. doi: 10.5114/pg.2015.49003

20. Sasaki Y, Iwai N, Kimura O, Hibi M. The treatment of rectal prolapse in children with phenol in almond oil injection. *Eur J Pediatr Surg.* (2004) 14:414–7. doi: 10.1055/s-2004-821151
21. Shah A, Parikh D, Jawaheer G, Gornall P. Persistent rectal prolapse in children: sclerotherapy and surgical management. *Pediatr Surg Int.* (2005) 21:270–3. doi: 10.1007/s00383-005-1384-y
22. Zganjer M, Cizmic A, Cigit I, Zupancic B, Bumci I, Popovic L, et al. Treatment of rectal prolapse in children with cow milk injection sclerotherapy: 30-year experience. *World J Gastroenterol.* (2008) 14:737–40. doi: 10.3748/wjg.14.737
23. Knobloch K, Yoon U, Vogt PM. Preferred reporting items for systematic reviews and meta-analyses (PRISMA) statement and publication bias. *J Craniomaxillofac Surg.* (2011) 39:91–2. doi: 10.1016/j.jcms.2010.11.001
24. Hintz GC, Zou VZ, Baird R. Sclerotherapy for rectal prolapse in children: a systematic review and meta-analysis. *J Pediatr Surg.* (2019) 54:1083–8. doi: 10.1016/j.jpedsurg.2019.01.033
25. Morrison ZD, LaPlant M, Hess D, Segura B, Saltzman D. A systematic review of management options in pediatric rectal prolapse. *J Pediatr Surg.* (2019) 54:1782–7. doi: 10.1016/j.jpedsurg.2019.03.002

24

Inflow Occlusion Combined with Bleomycin Sclerotherapy for Management of Macro/Mixed Cystic Lymphatic Malformation in Children

*Tao Han, Yi Ji, Jie Cui and Weimin Shen**

Department of Burns and Plastic Surgery, Children's Hospital of Nanjing Medical University, Nanjing, China

***Correspondence:**
Weimin Shen
swmswmswm@sina.com

Background: The link between cystic lymphatic malformation (cLM) and normal lymphatic system has become the focus of research. This study aimed to assess the outcomes of indocyanine green (ICG) lymphography-guided inflow occlusion combined with bleomycin sclerotherapy for the management of macro or mixed cLM in children.

Methods: Between June 2018 and October 2020, inflow occlusion combined with bleomycin sclerotherapy was performed in 81 cLM patients (age range from 6 months to 8 years). All cases were evaluated by the following parameters: cLM location, histological typing, number of afferent lymph vessels, dermal backflow, curative effects, treatment frequency, and postoperative complications. The duration of postoperative follow-up was from 10 to 16 months.

Results: All cLM cases could be found with at least one lymphatic inflow. Excellent outcomes were observed in 68 cases (84.0%), 11 cases (13.6%) experienced good outcomes, and two (2.5%) cases had fair outcome. No case experienced repeated treatment for more than three times. Wound infection, fever, and scar hyperplasia were the independent adverse events, which were managed by symptomatic treatment.

Conclusion: Inflow occlusion combined with bleomycin sclerotherapy renders a safe and efficient approach for the management of macro or mixed cLM.

Keywords: cystic lymphatic malformation, inflow occlusion, bleomycin, indocyanine green, lymphography

INTRODUCTION

Cystic lymphatic malformations (cLM) are nonmalignant vascular malformations of the lymphatic system, characterized by the dilated cysts lined by lymphatic endothelial cells (1, 2). According to the classification system of the International Society for the Study of Vascular Anomalies (ISSVA), cLM can be histologically categorized into three subtypes, including macrocystic, microcystic, and mixed cystic. It may change in size resulting from local infection, intracapsular hemorrhage or trauma, and even resolve spontaneously in rare cases (3–5). cLM has been managed by multidisciplinary teams worldwide, each according to their own preferences regarding therapeutic intervention approaches, including surgical resection, sclerotherapy, oral sirolimus, radiofrequency ablation, and laser therapy (6–11). In recent years, sclerotherapy plays a main role in the management of macro cLM in terms of safety and aesthetics.

However, given that some of cLMs with inflow pattern are connected to lymphatic system, posttreatment accumulation of lymph in the lesion could always be observed, which may eventually lead to local recurrence and repeated sclerotherapy (12, 13). For improved outcomes, the link between cLM and normal lymphatic system has gradually become the focus of research nowadays. Recently, indocyanine green (ICG) fluorescence imaging system has gained increasing interest with its significant detection of both inflow and outflow of cLM and is considered to be useful for the interventions of cLM (14).

With our previous ICG lymphography study, we found that only one afferent lymph vessel was detected in most cases of macro cLM and mixed cLM, while all micro cLM cases had more than two inflows. Based on our experience and relevant literatures, we herein hold the thought that it is feasible for macro/mixed cLM cases to perform inflow occlusion for blocking the link to the lymphatic system, which could be beneficial for reducing lymph accumulation postoperatively. The purpose of this study was to present our experience in performing inflow occlusion combined with bleomycin sclerotherapy as an alternative management of macro/mixed cLM in children.

PATIENTS AND METHODS

Patients

Between June 2018 and October 2020, we conducted a prospective research for this treatment in 81 children diagnosed with macro or mixed cystic LM in our center. The male-to-female ratio was 48:33, with an age range of from 6 months to 8 years. Preoperative physical examination and MRI were performed to determine both region and extent of cLM lesions. All patients were evaluated by the following parameters: cLM location, histological typing, number of afferent lymph vessels, dermal backflow, curative effects, treatment frequency, and postoperative complications. Adverse events included wound infection, fever, scar hyperplasia, and temporary ICG-related pigmentation. The inclusion criteria included the following: (1) no previous intervention (including surgery or sclerotherapy), (2) rapidly involving symptoms, (3) macro/mixed cLM confirmed by preoperative MRI and postoperative pathology, and (4) inflows from lymphatic system confirmed by ICG lymphography. The exclusion criteria included the following: (1) history of iodine allergy, (2) micro cLM, (3) syndromic cLM (e.g., Klippel–Trenaunay syndrome, Gorham-Stout disease), and (4) isolated cLM (no inflow detected). All study protocols were conducted subsequent to receiving consents from the parents of cLM patients. This clinical study was approved by the Ethics Committee of the Children's Hospital of Nanjing Medical University.

Surgical Technique

Bleomycin powder (15 mg, Hisun Pfizer Co., Ltd., Hangzhou, China) was reconstituted with 15 ml of normal saline, yielding a 1-mg/ml concentration. The amount of bleomycin injection depended on the size of cLM. The dose of injection was 0.5–1 mg/kg, and the maximum dose was limited to 15 mg per session.

Under general anesthesia, both intradermal and subcutaneous injections of ICG were performed in multipoints distal to the cLM lesion. At each injection site, 0.05 to 0.1 ml of ICG solution (concentration: 2.5 mg/ml, Dandong Yichuang, China) was administered. The maximum dose of ICG was 0.5 mg/kg per session. To minimize the possibility that injected ICG does not enter the lesion and stays in the soft tissue around the injection site or in the lymph node, we routinely performed a 10-min local massage from the distal to proximal regions. ICG lymphography was performed by using near-infrared fluorescence imaging system (Mingde Medical Diagnosis Inc., Langfang, China) with its optical handheld probe. The probe, perpendicular to the skin, was covered with a sterile drape for adjusting its position at a distance of 10 cm. The tissue penetration was limited to 10 mm for visualization, and real-time video images captured during the procedure were stored for later review. The injection points for detecting inflows of cLM at specific locations were summarized as follows: (1) cLM at the cervicofacial region: temporal scalp, (2) cLM at the chest: ipsilateral para-areolar area, (3) cLM at the abdomen or back: midline area, 3–5 cm distal to the cLM, (4) cLM at the upper extremities: first and third web spaces, ulnar and radial volar wrist area, (5) cLM at the lower extremities: first and third web spaces, and (6) cLM at digits: both sides of the tiptoe/fingertip, nail bed (**Figure 1**).

With completion of ICG injections and observations, we confirmed both location and number of inflows. The detected inflows were visualized gradually from distal to proximal region, and a skin incision was performed in the region where afferent lymph vessels drained into the cLM lesion. The lymph vessels were separated from the incision and confirmed by ICG lymphography (**Figure 2A**). Subsequently, identified inflows

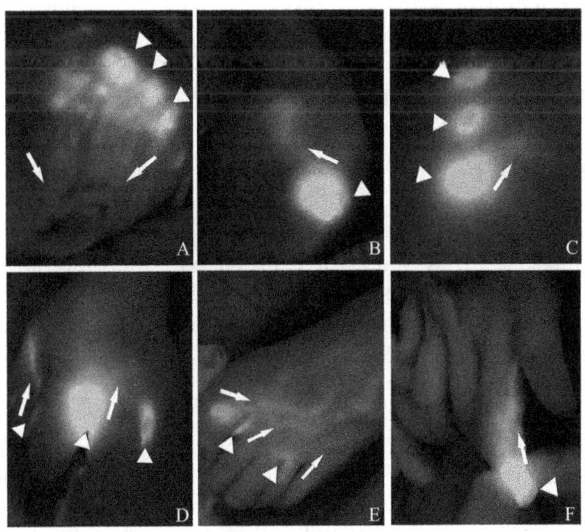

FIGURE 1 | The selection of indocyanine green (ICG) injection points for detecting inflows of cystic lymphatic malformations (cLM) at the **(A)** cervicofacial region, **(B)** chest, **(C)** abdomen or back, **(D)** upper extremities, **(E)** lower extremities, and **(F)** digits. *Arrow head*, lymph vessel; *triangle*, ICG injection point.

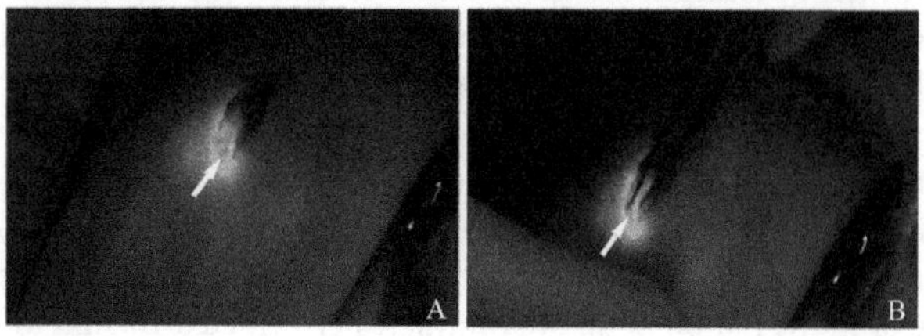

FIGURE 2 | (A) ICG lymphography indicates the localization of the afferent lymph vessels. **(B)** Inflow occlusion is conducted by bipolar electrocoagulation. *Arrow head*, lymph vessel.

were occluded by bipolar electrocoagulation with the power of 50 W (**Figure 2B**). A pair of scissors was used to pass through the cystic wall, and lymph in the lesion was drained by suction, and then a small part of the cystic tissue was resected for postoperative pathology. For reducing the postoperative accumulation of lymph, fluorescence imaging probe (without another ICG injection) was used again to rule out both inflow visualization and lymphatic leak with the focus on the previous detected site.

Thereafter, we placed a drainage tube into the cyst from the incision, and bleomycin was then administered through this tube. After 2 h, a syringe of negative pressure was then connected to the intralesional drainage tube. It was removed on the fifth to seventh day of postoperation when no lymph could be aspirated. For all patients enrolled in our study, the duration of postoperative follow-up was from 10 to 16 months (mean length: 12.4 months).

Curative Effect Evaluation

Both physical examination and MRI images were compared preoperatively and postoperatively; the effective response was evaluated by assessing the reduction rate of the lesion (reduced size/pre-op size × 100%) as follows: (1) excellent, defined as a reduction rate of more than 90%, (2) good, defined as a reduction rate from 75 to 90%, (3) fair, defined as a reduction rate from 50 to 75%, and (4) poor, defined as a reduction rate of <50% (15).

RESULTS

The characteristics and outcomes of all 81 cases with macro or mixed cLM are summarized in **Table 1**. After injection of ICG, the afferent lymph vessels were gradually visualized from the distal to proximal region, and eventually drained into cLM lesions. As shown by ICG lymphography, no morphological or structural abnormality in afferent lymph vessels was detected. Remarkably, all cLM cases could be found with at least one lymphatic inflow, but without outflow. After occlusion, the afferent lymph vessels could not be visualized on the previous detected site. Neither lymphatic leak nor regeneration of the collateral pathway was observed postoperatively. One mixed cLM case with lymphatic dermal backflow was revealed in this study. This might be caused by the high pressure or dysfunction of lymph vessels, and ICG/lymph flowed back abnormally to the dermal tissue space. Sixty-eight cases (84.0%) with excellent clinical outcomes resulted in notably improved appearance

TABLE 1 | Characteristics and outcomes of patients.

Demographics	Patients (n = 81)	%
Gender		
Male	48	59.3
Female	33	40.7
Age group (years)		
<1	27	33.3
1~3	40	49.4
>3	14	17.3
Location		
Cervicofacial region	41	50.6
Trunk	29	35.8
Extremities	11	13.6
Histological typing		
Macro cLM	50	61.7
Mixed cLM	31	38.3
Inflow (no.)		
1	74	91.4
2	7	8.6
Dermal backflow	1	1.2

cLM, cystic lymphatic malformation.

(**Figures 3–5**), 11 cases (13.6%) experienced partial reduction in the size of cLM lesion, two cases (2.5%, one at the right scapular region, one at the right upper extremity) with fair outcomes required subsequent treatment, and their follow-up was still in progress. Besides, majority of our cases (91.4%) experienced only one session of this treatment. Repeated treatments were needed in 8.6% of cases, in which inflow was no longer visualized by ICG lymphography. Therefore, inflow occlusion was not necessary to perform again, and only bleomycin sclerotherapy was repeated in a subsequent procedure. It is worth noting that no case in our research was treated for more than three times (**Table 2**).

In this study, fever (8.3%) and scar hyperplasia (8.3%) were the independent adverse events, which were managed by symptomatic treatment. All patients experienced temporary ICG-related pigmentation in the injection sites, which faded away gradually within 1 month postoperatively. There was no ICG allergy or secondary lymphedema occurring in all cases (**Table 3**).

DISCUSSION

Given a localized lesion, surgery resection and sclerotherapy are always the main choices for the management of both macro and mixed cLM (3, 16–19). However, a series of cLM cases treated by surgery or sclerotherapy suffer from limited efficacy or local recurrence, especially for the cLM at the cervicofacial region, axilla, and joints. The uncertain border of cLM at these regions makes radical resection very difficult, and the lymph from afferent vessels accumulates again after sclerotherapy, leading to multiple sessions and even focal relapse of cLM (20, 21). Therefore, exploring the link between cLM and the lymphatic

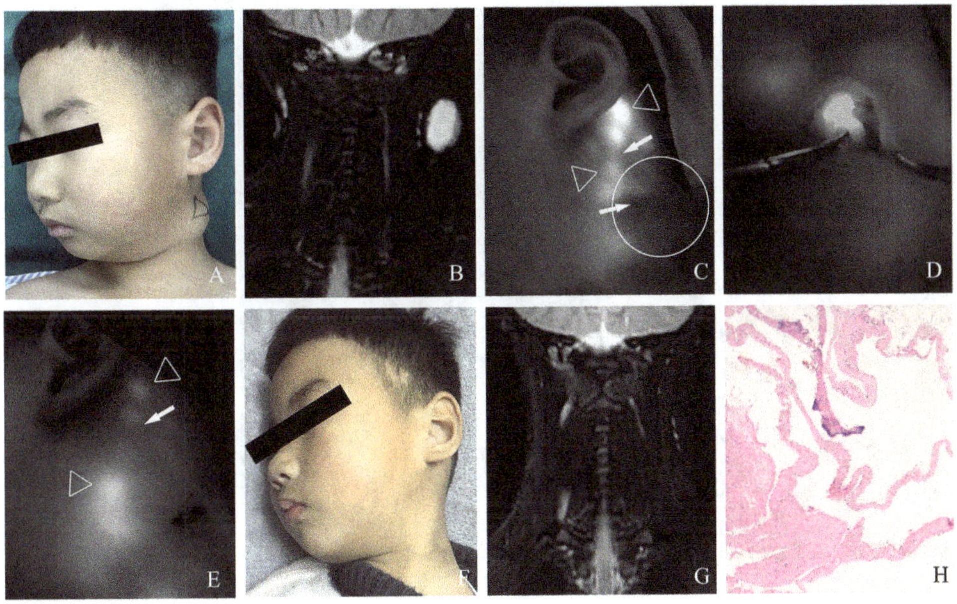

FIGURE 3 | (A) A 4-year-old male patient with macro cLM of left neck preoperatively. **(B)** MRI preoperatively. **(C)** A normal lymph vessel from the left temporal scalp ran into the posterior auricular region, from which another afferent lymph vessel was observed flowing into the lesion cite. **(D)** The cLM lesion confirmed by ICG lymphography during surgery. **(E)** No inflow visualization or lymphatic leak on the previous detected site after inflow occlusion. **(F)** Ten months postoperatively, complete regression of cLM met the criterion of excellent curative effect. **(G)** MRI postoperatively. **(H)** Pathology postoperatively. *Arrow head*, lymph vessel; *circle*, region of cLM; *hollow triangle*, lymph node.

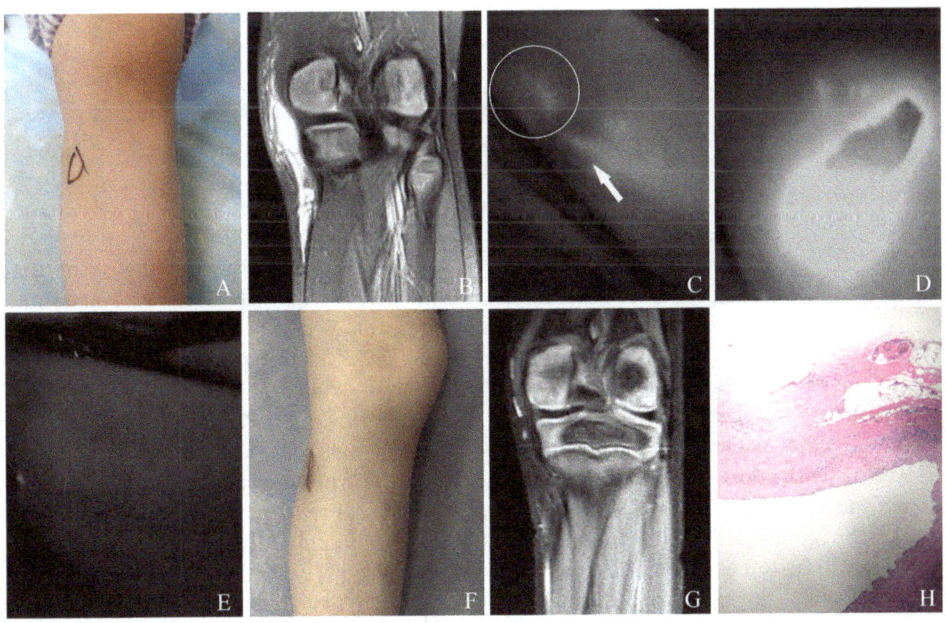

FIGURE 4 | (A) A 5-year-old female patient with mixed cLM of left knee preoperatively. **(B)** MRI preoperatively. **(C)** ICG finding with one afferent lymph vessel draining into a lesion. **(D)** The cLM lesion confirmed by ICG lymphography during surgery. **(E)** No inflow visualization or lymphatic leak on the previous detected site after inflow occlusion. **(F)** Twelve months postoperatively, complete regression of cLM met the criterion of excellent curative effect. Remarkably, this patient suffered from skin scar hyperplasia. **(G)** MRI postoperatively. **(H)** Pathology postoperatively. *Arrow head*, lymph vessel; *circle*, region of cLM.

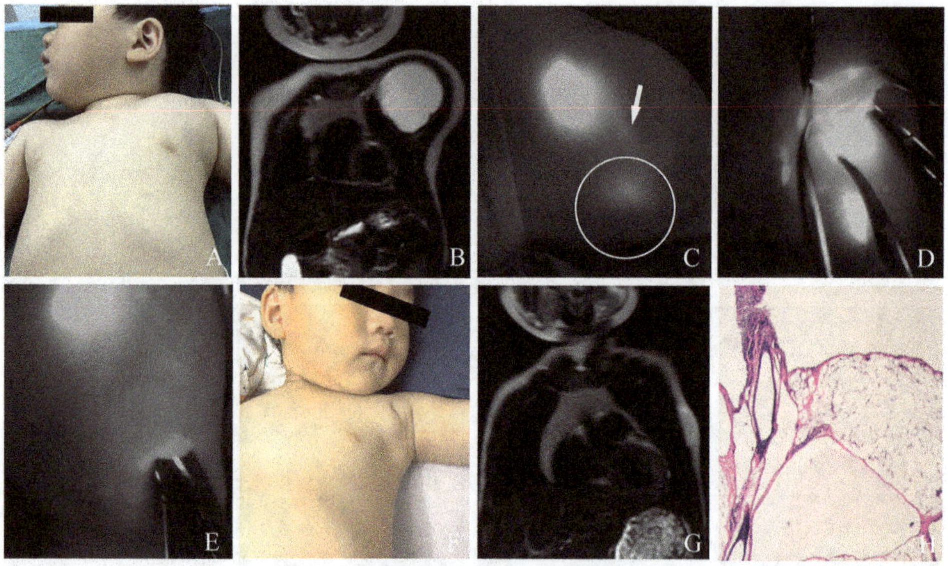

FIGURE 5 | (A) A 2-year-old male patient with macro cLM of the left chest preoperatively. **(B)** MRI preoperatively. **(C)** ICG finding with one afferent lymph vessel draining into a lesion. **(D)** The cLM lesion confirmed by ICG lymphography during surgery. **(E)** No inflow visualization or lymphatic leak on the previous detected site after inflow occlusion. **(F)** Ten months postoperatively, complete regression of cLM met the criterion of excellent curative effect. **(G)** MRI postoperatively. **(H)** Pathology postoperatively. *Arrow head*, lymph vessel; *circle*, region of cLM.

TABLE 2 | Outcomes of the postoperative period.

Results	Patients ($n = 81$)	%
Curative effects		
Excellent	68	84.0
Good	11	13.6
Fair	2	2.5
Poor	0	0
Treatment frequency (times)		
1	74	91.4
2–3	7	8.6
>3	0	0

TABLE 3 | Postoperative complications.

Subject	Patients ($n = 81$)	%
Fever	2	2.5
Scar hyperplasia	2	2.5
Temporary ICG-related pigmentation	81	100

ICG, indocyanine green.

system, could gain insight into its pathogenesis and, furthermore, offers a new thought for targeted therapeutic approaches.

MRI examination, as the principal method of diagnosing cLM, is widely employed in evaluation of the lesion and its relationship with adjacent structures (22, 23). MRI is particularly useful for indicating its border, septum, lesion range, and content within the cysts, with low-signal intensity on T1 and high-signal intensity on T2. However, the peripheral lymph flow around cLM cannot be demonstrated by MRI, which hinders the understanding of changes in the local lymphatic drainage in cLM patients. Therefore, it is necessary to combine lymphography imaging to improve the assessment of cLM.

ICG, as a safe and stable fluorescent dye, can be easily absorbed by lymphatic capillaries (24). The original applications of ICG lymphography in the field of lymphatic surgeries were to detect lymph flow patterns or to confirm the treatment outcomes in both primary and secondary lymphedema (25–27). Recently, its capability to penetrate deep into soft tissue (up to 10 mm for visualization) opens the door to real-time intraoperative navigation for the management of cLM. Kato et al. (13, 14, 28) reported that the flow patterns of cLM can be classified into four types, and flow-oriented venous anastomosis for creating drainage bypass was considered an effective surgical approach for micro or mixed cLM. Kubota et al. (29) reported an adult case with axillary cLM that was successfully treated with ICG lymphography for visualization of lymph vessel and lesion. Additionally, Shirota et al. (30) revealed that following ICG injection into the skin above the lesion, the precise surgical margins of cLM could be identified, which, in turn, aid in complete resection.

In the study presented here, we performed intraoperative ICG lymphography to detect afferent lymph vessels. The skin incision was selected in the region where afferent lymph vessels drained into the lesion, so that it was beneficial for exposure of both inflow and cLM. For stable postoperative outcome, we performed inflow occlusion combined with bleomycin sclerotherapy, which had not been previously reported in the treatment of macro or mixed cLM. The principle behind this technique is to block the communication between the lesion and lymphatic system, and to induce shrinkage of the cysts. Fluorescence imaging probe was intraoperatively used to assess inflow occlusion and ruled out lymphatic leak, so as to reduce the postoperative accumulation of lymph in the lesion.

It is worth mentioning that, it is not feasible to ligate the inflow without lesion resection, which may lead to a regeneration of the collateral pathway postoperatively (13). Besides, for patients with micro cLM, our technique is not the ideal treatment modality of choice. Due to multiple small inflows observed in most micro cLM cases, occluding all of them may impede normal lymphatic drainage and cause secondary lymphedema subsequently.

The selection of management of cLM relies on lesion location, patient preference, and experience of the surgeon. Sclerotherapy has emerged as a first-line treatment for macro cLM in the cervicofacial region with its advantages, including simple operation, less trauma, and fewer side effects (31, 32). Bleomycin, an antibiotic derivative with cytostatic properties, induces obliteration and fibrosis of cysts by its sclerosant effect on lymphatic endothelium (33, 34). However, therapeutic responses of bleomycin are always delayed for >3 months after initial treatment, and posttreatment accumulation of lymph may cause multiple sessions of treatment (35–37). Thus, for cLMs connecting to the lymphatic system, we think that inflow occlusion can inhibit lymph accumulation after sclerotherapy, so as to improve curative effect and reduce treatment frequency. Two hours after bleomycin sclerotherapy, we applied negative pressure for continuous drainage to promote cyst shrinkage and reduce posttreatment accumulation of the remaining lymph. Our technique provided rapid results, and 91.4% of cases did not need extra treatment postoperatively. Therefore, we believe that it could be an effective alternative for the management of macro or mixed cLM.

Our research has several limitations. Because ICG tissue penetration was limited to 10 mm for visualization, we cannot assure inflow occlusion in the deep tissue. Postoperative accumulation of lymph from deep inflows might be the cause of two cases with fair outcomes. In addition, further investigations with both larger sample sizes and longer follow-up period (1.5–2 years) would provide more concrete evidence for the effectiveness of this new technique.

In conclusion, this research introduces a novel technique, which combines inflow occlusion and bleomycin sclerotherapy based on intraoperative ICG lymphography. This procedure is performed with easy operation, satisfactory curative effect, and favorable treatment frequency. We therefore believe that the findings of this study could offer an effective and safe alternative for the management of macro or mixed cLM.

ETHICS STATEMENT

The studies involving human participants were reviewed and approved by Ethics Committee of the Children's Hospital of Nanjing Medical University. Written informed consent to participate in this study was provided by the participants' legal guardian/next of kin. Written informed consent was obtained from the minor(s)' legal guardian/next of kin for the publication of any potentially identifiable images or data included in this article.

AUTHOR CONTRIBUTIONS

WS and JC performed the surgery and conducted the data analyses. YJ performed postoperative follow-up, analyzed the data, wrote sections of the article, and edited the figures. TH wrote a draft of the article and edited the figures. All authors contributed to the article and approved the submitted version.

REFERENCES

1. Wassef M, Blei F, Adams D, Alomari A, Baselga E, Berenstein A, et al. Vascular anomalies classification: recommendations from the international society for the study of vascular anomalies. *Pediatrics.* (2015) 136:e203–14. doi: 10.1542/peds.2014-3673
2. Hanif AM, Saunders JA, Hawkins CM, Wojno TH, Kim HJ. Use of percutaneous bleomycin sclerotherapy for orbital lymphatic malformations. *Orbit.* (2019) 38:30–6. doi: 10.1080/01676830.2018.1480636
3. Bagrodia N, Defnet AM, Kandel JJ. Management of lymphatic malformations in children. *Curr Opin Pediatr.* (2015) 27:356–63. doi: 10.1097/MOP.0000000000000209
4. Perkins JA, Maniglia C, Magit A, Sidhu M, Manning SC, Chen EY. Clinical and radiographic findings in children with spontaneous lymphatic malformation regression Otolaryngol. *Head Neck Surg.* (2008) 138:772–7. doi: 10.1016/j.otohns.2008.02.016
5. Mestak O, Mestak J, Pokorna K, Bruna J, Sukop A. Unusual regression of severe recurrent lymphatic malformation of a face after contraception and pregnancy. *Gynecol Endocrinol.* (2012) 28:764–6. doi: 10.3109/09513590.2012.664190
6. Cheng J, Liu B, Lee HJ. 30-Day outcomes analysis of NSQIP-pediatric for surgical management of head and neck lymphatic malformations in children. *Int J Pediatr Otorhinolaryngol.* (2019) 118:21–4. doi: 10.1016/j.ijporl.2018.12.008
7. Dubois J, Thomas-Chausse F, Soulez G. Common (Cystic) lymphatic malformations: current knowledge and management. *Tech Vasc Interv Radiol.* (2019) 22:100631. doi: 10.1016/j.tvir.2019.100631
8. Tian R, Liang Y, Zhang W, Wang J, Shan Y, Gao H, et al. Effectiveness of sirolimus in the treatment of complex lymphatic malformations: Single center report of 56 cases. *J Pediatr Surg.* (2020) 55:2454–8. doi: 10.1016/j.jpedsurg.2019.12.021
9. Chaudry G, Guevara CJ, Rialon KL, Kerr C, Mulliken JB, Greene AK, et al. Safety and efficacy of bleomycin sclerotherapy for microcystic lymphatic malformation. *Cardiovasc Intervent Radiol.* (2014) 37:1476–81. doi: 10.1007/s00270-014-0932-z
10. Thottam PJ, Al-Barazi R, Madgy DN, Rozzelle A. Submucosal resection of a microcystic oropharyngeal lymphatic malformation using radiofrequency ablation. *Int J Pediatr Otorhinolaryngol.* (2013) 77:1589–92. doi: 10.1016/j.ijporl.2013.05.037
11. Horbach SE, Rigter IM, Smitt JH, Reekers JA, Spuls PI, van der Horst CM. Intralesional Bleomycin Injections for Vascular Malformations: A Systematic Review and Meta-Analysis. *Plast Reconstr Surg.* (2016) 137:244–56. doi: 10.1097/PRS.0000000000001924

12. Perkins JA, Manning SC, Tempero RM, Cunningham MJ, Edmonds JL Jr, Hoffer FA, et al. Lymphatic malformations: current cellular and clinical investigations. *Otolaryngol Head Neck Surg.* (2010) 142:2789–94. doi: 10.1016/j.otohns.2010.02.025
13. Kato M, Watanabe S, Watanabe A, Iida T. Flow-oriented venous anastomosis to control lymph flow of lymphatic malformation. *Plast Reconstr Surg Glob Open.* (2019) 7:e2199. doi: 10.1097/GOX.0000000000002199
14. Kato M, Watanabe S, Iida T, Watanabe A. Flow pattern classification in lymphatic malformations by indocyanine green lymphography. *Plast Reconstr Surg.* (2019) 143:558e–64e. doi: 10.1097/PRS.0000000000005362
15. Yang X, Jin Y, Lin X, Chen H, Ma G, Hu X, et al. Management of periorbital microcystic lymphatic malformation with blepharoptosis: Surgical treatment combined with intralesional bleomycin injection. *J Pediatr Surg.* (2015) 50:1393–97. doi: 10.1016/j.jpedsurg.2014.12.011
16. Bajaj Y, Hewitt R, Ifeacho S, Hartley BE. Surgical excision as primary treatment modality for extensive cervicofacial lymphatic malformations in children. *Int J Pediatr Otorhinolaryngol.* (2011) 75:673–7. doi: 10.1016/j.ijporl.2011.02.009
17. Cheng J. Doxycycline sclerotherapy in children with head and neck lymphatic malformations. *J Pediatr Surg.* (2015) 50:2143–6. doi: 10.1016/j.jpedsurg.2015.08.051
18. Shergill A, John P, Amaral JG. Doxycycline sclerotherapy in children with lymphatic malformations: outcomes, complications and clinical efficacy. *Pediatr Radiol.* (2012) 42:1080–8. doi: 10.1007/s00247-012-2406-2
19. Vlahovic A, Gazikalovic A, Adjic O. Bleomycin sclerotherapy for lymphatic malformation after unsuccessful surgical excision: case report. *Acta Otorhinolaryngol Ital.* (2015) 35:365–7. doi: 10.14639/0392-100X-105513
20. Lerat J, Mounayer C, Scomparin A, Orsel S, Bessede JP, Aubry K. Head and neck lymphatic malformation and treatment: Clinical study of 23 cases. *Eur Ann Otorhinolaryngol Head Neck Dis.* (2016) 133:393–96. doi: 10.1016/j.anorl.2016.07.004
21. Fliegelman LJ, Friedland D, Brandwein M, Rothschild M. Lymphatic malformation: predictive factors for recurrence. *Otolaryngol Head Neck Surg.* (2000) 123:706–10. doi: 10.1067/mhn.2000.110963
22. Colbert SD, Seager L, Haider F, Evans BT, Anand R, Brennan PA. Lymphatic malformations of the head and neck-current concepts in management. *Br J Oral Maxillofac Surg.* (2013) 51:98–102. doi: 10.1016/j.bjoms.2011.12.016
23. Romeo V, Maurea S, Guarino S, Sirignano C, Mainenti PP, Picardi M, et al. A case of lower-neck cystic lymphangioma: correlative US, CT and MR imaging findings. *Quant Imaging Med Surg.* (2013) 3:224–7. doi: 10.3978/j.issn.2223-4292.2013.08.03
24. Kraft JC, Treuting PM, Ho RJY. Indocyanine green nanoparticles undergo selective lymphatic uptake, distribution and retention and enable detailed mapping of lymph vessels, nodes and abnormalities. *J Drug Target.* (2018) 26:494–504. doi: 10.1080/1061186X.2018.1433681
25. Medina-Rodriguez ME, de-la-Casa-Almeida M, Gonzalez Martin J, Hermida Anllo M and Medrano-Sanchez EM. Changes in indocyanine green lymphography patterns after physical treatment in secondary upper limb lymphedema. *J Clin Med.* (2020) 9:306. doi: 10.3390/jcm9020306
26. Frojo G, Castro O, Tadisina KK, Xu KY. Lymphovenous Bypass Using Indocyanine Green Mapping for Successful Treatment of Penile and Scrotal Lymphedema. *Plast Reconstr Surg Glob Open.* (2020) 8:e2938. doi: 10.1097/GOX.0000000000002938
27. Li K, Min P, Sadigh P, Grassetti L, Lazzeri D, Torresetti M, et al. Prefabricated cervical skin flaps for hemi-facial resurfacing: elucidating the natural history of postoperative edema using indocyanine green. *Lymphat Res Biol.* (2018) 16:100–08. doi: 10.1089/lrb.2015.0043
28. Kato M, Watanabe S, Iida T, Watanabe A, Megumi F. Peri-orbital lymphangioma treated by lymphatic-venous anastomosis with indocyanine green lymphography analysis. *J Pediatric Surg Case Rep.* (2017) 23:9–14. doi: 10.1016/j.epsc.2017.05.008
29. Kubota O, Uchiyama T, Nakamura K, Hayashi Y, Onuki Y, Baba S. Adult axillary lymphangioma removal using indocyanine green fluorescence imaging system: A case report. *Int J Surg Case Rep.* (2020) 72:255–59. doi: 10.1016/j.ijscr.2020.05.090
30. Shirota C, Hinoki A, Takahashi M, Tanaka Y, Tainaka T, Sumida W, et al. New navigation surgery for resection of lymphatic malformations using indocyanine green fluorescence imaging. *Am J Case Rep.* (2017) 18:529–31. doi: 10.12659/ajcr.903465
31. Wang Y, Tang W, Li X. Safety and efficacy of surgery combined with bleomycin irrigation for complex cervical-facial lymphatic malformations of children. *Int J Pediatr Otorhinolaryngol.* (2020) 128:109724. doi: 10.1016/j.ijporl.2019.109724
32. Ardicli B, Karnak I, Ciftci AO, Tanyel FC, Senocak ME. Sclerotherapy with bleomycin versus surgical excision for extracervical cystic lymphatic malformations in children. *Surg Today.* (2016) 46:97–101. doi: 10.1007/s00595-015-1128-0
33. Anggreyni G, Agustriani N, Agustriani N, Gunadi. Comparison of different therapeutic approaches for children with common lymphatic malformation. *Med J Malaysia.* (2020) 75:32–6.
34. Sainsbury DCG, Kessell G, Fall AJ, Hampton FJ, Guhan A, Muir T. Intralesional bleomycin injection treatment for vascular birthmarks: a 5-year experience at a single United Kingdom unit. *Plast Reconstr Surg.* (2011) 127:2031–44. doi: 10.1097/PRS.0b013e31820e923c
35. Trenor CC. 3rd, Chaudry G. Complex lymphatic anomalies. *Semin Pediatr Surg.* (2014) 23:186–90. doi: 10.1053/j.sempedsurg.2014.07.006
36. Basaran MM, Karatayli SO, Pampal A, Akmansu SH. Successful treatment of a case with cervical lymphatic malformation: repeated bleomycin sclerotherapy. *Turk Arch Otorhinolaryngol.* (2017) 55:180–83. doi: 10.5152/tao.2017.2360
37. Leung M, Leung L, Fung D, Poon WL, Liu C, Chung K, et al. Management of the low-flow head and neck vascular malformations in children: the sclerotherapy protocol. *Eur J Pediatr Surg.* (2014) 24:97–101. doi: 10.1055/s-0033-1354585

25

Primary Omental Lipoma in a Child

*Qiang Yuan, Xufei Duan and Xueqiang Yan**

Department of Pediatric Surgery, Wuhan Children's Hospital (Wuhan Maternal and Child Healthcare Hospital), Tongji Medical College, Huazhong University of Science and Technology, Wuhan, China

***Correspondence:**
Xueqiang Yan
yanxueqiang1@163.com

Background: Lipoma is a common benign tumor derived from adipose tissue, with an incidence of nearly 10%. It is the most common mesenchymal tumor throughout the body. However, the pathogenesis of lipoma is not clear yet, and the increased incidence is attributable to obesity, elevated serum cholesterol, diabetes, trauma, radiation, familial predisposition, and chromosome. Primary omental tumor is a rare lipoma occurring in the greater omentum, most of which is reported in the form of clinical case reports. Nevertheless, primary omental tumor is even rarer in children. To date, there have been few reports of clinical cases.

Case Presentation: We report a rare case of primary omental lipoma in a 6-year-old boy. After an accidental fall, a CT scan found that he had a tumor in the left upper abdomen. He had no history of abdominal pain, abdominal mass, vomiting, etc. The boy was admitted to the hospital within 3 days, and was diagnosed with an intra-abdominal tumor. After admission, abdominal ultrasound and enhanced CT showed a 71 ×40 × 60 mm mass in the left middle abdomen, which was considered a lipoma. There was no abnormality in tumor markers. Through laparoscopic surgery, intraoperative exploration revealed that the tumor was located in the left mid-upper abdomen, and was yellow, solid, soft, and isolated. The intraoperative diagnosis was an omental lipoma. We used an ultrasonic knife to resect the omentum close to the base of the tumor. The tumor was completely resected, put in a retrieval bag and sealed. Finally, the left and right sides of the umbilical incision were extended to take out the tumor tissue. The child received liquid food 6 h after the operation and was discharged 3 days later. The postoperative pathological diagnosis was an omental lipoma. He was seen at follow-up 3 months after discharge and had no complaints, an abnominal ultrasound showed no tumor recurrence.

Conclusion: Primary omental lipoma in children is a rare benign tumor of the omentum. Its etiology and pathology are not clear. US, CT, and MRI can facilitate clinical diagnosis and preoperative evaluation. Laparoscopic surgery is an effective treatment, and the prognosis of children is favorable. This case is beneficial to improve the clinical knowledge of pediatric surgeons about this rare disease.

Keywords: primary omental lipoma, laparoscopy, child, US, resect

INTRODUCTION

Primary omental lipoma is a rare benign tumor of the omentum. The pathogenesis is not clear, and there is no statistical data on its incidence. This lipoma in children is even rarer, most of which are reported in the form of clinical case reports. This study reports the diagnosis and treatment of a 6-year-old boy with primary omental lipoma. Meanwhile, it discusses the clinical characteristics as well as methods of diagnosis and treatment of primary omental lipoma based on previous literature data. This study was approved by the Research and Ethics Committee of our institution, and written informed consent was obtained from the patient's family.

CASE PRESENTATION

A 6-year-old male child was found to have a tumor in the left mid-upper abdomen on a CT examination of his abdomen after an accidental fall. The boy had no history of abdominal pain, abdominal mass, and vomiting. He was admitted to the hospital with an abdominal tumor within 3 days. The initial diagnosis was an intraperitoneal tumor. After admission, laboratory tests showed no abnormality in blood cell count, biochemical analysis, and tumor markers. Abdominal ultrasound and enhanced CT showed a mass in the left middle abdomen, which size was 71 × 40 × 60 mm. Intra-abdominal lipoma should be considered, and the blood-supplying vessels were derived from branches of the omental artery (**Figures 1A,B**).

We performed laparoscopy surgery on the child: three incisions for 5 mm trocars were made on the insufflated abdomen respectively at the left and right sides of the umbilicus and at the anti-Mc Burney's point. Intraoperative laparoscopic exploration revealed a tumor in the left part of middle and upper abdomen, with a size of about 70 × 60 × 50 mm. It was yellow, solid, soft, isolated, and its base was derived from the greater omentum without torsion (**Figure 2A**). Preoperative and intraoperative assessments revealed that the tumor could be successfully and completely resected by laparoscopic surgery. The ultrasound

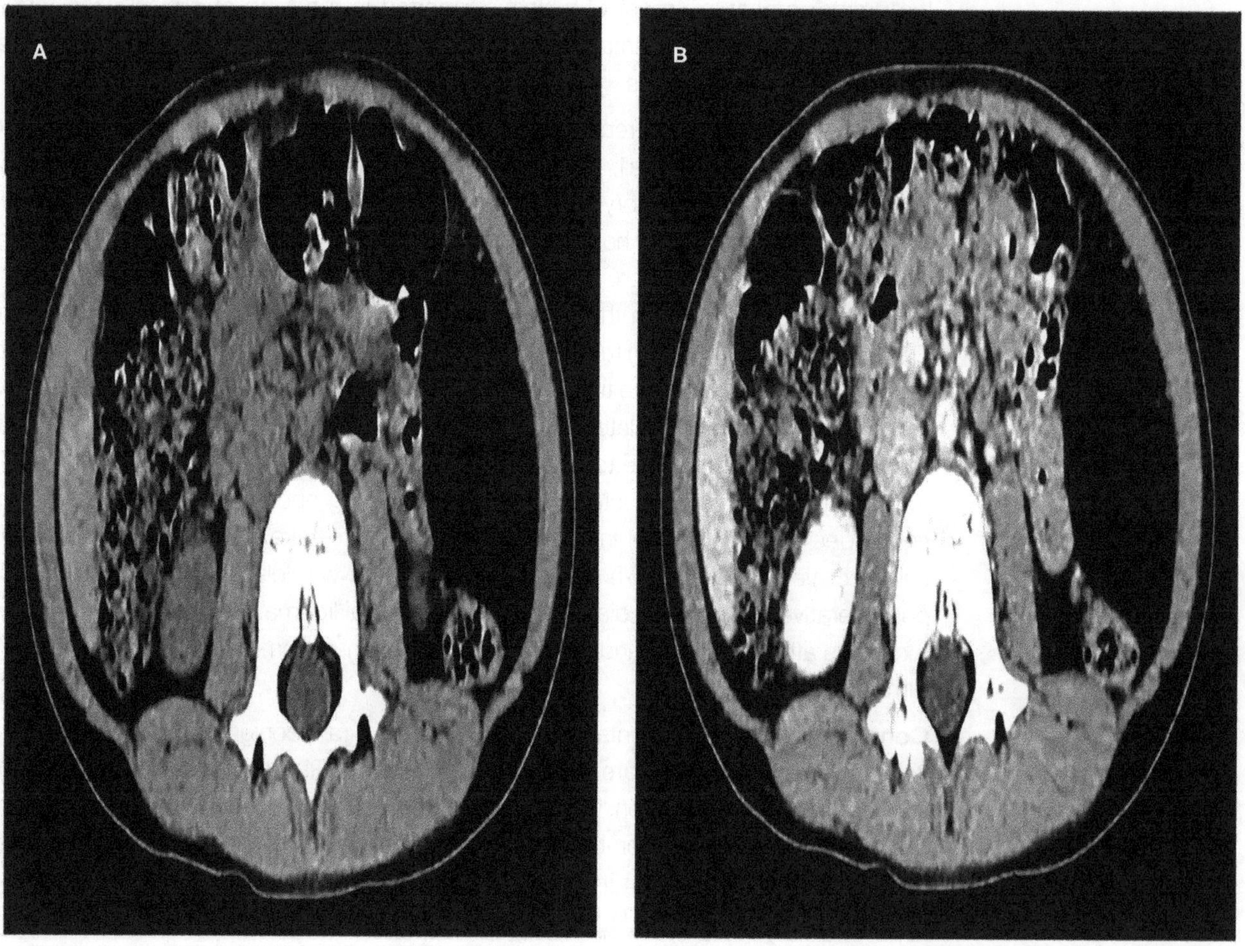

FIGURE 1 | (A), Computed tomography (CT) scan shows an elliptical, very low-density mass in the left middle abdomen, which is wrapped in the left abdominal cavity, and the surrounding intestine is slightly compressed and displaced. **(B)**, The tumor was not enhanced on enhanced CT scan, and its blood supply arteries were not shown.

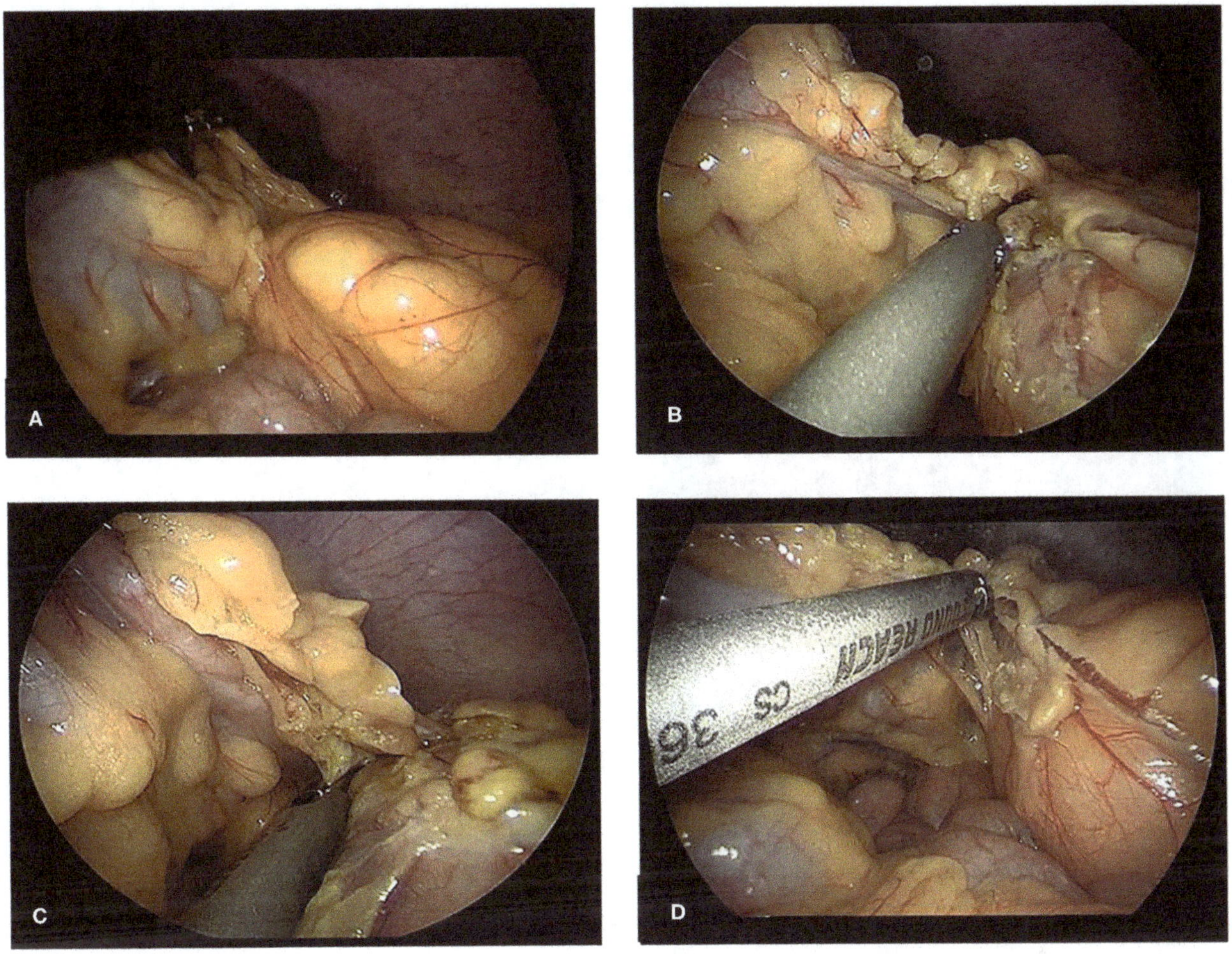

FIGURE 2 | (A), Laparoscopic examination of the left mid-upper abdominal tumor, which was yellow, solid, isolated, derived from the greater omentum, without torsion. **(B,C)**, Ultrasonic knife separates the omentum and the tumor. **(D)**, Ultrasonic scalpel coagulates the tumor blood supply artery.

knife cut off the greater omentum and the blood-supplying vessels at the base of the tumor. The tumor was completely removed and was placed in the specimen retrieval bag which was then closed. The ultrasound knife coagulated the residual end of the greater omentum to stop bleeding. No other abnormality was found in the abdominal cavity below the umbilicus to take out the tumor tissue completely (**Figures 2B–D**).

The operation time was 27 min. The weight of the excised tumor tissue was 295 g, size of about 80 × 55 × 30 mm with; the tumor capsule intact; and the cut surface is grayish-yellow and soft (**Figure 3A**). Microscopic examination showed that the tumor was composed of mature adipocytes without atypia (**Figure 3B**); and the diagnosis was of a benign omental lipoma. The patient was discharged 3 days postoperatively without further complication, follow-up abdominal ultrasonography after 3 months showed no recurrence of lipoma.

Pubmed, Springer Link, CNKI, and Wanfang databases were searched before June 2021 to retrieve the related literature of omental lipoma, a total of 12 clinical reports of primary omental lipoma in children were retrieved in the previous literature (**Table 1**).

DISCUSSION AND CONCLUSIONS

Lipoma is a common benign tumor derived from adipose tissue, with an incidence of nearly 10% (1). It is the most common mesenchymal tumor throughout the body. However, the pathogenesis of lipoma is not clear yet, and the increased incidence is attributable to obesity, elevated serum cholesterol, diabetes, trauma, radiation, familial predisposition, and chromosome abnormality (2, 3). The omentum is a double-layer membrane composed of peritoneum and adipose tissue, which is attached to the greater curvature of the stomach and transverse colon. It covers the abdominal organs in the abdominal cavity in the shape of a skirt, including blood vessels, nerves, lymphatic vessels, and connective tissue (4, 5). Primary omental lipoma is very rare, and most of which is described in the form of case reports.

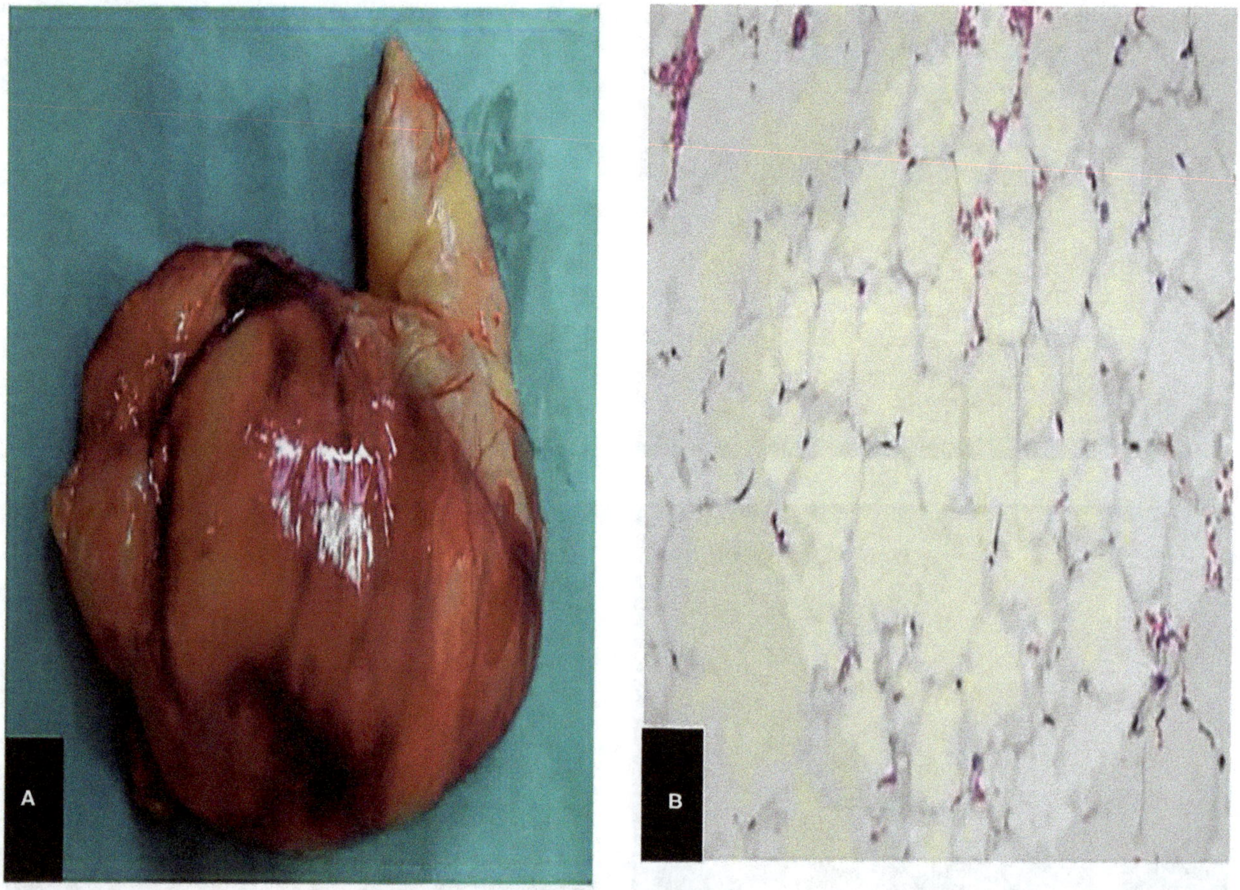

FIGURE 3 | (A), A piece of yellow tissue can be seen with the naked eye, 295g in weight, about 80mm* 55mm * 30mm in size, with intact capsule, solid and soft. **(B)**, Microscopically, the tumor is composed of mature adipocytes without atypia.

TABLE 1 | Cases of children reported to have omental lipoma found in the available literature.

Case	Authors	Year	Age	Sex	Clinical presentation	Weigh (g)	Size (cm)	Treatment
1	Haller	1978	3y	F	NR	NR	8*5*4	Excision
2	Giubilei	1980	8y	M	NR	NR	18*15*8	Excision
3	Joulak	1998	3y	M	NR	NR	13*9*6	Excision
4	Barauskas	2004	8y	F	NR	720	11*10*8	Excision
5	Luo	2005	11m	M	Abdominal distention	1820	21*15*12	Excision
6	Srinivasan	2009	9m	NR	NR	1500	NR	Excision
7	Abubakar	2009	13y	F	NR	12300	34*26*22	Excision
8	Chaudhary	2011	2y	M	NR	NR	NR	Excision
9	Cascini	2012	19m	M	Abdominal distention	1185	22*18*8	Excision
10	Cascini	2012	7y	F	Abdominal distention	2070	25*22*10	Excision
11	Cascini	2012	10y	F	Abdominal pain	1370	18*12*10	Excision
12	Kinjo	2014	5y	F	NR	335	8*6*3	Excision
13	Present case (2021)	2021	6y	M	NR	295	8*5.5*3	Excision

NR, not reported; y, years; m, moths.

A variety of pathologies have been reported in the clinic, such as leiomyosarcoma, fibrosarcoma, hemangiopericytoma, liposarcoma, leiomyoma, lipoma, fibroma, and mesothelioma tumors. Lipoma may be the rarest of all the above forms, with an extremely low incidence, accounting for about 7–9% of omental tumors (6, 7).

Review-of the retrieved literature of 12 cases of primary omental lipoma in children, found that children with omental lipoma are usually asymptomatic and are discovered incidentally during medical examination, trauma, or abdominal diseases. The main symptoms of these children include abdominal pain, abdominal distention, and abdominal mass. Nausea, weight loss, and intraperitoneal hemorrhage occurred occasionally, and a few children were admitted to the emergency department due to torsion of the omentum. It has been reported that adult patients were hospitalized due to intussusception and intestinal obstruction (8, 9).

Common imaging methods for diagnosing omental tumors include ultrasound, CT, and MRI. It is clinically difficult to discriminate benign and malignant omental tumors. The differential diagnosis of omental lipoma includes lymphangioma, lymphoma, duplication of the digestive tract, and neuroblastoma. However, the main differential diagnosis is lipoblastoma (10). Omental lipoma is easily found by ultrasound examination. Ultrasound can show that the tumor has heterogeneous echo and abundant blood flow signals, it also reveals the size of the tumor. Smaller omental lipomas are sometimes misdiagnosed as normal mesenteric fat (11). Ultrasound elastography is a non-invasive imaging technology based on different tissue hardness which have been developed in recent years. It can measure the elasticity of the tissue, according to the various performance of the tissue under different external pressure, then to distinguish benign and malignant lesions. Zhang et al. (12) explored whether ultrasound elastography is effective in the diagnosis of benign and malignant omentum thickening. The results showed that the elasticity score of the malignant omentum thickening group was higher than that of the benign omentum thickening group ($P < 0.01$). In addition, ultrasound-guided percutaneous needle biopsy has been a commonly used method for the diagnosis of intra-abdominal lesions, such as liver, kidney, pancreas lesions, and other solid organs, but it is not commonly used for peritoneal and omental lesions. It may cause controversy by seeding tumor cells along the needle path (13). CT examination can show clear, uniform, and low-density intra-abdominal mass, which may have fibrous partitions and a few calcification points inside. Enhanced CT helps to assess the relationship between the tumor and surrounding organs, and also helps to identify the blood-supplying arteries of the tumor (14). MRI has high specificity for the diagnosis of simple lipoma and can distinguish it from well-differentiated liposarcoma. By using an MRI pulse sequence, lipomas show signal intensity similar to that of fat on high T1 signal and intermediate T2 signal. If there are thicker intervals inside the tumor, nodules, and non-fat-like masses, the proportion of fat in the lesion will decrease. It suggests the diagnosis of liposarcoma (15, 16).

Laparoscopic exploration is an important method to confirm that lipomas originate from the greater omentum during the operation, and surgical resection is an effective treatment for the lipoma of the greater omentum. The tumor can be completely resected under laparoscopy.When a patient is admitted to the hospital due to torsion of the greater omentum, laparoscopic exploration can be performed in the emergency department, both laparoscopic tumor resection and the greater omentum resection can be performed at the same time. According to previous reports in the literature, the recurrence rate after resection is $<5\%$, mainly due to incomplete resection (17).

In conclusion, we reported a rare case of primary omental lipoma in children. By reviewing the previous literature, we found that primary omental lipoma in children is very rare. Preoperative ultrasound and enhanced CT can determine intra-abdominal lipoma, which can also help to identify the origin of the tumor's blood vessels. Intraoperative exploration of laparoscopic surgery can confirm that the lipoma originates from the greater omentum. The lipoma can be completely resected under laparoscopic surgery. If combined with torsion of the greater omentum, partial resection of the greater omentum can be performed at the same time. Laparoscopic surgery is minimally invasive and generally without complications. The prognosis of the child is good.

ETHICS STATEMENT

The studies involving human participants were reviewed and approved by Wuhan Children's Hospital (Wuhan Maternal and Child Healthcare Hospital), Tongji Medical College, Huazhong University of Science and Technology. The patients/participants provided their written informed consent to participate in this study. Written informed consent was obtained from the individual(s), and minor(s)' legal guardian/next of kin, for the publication of any potentially identifiable images or data included in this article.

AUTHOR CONTRIBUTIONS

QY and XY designed the study, collected the clinical data, performed the statistical analysis, participated in the operation, and drafted the manuscript. XD participated in the operation and revised the article. All authors read and approved the final manuscript.

REFERENCES

1. Sanchez MR, Golomb FM, Moy JA, Potozkin JR. Giant lipoma: case report and review of the literature. *J Am Acad Dermatol.* (1993) 28(2 Pt 1):266–8. doi: 10.1016/S0190-9622(08) 81151-6
2. Enzinger FM, Weiss SW. *Soft Tissue Tumors.* 3rd ed. St Louis (Mo): Mosby (1995). p. 384–405.
3. Weiss SW. Lipomatous tumors. *Monogr Pathol.* (1996) 38:207–39.
4. Koppe MJ, Nagtegaal ID, de Wilt JH, Ceelen WP. Recent insights into the pathophysiology of omental metastases. *J Surg Oncol.* (2014) 110:670–5. doi: 10.1002/jso.23681
5. Krist LF, Koenen H, Calame W, van der Harten JJ, van der Linden JC, Eestermans IL, et al.Ontogeny of milky spots in the human greater omentum: an immunochemical study. *Anat Rec.* (1997) 249:399–

404. doi: 10.1002/(SICI)1097-0185(199711)249:3<399::AID-AR11>3.0.CO;2-J

6. Dixon AY, Reed JS, Dow N, Lee SH. Primary omental leiomyosarcoma masquerading as hemorrhagic ascites. *Hum Pathol.* (1984) 15:233–7. doi: 10.1016/S0046-8177(84)80185-9
7. Tsurumi H, Okada S, Koshino Y, Oyama M, Higaki H, Shimokawa K, et al. A case of leiomyoblastoma (epithelioid leiomyosarcoma) of the greater omentum. *Gastroenterol Jpn.* (1991) 26:370–5. doi: 10.1007/BF02781927
8. Pintor-Tortolero J, Martínez-Núñez S, Tallón-Aguilar L, Padillo-Ruiz FJ. Colonic intussusception caused by giant lipoma: a rare cause of bowel obstruction. *Int J Colorectal Dis.* (2020) 35:1973–7.
9. Livne PM, Zer M, Shmuter Z, Dintsman M. Acute intestinal obstruction caused by necrotic mesenteric lipoma–a case report. *Am J Proctol Gastroenterol Colon Rectal Surg.* (1981) 32:19–22.
10. Abubakar AM, Mayun AA, Pindiga UH, Chinda JY, Adamu SA. Giant omental lipoma in a 13-year-old adolescent girl. *J Pediatr Surg.* (2009) 44:2230–2. doi: 10.1016/j.jpedsurg.2009.09.007
11. Cha JM, Lee JI, Joo KR, Choe JW, Jung SW, Shin HP, et al. Giant mesenteric lipoma as an unusual cause of abdominal pain: a case report and a review of the literature. *J Korean Med Sci.* (2009) 24:333–6. doi: 10.3346/jkms.2009.24.2.333
12. Zhang Y, Wang X, Tao C, Que Y, Zhao W, Chen B. Ultrasound elastography for differentiating benign from malignant thickened greater omentum. *Eur Radiol.* (2016) 26:2337–43. doi: 10.1007/s00330-015-4037-0
13. Beattie GC, Irwin ST. Torsion of an omental lipoma presenting as an emergency. *Int J Clin Pract Suppl.* (2005) 130–1. doi: 10.1111/j.1368-504X.2005.00457.x
14. Shiroshita H, Komori Y, Tajima M, Bandoh T, Arita T, Shiraishi N, et al. Laparoscopic examination and resection for giant lipoma of the omentum: a case report and review of related literature. *Surg Laparosc Endosc Percutan Tech.* (2009) 19:e217–20. doi: 10.1097/SLE.0b013e3181b97edd
15. Hamidi H, Rasouly N, Khpalwak H, Malikzai MO, Faizi AR, Hoshang MM, et al. Childhood giant omental and mesenteric lipoma. *Radiol Case Rep.* (2016) 11:41–4. doi: 10.1016/j.radcr.2015.12.003
16. Tirukonda P, Wu S, Brar J, Ng KS, Mirsadraee S. Trans arterial embolization of spontaneous intra-abdominal haemorrhage from omental lipoma. *Case Rep Radiol.* (2018) 2018:2926143. doi: 10.1155/2018/2926143
17. Squillaro AI, Chow MD, Arias F, Sadimin ET, Lee YH. A giant childhood mesenteric lipoblastoma with extensive maturation. *Front Pediatr.* (2020) 8:404. doi: 10.3389/fped.2020.00404

26

Preliminary Experiences with Robot-Assisted Choledochal Cyst Excision Using the Da Vinci Surgical System in Children Below the Age of One

Xiaolong Xie[†], *Yang Wu*[†], *Kewei Li, Chengbo Ai, Qi Wang, Chuan Wang, Jing Chen*[*] *and Bo Xiang*[*]

Department of Pediatric Surgery, West China Hospital, Sichuan University, Chengdu, China

***Correspondence:**
Jing Chen
jingchen@scu.edu.cn
Bo Xiang
xb_scu.edu@hotmail.com

The purpose of this study is to introduce our preliminary experiences with using the da Vinci surgical system to treat choledochal cysts in children under 1 year old and discuss the application of this robot-assisted surgery. We retrospectively analyzed all available clinical data of children below the age of 1 who underwent surgery for choledochal cysts using the da Vinci robotic surgical system between January 2015 and December 2020. Data collection mainly included demographic information, imaging data, perioperative details, and postoperative outcomes. Ten patients were included in this study. The average patient age was 8.5 months, and the average weight was 9.11 kg. Half of these patients suffered from abdominal pain, while 30% exhibited vomiting and 10% jaundice. Eight of them were type Ia, and two were Ic. The average operation time among the patients was 219.5 min. None of the 10 patients had to receive a blood transfusion or conversion. The average time of the patients' subsequent fluid diet was 3.28 days, and the solid diet was 3.76 days. Meanwhile, the average length of hospital stay was 7.6 days. All 10 patients recovered and were eventually discharged. We believe that the da Vinci surgical system is a safe and feasible form of treatment for choledochal cysts in children <1 year old.

Keywords: robot, choledochal cyst excision, da Vinci, children, 1 year old

INTRODUCTION

Choledochal cysts are the most common congenital malformation found in the biliary tract and are characterized by cystic or fusiform dilatation of the common bile duct. These have also been known to simultaneously appear alongside intrahepatic bile duct dilatation (1–3). Without effective treatment, patients with choledochal cysts may suffer from cyst perforation, recurrent pancreatitis, cancer, or even severe cholestasis, which can then lead to liver cirrhosis, portal hypertension, and eventually liver failure (4).

The best option for treatment of choledochal cysts is surgery, which mainly involves choledochal cyst resection, cholecystectomy, and hepaticojejunostomy (5). Minimally invasive approaches toward choledochal cysts are currently the mainstream method, and this includes both laparoscope-assisted and robot-assisted surgeries. However, the laparoscopic procedure is as of yet not widely promoted throughout the world because a laparoscopic choledochojejunostomy is technically demanding, as well as requiring a certain learning curve. Therefore, robotic procedures are usually proposed an alternative form of minimally invasive surgery on choledochal cysts due to their unique three-dimensional (3D) imaging and the flexible design of their simulation manipulator, which significantly improve operability and accuracy (6). Woo et al. reported the first robot-assisted choledochal cyst resection in children and their success with it in 2006 (7). The technology has been reported time and time again since then, with several other successful operations taking place (6, 8, 9). However, there are still few reports regarding robot-assisted choledochal cyst resection in the under 1-year-old age group available in the literature (8). Our department alone completed 134 operations on choledochal cyst resection using the da Vinci surgical system between January 2015 and December 2020. Of these, 10 cases were in children below the age of 1, and in this study, we present our experiences and discuss the relevant technical points.

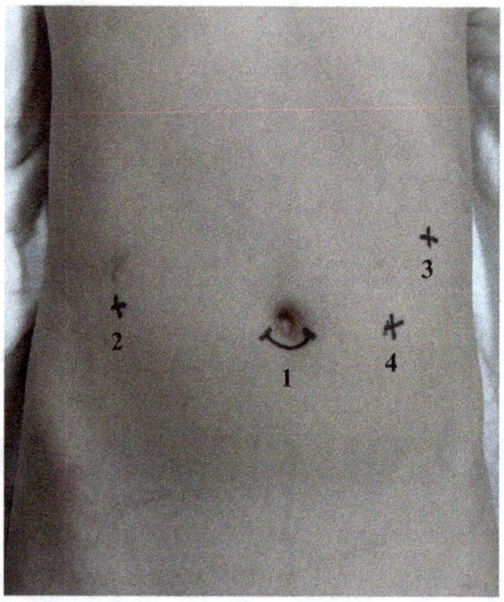

FIGURE 1 | Port placement in robot-assisted surgery for choledochal cysts. (1) Camera port. (2) Port I. (3) Port II. (4) Assistant port.

METHODS

Study Population

We retrospectively analyzed clinical data from patients below the age of 1 year who had undergone robot-assisted surgery to treat choledochal cysts from January 2015 to December 2020 in the West China Hospital of Sichuan University. Informed consent was naturally obtained from the children's parents. The study passed the ethics review of our hospital ethics committee (No. 1082). Candidates for inclusion in the study were based on the following requirements: (1) patients were diagnosed with choledochal cysts through preoperative history, physical examination, B-ultrasound, computed tomography (CT), or magnetic resonance cholangiopancreatography (MRCP); (2) patients would be able to tolerate CO_2 pneumoperitoneum during general anesthesia and robotic surgery; and (3) the patient's coagulation function was normal, and they had no serious organ dysfunction. Conversely, exclusion criteria included secondary operations, cyst perforation, and malignant transformation of the choledochal cyst before the operation.

Procedure of the Operation

A gastric tube was first set in place for gastrointestinal decompression after general anesthesia had been induced. The patient's right upper abdomen should be raised with his/her head elevated 15° with a left incline of 15°. End-to-side anastomosis of the jejunum was performed extracorporeally with a 1.2- to 1.5-cm incision below the umbilicus, and the intestine was returned to the abdominal cavity. A 12-mm trocar was then set as a 3D endoscopic port at the subumbilical incision and constructing pneumoperitoneum with a 12-mmHg pressure (**Figure 1**). With the use of images from the camera, two 8-mm trocars were placed in the right upper abdomen 5–8 cm away from the umbilicus and 4 cm below the front rib of the left axillary line. Following this, No. 1 and No. 2 arms were introduced, and a 5-mm trocar was placed between the endoscopic port and No. 1 arm as an auxiliary port. The ligamentum teres hepatis and the middle part of the gallbladder were suspended with a 3-0 sliding line to expose the cyst and hilar (**Figure 2A**). If the cyst was large, decompression was performed first. The anterior and posterior walls of the cyst were dissected using an electric hook close to the cyst wall. The distal end would then be dissected to the proximal pancreaticobiliary junction, and the distal end ligated with a 5-0 synthetic clip (JY1004-2103005; Zhejiang Wedu Medical; No. 3766, South Circular Road, Binjiang District, Hangzhou, China) (**Figure 2B**). This led to the dissection of the triangle of the gallbladder and ligation of the cystic artery and cystic duct. The proximal end of the cyst was dissected in reverse along the cyst wall to the hepatic duct of the hilar part and was removed (**Figure 2C**). After this, the biliary loop was lifted up to the hepatic hilum through the right mesentery of transverse colon. A 4-0 StratafixTM (SXMD1B402; Surgical Specialties Corporation; 247 Station Drive, NE1 Westwood, MA, USA) was used for end-to-side choledochojejunostomy. The anastomosis was performed from the posterior wall to the anterior wall and from the right side to the left side of the child (**Figure 2D**). The transverse mesocolonic hiatus was closed with a 3-0 absorbable suture, and the gallbladder was removed with the electric hook. Wrapping up the operation, a drainage tube was placed around the anastomotic site.

Intraoperative and Postoperative Observations and Recording Indicators

A liquid diet was initiated following the recovery of intestinal function. Discharge would only be arranged when a patient could eat normally without abdominal pain or any other discomfort. Demographic information was monitored and recorded, as well as clinical manifestation, cyst type, diameter of cyst, operation time, anesthesia time, intraoperative bleeding, transfusion, time to taking water, hospital stay, and postoperative complications.

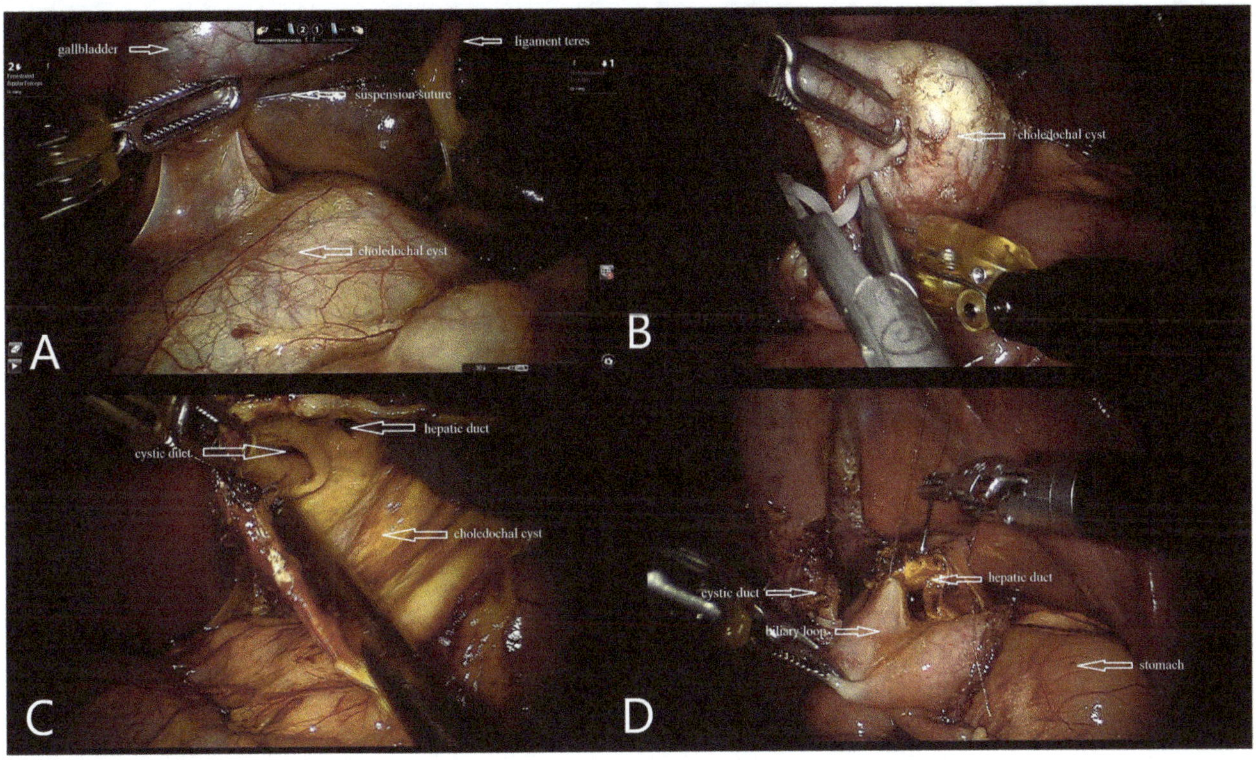

FIGURE 2 | Intraoperative photographs. **(A)** Suspension of gallbladder and ligamentum teres. **(B)** Ligation of the distal end of the cyst. **(C)** Confirm cystic duct and hepatic duct. **(D)** Hepaticojejunostomy with robotic instruments

Statistical Analyses

The statistical data were entered into Excel 2007 and analyzed using SPSS 23.0 software. The numerical variables were expressed by both the mean and standard deviation, and the categorical variables were expressed by counts (N) and percentage (%).

RESULTS

Ten patients below the age of 1 year and diagnosed with choledochal cysts were treated with robot-assisted procedures and subsequently analyzed in our study. The average follow-up time was 24 months. The baseline data of the 10 children are shown in **Table 1**. Three of the patients were male and two were female. The children's average age was 8.5 months, and the average weight was 9.11 kg. About 50% of these patients suffered from abdominal pain, while 30% experienced vomiting and 10% jaundice. Palpable abdominal masses were observed in 40% of the patients. Eight of them were Todani type Ia, and two were Todani type Ic. The average diameter of the choledochal cyst was 4.26 cm.

Perioperative details and postoperative outcomes are presented in **Table 2**. The total average operation time was 219.5 min. The average docking time was 15.6 min, and the console time was 178.5 min. The average volume of blood loss was 17 ml. None of the 10 patients received blood transfusions or conversions. The average time of their fluid diet was 3.28 days and solid diet 3.76 days. Meanwhile, the average length of hospital stay was 7.6 days. Only one patient developed an incomplete intestinal obstruction following the operation, and this was dealt with using conservative treatment. All 10 patients eventually recovered and were discharged.

DISCUSSION

Our team has previously published papers regarding our experiences with total robot-assisted resections of choledochal cysts in children (10). The purpose of this article is to summarize and share our valuable experience with robot surgery for choledochal cysts in children below the age of 1 year. At present, the main methods of surgery for choledochal cysts include the open approach, laparoscopic approach, and robotic approach. Laparoscopic procedures and robot-assisted procedures are both minimally invasive and thus have the advantage of being more cosmetic, leading to a faster recovery and providing a better view of deep anatomical structures such as the bile duct, portal vein, and hepatic artery than open procedures (11). However, laparoscopic surgery has not been widely used thus far because of its high technical requirements, and this is especially true for the laparoscopic hepaticojejunostomy. A steep learning curve is needed in the initial stage due to the limited operation space, limited movement of the operating instruments, and instability of the two-dimensional imaging platform. However, along with the progress of surgical technology and increased experience with

TABLE 1 | Characteristics of the patients.

N = 10	Sex (M/F)	Age (month)[a]	Weight (Kg)[b]	Abdominal pain	Vomiting	Distension	Jaundice	Palpable mass	WBC (/mm^3)[b]	N (%)[b]	ALT (IU/L)[b]	AST (IU/L)[b]	TBIL (umol/l)[b]	DBIL (umol/l)[b]	IBIL (umol/l)[b]	Cyst type	Diameter of cyst (cm)[b]
Case 1	Female	6	8.3	No	No	No	No	No	9.82	25.6	38	41	23.3	11.6	11.7	Ia	4
Case 2	Male	8	8.9	Yes	Yes	No	No	No	12.19	17.3	39	56	33.4	28.1	5.3	Ia	4.5
Case 3	Male	8	8.5	No	No	No	No	Yes	5.58	33.3	15	33	7.7	2.6	5.1	Ia	6.4
Case 4	Female	9	9.5	Yes	No	No	Yes	Yes	7.14	33.7	11	29	2.8	1.3	1.5	Ia	5.5
Case 5	Female	10	9.9	Yes	No	No	Yes	No	8.9	22.8	39	86	13.4	18.1	5.3	Ia	3.9
Case 6	Female	11	9.7	No	Yes	No	No	Yes	11.38	17.6	52	70	14	3.8	11.2	Ia	5.8
Case 7	Female	11	9.8	No	No	No	No	No	10.88	29.9	19	29	3	1	2	Ic	1.5
Case 8	Female	7	8.5	Yes	No	No	No	No	6.79	25.4	33	34	7.6	2.9	4.7	Ia	2.5
Case 9	Male	8	8.8	No	Yes	Yes	No	No	7.16	24.1	36	41	10.1	3.1	7	Ic	2.1
Case 10	Female	10	9.2	Yes	No	No	No	Yes	6.37	28.1	16	33	2.4	1.4	1	Ia	6.4
N = 10	3/7	8.50 (7.75–10.25)	9.11 (0.59)	5 (50%)	3 (30%)	1 (10%)	2 (20%)	4 (40%)	8.62 (2.33)	25.78 (5.70)	29.80 (13.57)	45.20 (19.38)	11.77 (9.95)	7.39 (8.13)	5.48 (3.69)	8/2	4.26 (1.79)

[a]*Median, interquartile range;* [b]*mean, standard deviation. WBC,White blood cell count; N,Neutrophils; ALT, Alanine transferase; AST, Aspartic aminotransferase; TBIL, Total bilirubin; DBIL, Direct bilirubin; IBIL, Indirect bilirubin.*

TABLE 2 | Intraoperative and postoperative outcomes and complications.

N = 10	Operation time (min)[a]	Docking time	Console time	Anesthesia time (min)[a]	Intraoperative bleeding (mL)[a]	Transfusion rate[a]	Conversion to open surgery	Time to taking water (days)[a]	Time to starting solids diet (days)[a]	Complications	Hospital stay (days)[a]
Case 1	219	17	175	244	20	0	0	3	3.7	/	7.4
Case 2	222	17	178	252	10	0	0	3.1	3.8	/	7.1
Case 3	213	15	169	234	20	0	0	3.2	3.5	/	8
Case 4	219	15	180	250	25	0	0	3.4	3.6	/	7.2
Case 5	195	16	161	236	10	0	0	3.3	3.5	/	8
Case 6	219	16	176	252	20	0	0	3.7	4	/	7.3
Case 7	212	17	177	247	20	0	0	3.5	3.7	/	7
Case 8	233	15	189	267	15	0	0	2.9	3.9	/	6
Case 9	228	14	187	260	10	0	0	3.5	3.9	Intestinal obstruction	1
Case 10	235	14	193	259	20	0	0	3.2	4	/	8
N = 10	219.50 (11.55)	15.60 (1.17)	178.50 (9.50)	250.10 (10.41)	17.00 (5.38)	0 (0.00%)	0 (0.00%)	3.28 (0.25)	3.76 (0.19)	1 (10.00%)	7.60 (1.04)

[a]*mean, standard deviation.*

this procedure, the possibility of conversion to open surgery and postoperative complications is significantly reduced. When compared with laparoscopic surgery, robotic surgery has some obvious advantages (12). Firstly, a 3D three-dimensional field of vision with magnification of up to 10 times can reveal the deep anatomical structure more clearly. In addition to this, surgeons can adjust the depth and angle of the lens according to their own preference and requirements (13). Secondly, the da Vinci robotic surgery system can completely remove the choledochal cyst to its maximum extent, from the pancreaticobiliary junction to the hilar bile duct. Moreover, the da Vinci robot surgery system's simulation manipulator is highly flexible and can simulate the translation, bending, opening, closing, rotation, and other operations of the human hand (14). It can even rotate 540° to accurately grasp, free, cut, and sew all while eliminating the problem of shakiness and providing advanced motion calibration (15). Altogether, the advantages of robotic surgery significantly reduce the difficulty of surgery. Of course, robotic surgery is not without its drawbacks though. Firstly, generally speaking, the cost of robotic procedures can be prohibitive, as it is significantly higher than that of other techniques. Yoon et al. reported that the total hospital and operation charges of robotic surgery are about 1,000 USD higher than those of laparoscopic surgery. However, making matters even worse, the patient's actual bill for robotic surgery is 4,000 USD higher than that of laparoscopic surgery (16). Moreover, in a country such as China, for example, the cost of robotic surgery rises by 20,000–40,000 RMB (the equivalent of roughly 3,000 6,000 USD) compared with open and laparoscopic methods, as evidenced from our hospital's experiences. Further making matters more complicated, the da Vinci surgical system does not allow for tactile feedback; that is, the operator cannot directly feel the mechanical response when separating, suturing, or knotting. However, it is hoped that with the overcoming of the learning curve, visual feedback through hand–eye coordination can make up for this lack of tactile feedback.

Kim et al. reported on one patient and Alizai et al. reported on five patients who after initially undergoing robotic procedures were converted to open procedures shortly thereafter (9, 17). Although the patients in our study are younger than those reported in these studies, we found no similar experience of such conversion to open surgery. Through our preliminary experiences, there are some measures that can be taken to maximize the working space in these younger and smaller children, which we would like to make clear in this following section, as it would allow for smoother surgery. (1) Creating an incision below the umbilicus offered a better visual field of the cyst than from above the umbilicus. And a 1.5-cm subumbilical incision provided enough space to perform intestinal anastomosis extracorporeally and place the camera. Port I and port II were placed in the right upper abdomen at least 5–8 cm away from the umbilicus and 4 cm below the front rib of the left axillary line. And the position of the assistant port was on the triangle diagonal line with the cyst as the apex with the 3D camera port and port II forming the bottom line. The assistant port was lower than the umbilical plane to reduce any interference with the camera port and port II (No. 2 arm). The 3D camera port and operative ports only need to be inserted into a few millimeter port to maximize the working space between the head of scope and the operating area. (2) The cysts found in patients who were <1 year old were frequently large, and cyst decompression could provide sufficient operating space. (3) In the end, it is suggested to remove the gallbladder because the middle part of the gallbladder should be suspended to allow for a clear visual field. Besides, it is not so suitable to remove the gallbladder from the abdominal cavity during operation after coming into contact with the machine.

In addition to our tips for increasing the operating space as much as possible, we would also like to offer some additional advice to ensure that the operation runs smoothly. (1) It is strongly suggested that the cyst be free as a whole without being transected. Dissect the anterior side of the cyst first and then the distal part of the cyst to the pancreatic segment close to the wall afterwards. After distal ligation, the posterior wall of the cyst can be dissected in reverse, and the direction and dissociation should be from the lower side of cyst to the upper side. (2) It needs to be remembered that there is a learning curve in robot-assisted choledochal cyst resection. Dealing with older patients is recommended in the early stages of one's operation of this procedure to become more familiar and confident with it. Then, with the accumulation of experience and the flattening of the learning curve, the age of patient being operated on could be gradually lowered. In our study, the youngest patient was 6 months old. Our initial experience suggested that robotic surgery was not recommended in children under 6 months old for safety, chiefly due to lack of space and maneuverability. Along with improvements in the area of prenatal diagnosis though, there are more reports of the discovery of prenatal choledochal cysts (18, 19). However, there is still some controversy regarding the timing of surgery in this particular group of patients (19). On the one hand, one has to consider the gestational age, comorbidity of the patient, and the difficulty in performing complex reconstructive operations in infants (20). On the other hand, early surgery is advocated in view of the risks posed by the increase in size of the cyst, inflammation, or even ruptures while under observation (21). Our experience was that children under the age of 6 months with severe inflammation, severe liver injury, or a risk of perforation with a choledochal cyst can be operated on through open surgery or even traditional laparoscopy. (3) We used three ports to complete the operation without the need for a fourth port. Specifically, we made use of the camera port, ports 1 and 2, and ultimately completed the operation with the help of an assistant port. It is very important to cultivate a skilled team to prevent any complications potentially caused by robotic instruments, and a skilled assistant can ensure the successful completion of the operation and monitor the robot arm during the operation to avoid any injury to patients. During the cyst dissection process, the assistant can use wave forceps to form tension and expose the cyst and surrounding tissues. This is done so that the chief surgeon can dissect the free cyst with the No. 1 arm electric hook. If there is bleeding affecting the visual field, the assistant can then use the suction device alternately through the assistant port to suck up the blood to ensure a clear field of vision. Likewise, during a hepaticojejunostomy, the assistant mainly lifts the Stratafix with curved pliers through the assistant port to expose the visual field, so that the chief surgeon can perform a hepaticojejunostomy using No. 1 and No. 2 arms. And if intestinal fluid and bile affect the field of vision, the assistant can also use the suction device to suck up this intestinal fluid and bile. The whole process requires skilled cooperation and understanding between the assistant and chief surgeon.

However, our study also has some limitations. Firstly, the study includes a relatively small amount of samples of children below the age of 1 undergoing choledochal cyst resection using the da Vinci surgical system. Secondly, our study is a retrospective study. Multicenter and long-term follow-up data are needed to demonstrate the true benefits of robotic surgery for treating choledochal cysts in children below the age of 1. However, our overall experience thus far has found that robot-assisted choledochal cyst excisions in patients under 1 year old is safe and feasible in pediatrics.

CONCLUSION

The da Vinci surgical system is safe and feasible in the treatment of choledochal cysts in children below the age of 1.

ETHICS STATEMENT

The studies involving human participants were reviewed and approved by the West China Hospital of Sichuan University Ethics Committee (# 1,082). Written informed consent to participate in this study was provided by the participants' legal guardian/next of kin. Written informed consent was obtained from the minor(s)' legal guardian/next of kin for the publication of any potentially identifiable images or data included in this article.

AUTHOR CONTRIBUTIONS

BX and JC: study conception and design, analysis and data interpretation, and critical revision. XX: study concept and design, data analysis, drafting of the manuscript, and critical revision of the manuscript. YW: study conception, data collection, and analysis. KL: data collection, conducting a research, and investigation process. CA and QW: data collection, scrub data, and maintaining research data. CW: data collection. All authors contributed to the article and approved the submitted version.

REFERENCES

1. Olbourne NA. Choledochal cysts. A review of the cystic anomalies of the biliary tree. *Ann R Coll Surg Engl.* (1975) 56:26–32.
2. Howell CG, Templeton JM, Weiner S, Glassman M, Betts JM, Witzleben CL. Antenatal diagnosis and early surgery for choledochal cyst. *J Pediatr Surg.* (1983) 18:387–93. doi: 10.1016/S0022-3468(83)80187-0
3. Stringer MD, Dhawan A, Davenport M, Mieli-Vergani G, Mowat AP, Howard ER. Choledochal cysts: lessons from a 20 year experience. *Arch Dis Child.* (1995) 73:528–31. doi: 10.1136/adc.73.6.528
4. de Vries JS, de Vries S, Aronson DC, Bosman DK, Rauws EA, Bosma A. Choledochal cysts: age of presentation, symptoms, and late complications related to Todani's classifcation. *J Pediatr Surg.* (2002) 37:1568–73. doi: 10.1053/jpsu.2002.36186
5. Ishibashi H, Shimada M, Kamisawa T, Fujii H, Hamada Y, Kubota M, et al. Japanese study group on congenital biliary dilatation (JSCBD). Japanese clinical practice guidelines for congenital biliary dilatation. *J Hepatob Pancreat Sci.* (2017) 24:1–16. doi: 10.1002/jhbp.415
6. Meehan JJ, Elliott S, Sandler A. The robotic approach to complex hepatobiliary anomalies in children: preliminary report. *J Pediatr Surg.* (2007) 42:2110–4. doi: 10.1016/j.jpedsurg.2007.08.040
7. Woo R, Le D, Albanese CT, Kim SS. Robot-assisted laparoscopic resection of a type I choledochal cyst in a child. *J Laparoendosc Adv Surg Tech A.* (2006) 16:179–83. doi: 10.1089/lap.2006.16.179
8. Dawrant MJ, Najmaldin AS, Alizai NK. Robot-assisted resection of choledochal cysts and hepaticojejunostomy in children less than 10 kg. *J Pediatr Surg.* (2010) 45:2364–8. doi: 10.1016/j.jpedsurg.2010.08.031
9. Alizai NK, Dawrant MJ, Najmaldin AS. Robot-assisted resection of choledochal cysts and hepaticojejunostomy in children. *Pediatr Surg Int.* (2014) 30:291–4. doi: 10.1007/s00383-013-3459-5
10. Huo-Jian S, Ming X, Hong-Yi Z, Chao Y, Fu L, Ke-wei L, et al. Laparoscopic versus open surgery in children with choledochal cysts: a meta-analysis. *Pediatr Surg Int.* (2015) 31:529–34. doi: 10.1007/s00383-015-3705-0
11. Xiaolong X, Yujun L, Kewei L, Qi W, Bo X. Total robot-assisted choledochal cyst excision using da Vinci surgical system in pediatrics: report of 10 cases. *J Pediatr Surg.* (2021) 56:553–8. doi: 10.1016/j.jpedsurg.2020.07.019
12. Pier Cristoforo G, Andrea C, Marta A, Fabio S, Simone C, Tommaso B, et al. Robotics in general surgery: personal experience in a large community hospital. *Arch Surg.* (2003) 138:777–84. doi: 10.1001/archsurg.138.7.777
13. Sodergren MH, Darzi A. Robotic cancer surgery. *Br J Surg.* (2013) 100:3–4. doi: 10.1002/bjs.8972
14. Herron DM, Marohn M. SAGES-MIRA robotic surgery consensus group. A consensus document on robotic surgery. *Surg Endosc.* (2008) 22:313–25. doi: 10.1007/s00464-007-9727-5
15. Yang GZ, Kerr K, Darzi A. A special issue on selected papers from the 5th hamlyn symposium on medical robotics, 2012. *J Robot Surg.* (2013) 7:215. doi: 10.1007/s11701-013-0425-0
16. Jong HY, Ho KH, Woo JL, Chang MK. Minimally invasive surgery for choledochal cysts: laparoscopic versus robotic approaches. *Ann Hepatob Pancreat Surg.* (2021) 25:71–77. doi: 10.14701/ahbps.2021.25.1.71
17. Kim NY, Chang EY, Hong YJ, Park S, Kim HY, Bai SJ, et al. Retrospective assessment of the validity of robotic surgery in comparison to open surgery for pediatric choledochal cyst. *Yonsei Med J.* (2015) 56:737–43. doi: 10.3349/ymj.2015.56.3.737
18. Lee SC, Kim HY, Jung SE, Park KW, Kim WK. Is excision of a choledochal cyst in the neonatal period necessary? *J Pediatr Surg.* (2006) 41:1984–86. doi: 10.1016/j.jpedsurg.2006.08.023
19. Foo DC, Wong KK, Lan LC, Tam PK. Impact of prenatal diagnosis on choledochal cysts and the benefifits of early excision. *J Paediatr Child Health.* (2009) 45:28–30. doi: 10.1111/j.1440-1754.2008.01424.x
20. Okada T, Sasaki F, Ueki S, Hirokata G, Okuyama K, Cho K, et al. Postnatal management for prenatally diagnosed choledochal cysts. *J Pediatr Surg.* (2004) 39:1055–8. doi: 10.1016/j.jpedsurg.2004.03.054
21. Lugo-Vicente HL. Prenatally diagnosed choledochal cysts: observation or early surgery? *J Pediatr Surg.* (1995) 30:1288–90. doi: 10.1016/0022-3468(95)90486-7

27

Surgery-Related Quality of Life of Pediatric Patients with Crohn's Disease

*Valeria Dipasquale [1], Enrica Antonelli [2], Laura Cannavò [1], Giorgio Cavatoi [2], Carmelo Romeo [2], Giuseppe Trimarchi [3], Giuseppe Navarra [4] and Claudio Romano [1]**

[1] Pediatric Gastroenterology and Cystic Fibrosis Unit, Department of Human Pathology in Adulthood and Childhood "G. Barresi", University of Messina, Messina, Italy, [2] Pediatric Surgery Unit, Department of Human Pathology in Adulthood and Childhood "G. Barresi", University of Messina, Messina, Italy, [3] Department of Economy, University of Messina, Messina, Italy, [4] Surgical Oncology Division, Department of Human Pathology in Adulthood and Childhood "G. Barresi", University of Messina, Messina, Italy

***Correspondence:**
Claudio Romano
romanoc@unime.it

Objective: Up to 30% of pediatric patients with Crohn's disease (CD) require surgery. The aim of the study was to evaluate long-term health-related quality of life (HRQoL) outcome in children with CD who have had ileocolonic resection.

Materials and methods: This was a retrospective cross-sectional study on all pediatric patients who had undergone surgery for CD between January 2015 and December 2017 in the Pediatric Surgery and Gastroenterology Units of the University Hospital of Messina. Surgical treatment was represented by laparoscopic ileocecal resection with latero-lateral anastomosis. Patients were asked to fill in a modified version of the IMPACT III questionnaire made up of 15 closed questions before and after surgery. The questionnaire was scored on a five-point scale with 5 reporting "not a problem" and 1 "a very severe problem." The total score ranged from 15 (worst HRQoL) to 75 (best HRQoL). Frequency of relapses, reoperations, complications during follow-up, and postoperative bowel function were also studied.

Results: Data were obtained in 10 patients (9 males), who underwent surgery at a median age of 13.5 years (range 13–18), after a median post-diagnosis period of 2.5 years (range 0–8). Preoperative scores were low in all 4 domains of the questionnaire. Postoperatively, HRQoL measures improved significantly ($p < 0.05$) about symptoms, school attendance, social and emotional functioning. Overall, nearly all patients were completely satisfied with the surgical outcome.

Conclusions: HRQoL is low in CD children referred for possible operation, and surgery may positively affect the overall HRQoL. Collecting HRQoL data provides insight into the impact of treatment on children health status.

Keywords: Crohn's disease, inflammatory bowel disease, health-related quality of life, surgery, questionnaire, pediatrics

INTRODUCTION

Crohn's disease (CD) is a chronic, relapsing disease whose symptoms interfere with the daily activities of patients, especially in young patients who have a long life expectancy (1, 2). The incidence of pediatric CD, particularly in children 10–19 years of age, is increasing and the phenotype is often characterized by an aggressive disease course, higher risk of surgery (because of stenosis), and more extensive phenotypes compared with adults (1, 3). Quality of life (QoL) is considered the most important outcome for chronic conditions such as CD. In general, QoL is the feeling of overall life satisfaction, as determined by the mentally alert individual whose life is being evaluated. In health care, health-related QoL (HRQoL) is the assessment of how the individual's well-being may be affected by a disease, disability, or disorder (4, 5). Numerous physical and psychological factors contribute to the poor HRQoL in pediatric patients with CD, such as its relatively young age of onset, associated extraintestinal complications, disability, and debilitating symptoms (diarrhea, abdominal pain, gastrointestinal bleeding) that have the potential to cause significant psychosocial stress (1, 6). Even in the era of routine immunomodulator and biological therapies for moderate to severe CD, modifying the natural history of the disease remains a challenge, and about 20–30% of children require surgery within 10 years of diagnosis (1, 7, 8). Indications for surgery in CD include complications such as stricture, perforation, abscess, fistula, or severe perianal disease (1). Patients being referred for surgery experience a more aggressive disease and a poorer HRQoL (1, 9). Literature data mainly coming from adult studies showed that HRQoL in these patients seems to improve following resectional surgery (6, 10, 11). In pediatric patients with CD, the effects of small bowel resection on HRQoL have not been systematically studied. The aim of the present study was to evaluate the long-term health outcomes of children with CD and undergone ileocolonic resection and to compare preoperative and postoperative HRQoL with a disease-specific questionnaire.

MATERIALS AND METHODS

Patients

This retrospective cross-sectional study included all the pediatric patients (18 years or younger) followed up and undergone surgery for CD in the Pediatric Surgery, Pediatric Gastroenterology, and Adult Surgery Units of the University of Messina. Hospital records from January 2015 to December 2017 were reviewed. Patients with <1 year of follow-up were excluded. Data on demographics, age at diagnosis of CD, age at the time of surgery, the medication before surgery, indications for surgery, postoperative use of biologics, and possible surgical complications and re-resections were recorded from case notes. The diagnosis of CD was based on clinical features, laboratory tests, and endoscopic and histological findings. Disease activity was reported based on the Pediatric Crohn's Disease Activity Index (PCDAI) (12). Surgery was represented by laparoscopic-assisted ileocolonic resections with latero-lateral anastomosis. Disease relapse after surgery was defined as the presence of aphthous lesions according the Rutgeerts score (13) to predict postsurgical CD recurrence via ileocolonoscopy. This study was conducted in conformity with the principles and regulations of the Helsinki Declaration. The study was approved by the committee on research ethics of all participating sites and informed consent from participants and their parents, where necessary, was obtained.

Questionnaire

The instrument chosen to measure HRQoL in children affected by CD before and after surgery was a modified version of the IMPACT III questionnaire (14), which is a specific inflammatory bowel disease (IBD) questionnaire assessing the quality of life in an objective dimension. We modified the IMPACT III by decreasing the number of issues in order to make it easier to be completed by phone interview. The final version was made up of 15 closed questions of functional outcomes and HRQoL. All of the issues were grouped into 4 domains, such as systemic and IBD symptoms (7 questions), school functioning (2 questions), social functioning (3 questions), emotional functioning (3 questions) (**Supplementary Table 1**). The questionnaire was scored on a five-point scale with 5 reporting "not a problem" and 1 "a very severe problem." The total score ranged from 15 (worst HRQoL) to 75 (best HRQoL). The questionnaire also included an initial question asking the participants to comment on general satisfaction with surgery. Questionnaires were administered by the physician (pediatric surgeon or pediatric gastroenterologist) by telephone interview at 12 and 6 months before surgery and at 12 months following surgery. Respondents were patients or parents in case of minor patients.

Outcomes

Primary outcome was postoperative long-term HRQoL. Frequencies of relapses, reoperations, complications during follow-up, and postoperative bowel function were also studied.

Statistical Analysis

Continuous variables were presented as means and SD while the categorical variables were reported as percentages. The Shapiro–Whilk test showed variable distribution was asymmetric. The non-parametric Friedman test for paired data and the Conover *post-hoc* analysis (15) were used to compare the study times (6 months before vs. 12 months after surgery). Statistical analyses were performed in R version 3.5.3 (16) using the PMCMR plus (Calculate Pairwise Multiple Comparisons of Mean Rank Sums Extended) package. A $p < 0.05$ was considered significant.

RESULTS

Data were obtained in 10 patients (9 males), who underwent surgery at a median age of 13.5 years (range 13–18). The median amount of time that had elapsed after the operation was 4 years (range 1–9). The majority of patients underwent surgery because of active disease despite optimal medical therapy (4 with anti-TNF alpha). **Table 1** presents the background data of the patients.

HRQoL median scores were 43.2 and 34.5, 12 and 6 months before surgery, respectively. There was a significant improvement seen at 12 months postoperatively (median 65.4, $p < 0.001$).

TABLE 1 | Patients' demographic and clinical variables.

Variable	Total (*N* = 10)
Current age, y, median (range)	17.2 (12–23)
Age at diagnosis, y, median (range)	12.1 (6–16)
Ileocolonic disease, *n*	10
Disease duration before operation, y, median (range)	2.5 (0–8)
Age at surgery, y, median (range)	13.5 (13–18)
Follow up time after operation, y, median (range)	4 (1–9)
Moderate disease activity 12 months before surgery, *n**	9
PCDAI score 12 months before surgery, median	22
Moderate disease activity 6 months before surgery, *n**	10
PCDAI score 6 months before surgery, median	25
Remission 12 months after surgery, *n***	10
PCDAI score 12 months after surgery	9
Indications for surgery, *N*	
Bowel stricture	7
Bowel stricture with enteroenteric fistula	3
Medications at surgery, *N*	
Azathioprine	4
Anti-TNF (IFX, ADA)	4
None	2

**Pediatric Crohn's Disease Activity Index score 11–30.*
***Pediatric Crohn's Disease Activity Index score <10.*
IFX, infliximab; ADA, adalimumab.

This improvement was observed in all dimensions of HRQoL. About systemic and gastrointestinal symptoms (**Table 2**), a highly significant reduction ($p < 0.001$) of stool blood, abdominal pain, and fatigue was reported at 12 months after surgery. A significant improvement ($p < 0.001$) of appetite and weight was also reported, with less difficulty to perform the general activity of daily living ($p < 0.001$). Nonetheless, despite a slight reduction, stool frequency improvement was not significant in comparison to baseline.

Nearly all patients reported frequent school absences before surgery, with low scores both at 12 (median score 2.60 ± 1.26) and 6 months (1.60 ± 0.97). The most reported IBD-related problems which had caused an absence from school were abdominal pain, fatigue and diarrhea in 5, 3, and 2 patients both 12 and 6 months before surgery. School absences significantly reduced at 12 months after surgery (4.60 ± 0.84, $p < 0.001$).

Preoperatively, the scores showed markedly impaired social functioning (**Table 3**), including the ability to play and/or go out with friends, perform a sport, travel and/or go on holiday, with a significant recovery at 12 months from surgery ($p < 0.001$, $p < 0.008$, $p < 0.002$, respectively).

About the emotional functioning (**Table 4**), CD patients reported a significant reduction of feelings of anger, injustice and embarrassment due to their disease at 12-month follow-up ($p < 0.036$ and $p < 0.039$, respectively). On the contrary, surgery did not affect their concerns for future health problems ($p = 0.202$). Overall, nearly all patients were completely satisfied (score 5) with the outcome of the surgery at 12-month follow-up, with absolute score values of 75.

There were no operation-related mortality and complications. Two patients were started on biologics (adalimumab) for preventing postoperative recurrence. By the end of the follow-up, all patients were in clinical remission (PCDAI <10), and none of them experienced surgical complications and/or recurrences (Rutgeerts score <i2).

DISCUSSION

Surgery has a definite role in CD treatment protocols, and seems to positively impact the natural history of the disease (17). Some studies have demonstrated that the early use of biologics do not reduce the risk of surgery in CD (1, 18). Surgery can be a viable option in elective cases of CD, such as stricture or fistula, growth retardation, delayed puberty or a clinical condition unresponsive to medical treatment. It is also to be considered in urgent situations, such as occlusive syndrome, abscess or fistulas unresponsive to conservative treatment, massive hemorrhage or intestinal perforation (17).

In the present retrospective cross-sectional study, the long-term HRQoL and health-outcomes after surgery in pediatric CD median 4 years after bowel resection were studied, and it was showed that children and adolescents with CD have low HRQoL score and that HRQoL significantly improves postoperatively. A very limited number of studies evaluated the HRQoL in pediatric patients before and after surgery for CD (9, 19). In 2013 Piekkala et al. (19) carried out a retrospective study on 36 pediatric CD patients who had undergone intestinal resections during childhood between 1985 and 2008. Moreover, they selected 2 controls (with no IBD) per patient with CD matched for age and sex. All patients and controls answered questionnaires about health outcomes and QoL. Most patients had undergone surgery because of active disease despite optimal medical therapy (3 with infliximab) or steroid dependency (56%), as in the present study. The median follow-up after primary resection was longer than our study, with a median of 10 years (range 2–21). The different dimensions and overall HRQoL scores were similar between the patients and their matched controls. Similarly to our study, 96% were completely or moderately satisfied with the outcomes of the surgery (19). Notably, the overall HRQoL, physical and social functioning at follow-up were significantly lower among patients who had missed school or work because of surgery compared with patients who could normally attend school or work. Two other studies performed in the same center on limited number of patients (5 in each study) reported restricted sport activities in children due to stoma formation (20, 21). Permanent stoma had no impact on HRQoL in children compared to adults with a stoma who scored lower for general health and physical activity compared to controls (19, 22). In this study, no surgical complications were registered during the follow-up period. Data coming from pediatric literature are scarce and suggest that the number of complication in pediatric patients are higher if compared with adult data, but further studies are warranted. In the study by Piekkala et al. (19), nearly all patients had at

TABLE 2 | Systemic and IBD symptoms score preoperatively and 6 and 12 months after surgery.

Issue	12 months before surgery ($n = 10$)	6 months before surgery ($n = 10$)	12 months after surgery ($n = 10$)	p*
Stool blood, median	3.40 ± 1.26	3.20 ± 1.32	4.60 ± 0.70	<0.001
Increased stool frequency, median	4.80 ± 0.63	4.60 ± 0.84	5	0.223
Abdominal pain, median	2.20 ± 1.03	1.40 ± 0.84	4.60 ± 0.84	<0.001
Fatigue, median	1.40 ± 0.84	1	4.40 ± 0.97	<0.001
Reduced caloric intake, median	3.00 ± 1.89	2.20 ± 1.40	5	<0.001
Weight loss, median	2 ± 1.41	1.40 ± 0.84	4.80 ± 0.63	<0.001
Need to stop daily activities, median	3 ± 1.63	1.80 ± 1.40	4.60 ± 0.84	<0.001

**Comparison between 6 months before and 12 months after surgery.*
IBD, Inflammatory bowel disease.

TABLE 3 | Social activities score preoperatively and 6 and 12 months after surgery.

Issue	12 months before surgery ($n = 10$)	6 months before surgery ($n = 10$)	12 months after surgery ($n = 10$)	p*
Play and/or go out with friends, median	2.20 ± 1.40	1.60 ± 0.97	4.40 ± 1.35	<0.001
Play a sport, median	2.40 ± 1.35	1.80 ± 1.40	4 ± 1.41	<0.008
Travel and/or go on holiday, median	3.60 ± 1.65	2.60 ± 1.58	4.80 ± 0.63	<0.002

**Comparison between 6 months before and 12 months after surgery.*

TABLE 4 | Emotional functioning score preoperatively and 6 and 12 months after surgery.

Issue	12 months before surgery ($n = 10$)	6 months before surgery ($n = 10$)	12 months after surgery ($n = 10$)	p*
Feelings of anger or injustice related to the disease, median	3 ± 1.89	2.40 ± 1.65	4 ± 1.05	<0.036
Concerns for the future, median	4 ± 1.05	3.60 ± 1.35	4.20 ± 1.03	0.202
Embarrassment because of bowel condition, median	3.40 ± 1.84	3.20 ± 1.75	4.40 ± 1.35	<0.039

**Comparison between 6 months before and 12 months after surgery.*

least 1 surgical complication, mostly represented by strictures in the anastomosis.

About disease reactivation after surgery, literature data consistently report that about 50–60% of pediatric patients had a clinical relapse within 1.8–5 years postoperatively (7, 19, 23–26). On the other hand, the reoperation rates are very variable, ranging from 8–18% at 2 years (7, 27) to 29–50% at 10 years (17, 27). In this study, no disease re-activation after surgery was recorded, probably due to the small number of patients. One patient was started on anti-TNFα therapy soon after the intervention, as recommended in high-risk patients (extensive disease, short disease duration from diagnosis to surgery, recurrent surgery, long resected segment, surgery for fistulizing disease, disease complications, perianal disease, smoking) (1, 28).

Any conclusions drawn from the findings of this research study must be qualified in light of the study's limitations. First, the small number of patients, which precluded reliable statistical analysis (such as the evaluation of possible predictors of HRQoL after surgery); second, the retrospective design, so recruited cases and clinical management are the confounding variables; third, the lack of a control population, in order to compare life situation (and HRQoL) with that of patients with CD. Moreover, data were obtained by phone and not during a face to face consultation. The strength of the present study is being one of the limited number of studies reporting HRQoL outcome before and after surgery for CD in pediatric patients. Collection of HRQoL data provides insight into the impact of treatment on patient health status and well-being, especially in the pediatric group of age.

In conclusion, this study confirms that HRQoL is low in children and adolescents with complicated CD who previously failed medical therapy. Ileocecal resection for CD is safe and associated with significant and sustained improvement of the physical, psychological, and social dimensions of HRQoL in affected children. CD is a model of chronic disease, whose clinical and pharmacological management is crucial to gain an optimal HRQoL. On the other hand, the impact of therapy on HRQoL should be considered an integrative, "positive" step of the management strategy. The clinician should consider these HRQoL-related aspects, in comparison with pharmacological therapies-related concerns, such as the high infection risk carried out by high dose of biological or immunosuppressant drugs. This present study adds a contribution in this area, and confirms that surgery may positively affect HRQoL in pediatric patients with CD.

AUTHOR CONTRIBUTIONS

All authors have made substantial contributions to the design of the study, acquisition and interpretation of data, drafting the article and revising it critically for important intellectual content, and finally approved the version to be submitted.

REFERENCES

1. Amil-Dias J, Kolacek S, Turner D, Pærregaard A, Rintala R, Afzal NA, et al. IBD Working Group of ESPGHAN (IBD Porto Group). Surgical management of Crohn disease in children: guidelines from the Paediatric IBD Porto Group of ESPGHAN. *J Pediatr Gastroenterol Nutr.* (2017) 64:818–35. doi: 10.1097/MPG.0000000000001562
2. Guassora AD, Kruse C, Thomsen OO, Binder V. Quality of life study in a regional group of patients with Crohn disease. A structured interview study. *Scand J Gastroenterol.* (2000) 35:1068–74. doi: 10.1080/003655200451199
3. Vernier-Massouille G, Balde M, Salleron J, Turck D, Dupas JL, Mouterde O, et al. Natural history of pediatric Crohn's disease: a population-based cohort study. *Gastroenterology.* (2008) 135:1038–41. doi: 10.1053/j.gastro.2008.06.079
4. Centers for Disease Control and Prevention. *Measuring Healthy Days: Population Assessment of Health-Related Quality of Life.* Atlanta, GA: Centers for Disease Control and Prevention (2000).
5. Meeberg GA. Quality of life: a concept analysis. *J Adv Nurs.* (1993) 18:32–8. doi: 10.1046/j.1365-2648.1993.18010032.x
6. Wright EK, Kamm MA, De Cruz P, Hamilton AL, Ritchie KJ, Krejany EO, et al. Effect of intestinal resection on quality of life in Crohn's disease. *J Crohns Colitis.* (2015) 9:452–62. doi: 10.1093/ecco-jcc/jjv058
7. Pacilli M, Eaton S, Fell JM, Rawat D, Clarke S, Haddad MJ. Surgery in children with Crohn's disease refractory to medical therapy. *J Pediatr Gastroenterol Nutr.* (2011) 52:286–90. doi: 10.1097/MPG.0b013e3181e999af
8. Turunen P, Ashorn M, Auvinen A, Iltanen S, Huhtala H, Kolho KL. Long-term health outcomes in pediatric inflammatory bowel disease: a population-based study. *Inflamm Bowel Dis.* (2009) 15:56–62. doi: 10.1002/ibd.20558
9. Diederen K, de Ridder L, van Rheenen P, Wolters VM, Mearin ML, de Meij TG, et al. Quality of life and colorectal function in Crohn's disease patients that underwent ileocecal resection during childhood. *Eur J Pediatr.* (2019) 178:1413–21. doi: 10.1007/s00431-019-03427-3
10. Thirlby RC, Land JC, Fenster LF, Lonborg R. Effect of surgery on health-related quality of life in patients with inflammatory bowel disease: a prospective study. *Arch Surg.* (1998) 133:826–32. doi: 10.1001/archsurg.133.8.826
11. Thirlby RC, Sobrino MA, Randall JB. The long-term benefit of surgery on health-related quality of life in patients with inflammatory bowel disease. *Arch Surg.* (2001) 136:521–7. doi: 10.1001/archsurg.136.5.521
12. Hyams JS, Ferry GD, Mandel FS, Gryboski JD, Kibort PM, Kirschner BS, et al. Development and validation of a pediatric Crohn's disease activity index. *J Pediatr Gastroenterol Nutr.* (1991) 12(4):439–47. doi: 10.1097/00005176-199105000-00005
13. Rutgeerts P, Geboes K, Vantrappen G, Beyls J, Kerremans R, Hiele M. Predictability of the postoperative course of Crohn's disease. *Gastroenterology.* (1990) 99:956–63. doi: 10.1016/0016-5085(90)90613-6
14. Otley A, Smith C, Nicholas D, Munk M, Avolio J, Sherman PM, et al. The IMPACT questionnaire: a valid measure of health-related quality of life in pediatric inflammatory bowel disease. *J Pediatr Gastroenterol Nutr.* (2002) 35:557–63. doi: 10.1097/00005176-200210000-00018
15. Conover WJ. *Practical Nonparametric Statistics.* 3rd ed. Wiley & Sons (1999).
16. *R: A Language and Environment for Statistical Computing.* Vienna: R Foundation for Statistical Computing. Available online at: https://www.R-project.org/
17. Stewart D. Surgical care of the pediatric Crohn's disease patient. *Semin Pediatr Surg.* (2017) 26:373–8. doi: 10.1053/j.sempedsurg.2017.10.007
18. Schaefer ME, Machan JT, Kawatu D, Langton CR, Markowitz J, Crandall W, et al. Factors that determine risk for surgery in pediatric patients with Crohn's disease. *Clin Gastroenterol Hepatol.* (2010) 8:789–94. doi: 10.1016/j.cgh.2010.05.021
19. Piekkala M, Pakarinen M, Ashorn M, Rintala R, Kolho KL. Long-term outcomes after surgery on pediatric patients with Crohn disease. *J Pediatr Gastroenterol Nutr.* (2013) 56:271–6. doi: 10.1097/MPG.0b013e318279871c
20. Akobeng AK, Suresh-Babu MV, Firth D, Miller V, Mir P, Thomas AG. Quality of life in children with Crohn's disease: a pilot study. *J Pediatr Gastroenterol Nutr.* (1999) 28:S37–9. doi: 10.1097/00005176-199904001-00006
21. Rabbett H, Elbadri A, Thwaites R, Northover H, Dady I, Firth D, et al. Quality of life in children with Crohn's disease. *J Pediatr Gastroenterol Nutr.* (1996) 23:528–33. doi: 10.1097/00005176-199612000-00003
22. Andersson P, Olaison G, Bendtsen P, Myrelid P, Sjödahl R. Health related quality of life in Crohn's proctocolitis does not differ from a general population when in remission. *Colorectal Dis.* (2003) 5:56–62. doi: 10.1046/j.1463-1318.2003.00407.x
23. Besnard M, Jady O, Mougenot JF, Ferkdadji L, Debrun A, Faure C, et al. Postoperative outcome of Crohn's disease in 30 children. *Gut.* (1998) 43:634–8. doi: 10.1136/gut.43.5.634
24. Barrena S, Matinez L, Hernandez F, Lassaletta L, Lopez-Santamaria M, Prieto G, et al. Surgical treatment of chronic inflammatory bowel disease in children. *Pediatr Surg Int.* (2011) 27:385–90. doi: 10.1007/s00383-010-2809-9
25. El-Baba M, Chuan-Hao L, Klein M, Tolia V. Outcome after surgical intervention in children with chronic inflammatory bowel disease. *Am Surg.* (1996) 62:1014–7.
26. Baldassano RN, Han PD, Jeshion WC, Berlin JA, Piccoli DA, Lautenbach E, et al. Pediatric Crohn's disease: risk factors for postoperative recurrence. *Am J Gastroenterol.* (2001) 96:2169–76. doi: 10.1111/j.1572-0241.2001.03876.x
27. Boualit M, Salleron J, Turck D, Fumery M, Savoye G, Dupas J, et al. EPIMAD Group. Long-term outcome after first intestinal resection in pediatric-onset Crohn's disease: a population- based study. *Inflamm Bowel Dis.* (2013) 19:7–14. doi: 10.1002/ibd.23004
28. Splawski JB, Pffefferkorn MD, Schaefer ME, Day AS, Soldes OS, Ponsky TA, et al. NASPGHAN Clinical report on postoperative recurrence in pediatric Crohn disease. *J Pediatr Gastroenterol Nutr.* (2017) 65:475–86. doi: 10.1097/MPG.0000000000001606

Perioperative Respiratory Adverse Events Among Pediatric Surgical Patients in University Hospitals in Northwest Ethiopia

Desalegn Muche Wudineh[1], Yophtahe Woldegerima Berhe[2], Wubie Birlie Chekol[2], Habtu Adane[2] and Misganaw Mengie Workie[2]*

[1] *Felege-Hiwot Referral Hospital, Bahirdar, Ethiopia,* [2] *Department of Anesthesia, University of Gondar, Gondar, Ethiopia*

***Correspondence:**
Yophtahe Woldegerima Berhe
yophtii@gmail.com
orcid.org/0000-0002-0988-7723

Introduction: Perioperative respiratory adverse events (PRAEs) are frequent among pediatrics surgical patients and are accountable for 3/4th of perioperative critical incidents and 1/3rd of cardiac arrests.

Objective: Assess the prevalence and factors associated with PRAEs among pediatric surgical patients in University Hospitals in Northwest Ethiopia, 2020.

Methodology: After ethical approval obtained prospective observational study was conducted among 210 pediatric surgical patients. Perioperative respiratory adverse events were defined as the occurrence of any episode of single/combination of coughing, breath holding, hypoxemia, laryngospasm and bronchospasm. Bivariate and multivariate binary logistic regression analyses were performed and variables with $p < 0.05$ at 95% confidence interval were considered as statistically significant.

Results: The prevalence of PRAEs was 26.2% (CI: 20.5–30.9%). A total of 129 episodes of PRAEs were occurred and of them, 89 (69.0%) were occurred in the postoperative period. Desaturation was the predominant adverse event which was observed 61 (47.3%) times. Age $<$ 1 year (AOR: 3.6, CI: 1.3–10.0), ASA $\geq$ 3 (AOR: 5.2, CI: 1.9–22.9), upper respiratory tract infections (URTIs) (AOR: 7.6, CI: 1.9–30.2), secretions in the upper airway (AOR: 4.8, CI: 1.4–15.9) and airway related surgery (AOR: 6.0, CI: 1.5–24.1) were significantly associated with PRAEs.

Conclusions: Prevalence of PRAEs was high among pediatric surgical patients; the postoperative period was the most critical time for the occurrence of PRAEs and desaturation was the commonest PRAE. Age $<$ 1 year, URTIs (recent or active), secretions in the upper airways, ASA $\geq$ 3 and airway related surgery were significantly associated with PRAEs. Clinicians should perform effective risk assessment, preoperative optimization and preparation for the management of PRAEs.

Keywords: perioperative respiratory adverse events, perioperative complications, pediatric anesthesia, general anesthesia, adverse events

INTRODUCTION

Adverse event is defined as unanticipated and unwanted response to medical intervention during the perioperative period that can threaten patient wellbeing. Respiratory adverse events are any episodes of desaturation, partial or complete airway obstruction, persistent coughing, breath holding and bronchospasm (1–3). Despite improvements in pediatrics anesthesia, respiratory adverse events are still the most frequent cause of serious morbidity and mortality in the perioperative period. The 3/4th of all critical incidents and the 1/3rd of all perioperative cardiac arrests in pediatric anesthesia are caused by respiratory adverse events. Preoperative identification of those children at high risk is a challenging process (4, 5). Children are vulnerable to respiratory adverse events because of anatomical and physiological considerations and frequent respiratory tract infections (URTIs). The most common respiratory adverse events under anesthesia are desaturation, breath holding, laryngospasm, bronchospasm and coughing. Among these, laryngospasm, bronchospasm and persistent hypoxemia could result potentially devastating complication and death (6–8).

Inconsistent definitions of respiratory adverse events among studies make comparisons difficult and results in discrepancy on magnitude of the actual events (1). Despite introduction of new monitoring modalities, pharmacological products and new clinical practice guidelines, the prevalence of respiratory adverse events has remained high and increased length of hospital stay and medical costs (1, 9). The patient's age, techniques of anesthesia induction, comorbidities and airway surgery were strongly associated with increased occurrence of adverse events during surgery. Occurrence of respiratory adverse events differs according to timing of extubation whether awake or deep plane of anesthesia, airway device and urgency of procedures (10, 11). The severity of PRAEs and their complications depends on the nature of surgery, presence comorbidity, early detection, and prompt corrective measures. It may range from transient damage with full recovery to unanticipated morbidity and mortality (2). Risk assessment in the preoperative period is very important to decrease respiratory adverse events but still patient identification and selection are real challenges. If effective measures are not taken timely, serious complications and death would prevail. "*Critical respiratory incident recording and reporting system is poor particularly in the developing countries due to multiple reasons*" (12). The general objective of the current study was to assess the prevalence and factors associated with PRAEs among pediatrics surgical patients.

Abbreviations: AOR, Adjusted Odds Ratio; ASA, American Society of Anesthesiologist; COVID-19, Corona Virus Disease-2019; GA, General Anesthesia; LMA, Laryngeal Mask Airways; PRAEs, Perioperative Respiratory Adverse Events; SPO2, Peripheral Oxygen Saturation; SPSS, Statistical Package for Social Science; TGSH, Tibebe-Ghion Specialized Hospital; UoGCSH, University of Gondar Comprehensive and Specialized Hospital; URTIs, Upper Respiratory Tract Infections.

METHODOLOGY

A prospective observational study was conducted from March 1 to May 30, 2020 at the University of Gondar Comprehensive Specialized Hospital (UoGCSH) and Tibebe-Ghion Specialized Hospital (TGSH). The hospitals are located at Gondar and Bahirdar towns respectively in the Northwest Ethiopia. The source population was all pediatric surgical patients (0–12 years of age) that underwent surgery under general anesthesia and the study population was all pediatric surgical patients that underwent surgery under general anesthesia at UoGCSH and TGSH during the study period. All pediatric surgical patients whose parents/legal care-givers were volunteer were included and patients who had severe head injury, intubated patient, acute respiratory distress, hypoxia requiring mechanical ventilation in the preoperative period, operated for more than once, and transferred to intensive care unit for mechanical ventilation after operation were excluded.

Sample size was calculated by using single population proportion formula with 50% proportion, maximum acceptable difference (d) = 5%, and 95% confidence interval and found 385. We used a reduction formula to determine achievable sample size as the surgical registries showed that only 780 and 660 pediatrics surgical procedures were performed annually at UGCSH and TGCSH respectively. In-addition, due to COVID-19 pandemic, the flow of pediatric surgical patients was reduced. After reduction, the sample size became 195 and 15% non-response rate was added and the final sample size was 225.

All eligible pediatric surgical patients who received general anesthesia were included in the study. The dependent variables were PRAEs which were measured in terms of any episode of either coughing, breath holding, hypoxemia, laryngospasm, or bronchospasm. The independent variables were patient factors (history of prematurity, age, ASA classification, family history of asthma, URTIs, and other comorbidities), anesthetic factors (techniques of anesthetic induction, type of airway device, number of intubation attempts, muscle relaxant, depth of anesthesia, perioperative opioid use, and experience of the anesthesia providers), and surgical aspects (surgical site, duration, and urgency).

Operational Definitions

Perioperative respiratory adverse event: any episode of single/combination of coughing, breathe holding, hypoxemia, laryngospasm and bronchospasm (2, 3, 13–19). Detailed operational definitions were prepared accordingly.

Laryngospasm: complete airway obstruction with abdominal and chest muscle rigidity that require positive pressure ventilation or administration of succinylcholine (1).

Bronchospasm: increased work of breathing, particularly during expiration and wheezing on auscultation or requires bronchodilators (7, 13).

Desaturation or hypoxemia: peripheral arterial oxyhemoglobin saturation (SpO_2) < 95% more than 30 seconds measured by pulse oximetry regardless administrations

TABLE 1 | Perioperative respiratory adverse events severity scoring in pediatrics patients underwent surgery under general anesthesia.

Parameters	Severity score			
	1 (No adverse event)	2	3	4 (Serious adverse events)
SpO_2	95–100	90–94	80–89	< 80
Coughing (*n*)	None	1–2	3–4	Continuous
Breath holding (seconds)	None	< 15	15–30	> 30
Laryngospasm	None	Partial obstruction requires repositioning only	Partial obstruction requires CPAP	Complete obstruction requires muscle relaxant
Bronchospasm	None	Expiration phase only	Expiration and inspiration phase	Difficult to ventilate: treatment needed
Secretions	None	Minimal: no suctioning	Moderate: one suctioning	Copious: more than one suctioning

of 100% Oxygen or SpO_2 <90% in atmospheric air. Oxygen saturation was documented when pulse oximetry showed consistent readings with no artifacts (2, 7).

Coughing: a series of pronounced, persistent coughs lasting more than 5 s (7).

Breath holding or apnea: if the patient had apnea more than 15 s or irregular breathing or if the apnea is associated with bradycardia or cyanosis (13).

Partial upper airway obstruction: airway obstruction in the combination with snoring, inspiratory stridor or increased breathing efforts or paradoxical abdominal movement or both that can be effectively relieved by simple airway maneuvers (2).

Multiple intubation attempts: if required multiple intubation attempts ≥ 3 times (20). Active or current URTIs: the present of at least of two URTIs symptoms (rhinorrhea, sneezing, nasal congestion, sore or scratchy throat, cough, malaise, or fever > 38°C) at the time of surgery together with a confirmation by a parent (13).

Active/Recent URTIs: symptomatic URTIs during/within 2 weeks of the perioperative period was considered as active URTIs. If the URTIs occurred within 2–4 weeks before surgery but resolved at the time of surgery, it was considered as recent URTIs (13).

Acute respiratory distress: the presence of tachypnea, nasal flaring, grunting, intercostal and subcostal retractions, and cyanosis in room air and requires high flow Oxygen (21).

Light anesthesia: the presence of patient's movement with tachypnea, tachycardia and hypertension (change by more than 30% from baseline) (22).

Oropharyngeal secretions: the presence of secretion that requires suctioning of more than once (23).

Pulmonary aspiration: confirmed or suspected entrance of foreign materials such as gastric contents into the respiratory tract result in new/worsening respiratory signs such as hypoxia (24).

Airway related surgery: surgery that involve the airway which includes ENT and maxillofacial procedures such as adenotonsilectomy, cleft palate repair, direct laryngoscopy, and bronchoscopy (23, 25, 26).

All complications were scored according to severity from 1 (no complication) to 4 (serious complication). For patients who received anesthesia with endotracheal tubes or laryngeal mask airways, scores were multiplied by a constant factor of five. When facemask was used, scores were multiplied by a constant factor of three. Patients received a composite score of 5–20 for ETT or LMA and 3–12 facemask for each adverse event (**Table 1**) (23). The PRAEs were recorded starting from induction to the first postoperative hour. A patient experiencing PRAEs was counted just once independent of the numbers of events in perioperative period.

Ethical approval (**Reference No: PGC/587/07/2012**) was obtained from the Ethical Review Committee of School of Medicine, University of Gondar. Written informed consent was obtained from parents/legal care-givers of each child. When clinically significant PRAEs were noticed, data collectors reported for clinicians (Anesthetist, Surgeon or Nurse) to provide appropriate management. A pre-test was conducted on 20 (8%) patients whose data were not included in the main study. The data were analyzed by using SPSS version 20 (IBM Corporate). The normality was checked by using Shapiro-Wilk normality test. The Chi-squared or Fisher's exact tests were used when appropriate. The Hosmer-Lemeshow test was used to assess model fitness. The variance inflation factors and tolerance were used to diagnose multicollinearity. The associations between variables were determined by using bivariate and multivariate binary logistic regression. The cut-point of statistical significance was $p < 0.2$ for bivariate and < 0.05 for multivariate regression at 95% confidence interval. Odds Ratio were used to describe the strength of associations.

RESULTS

Two hundred ten (210) pediatric surgical patients who received general anesthesia were included in this study. The response rate was 93.3% and data from 15 patients were excluded due to incompleteness. The majority of the patients 115 (54.8%) were males. The median age (inter-quartile range) was 4.0 (1.1–8.0)

TABLE 2 | Clinical characteristics of pediatric surgical patients who underwent surgery under general anesthesia in UoGCSH and TGSH from March 1–May 30, 2020 (N = 210).

Variables	Frequency *n* (%)	Perioperative respiratory adverse events	
		Yes *n* (%)	No *n* (%)
Age			
< 1 year	52 (24.8)	22 (42.3)	30 (57.7)
≥ 1 year	158 (75.2)	33 (20.9)	125 (79.1)
Median (IQR) (years)	4.0 (1.1–8.0)		
Prematurity			
Yes	14 (6.7)	4 (28.6)	10 (71.4)
No	196 (93.3)	51 (26)	145 (74)
Preoperative hemoglobin			
< 11 g/dl	89 (42.4)	21(23.6)	68 (76.4)
≥ 11 g/dl	121 (57.6)	34 (28.1)	87 (71.9)
Surgical procedure			
ENT	25 (11.9)	12 (48)	13 (52)
Ophthalmic	34 (16.2)	4 (11.8)	30 (88.2)
Abdominal	75 (35.7)	17 (22.7)	58 (77.3)
Orthopedic	34 (16.2)	6 (17.6)	28 (82.4)
Neurosurgery	41 (20)	16 (38.1)	26 (61.9)
Airway device			
Endotracheal tube	136 (64.8)	40 (29.4)	96 (70.6)
Laryngeal mask airway	46 (21.9)	8 (17.4)	38 (82.6)
Facemask	28 (13.3)	7 (25.0)	21 (75.0)
Induction of anesthesia			
Intravenous	199 (94.8)	51 (22.6)	148 (74.4)
Inhalation	11 (5.2)	4 (36.4)	7 (63.6)
Muscle relaxant			
Yes	120 (57.1)	32 (26.7)	88 (73.3)
No	90 (42.9)	23 (25.6)	67 (74.4)
Time of extubation			
Awake extubation	175 (96.2)	46 (26.3)	129 (73.7)
Deep extubation	7 (3.8)	2 (28.6)	5 (71.4)
Intraoperative blood loss			
< 100 ml	72 (34.7)	18 (25)	54 (75)
100–500 ml	99 (46.2)	29 (29.9)	29 (29.9)
≥ 500 ml	41 (19.5)	8 (19.5)	33 (80.5)

IQR, Inter-quartile Range.

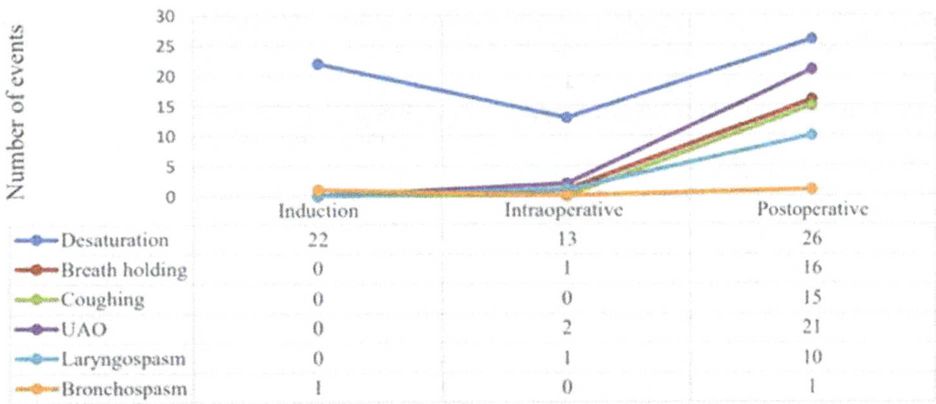

FIGURE 1 | Line graphs showing the frequency of respiratory adverse events among distinct phases of the perioperative period in pediatric surgical patients at UoGCSH and TGSH, Northwest Ethiopia; March 1–May 30, 2020 (N = 20).

TABLE 3 | Pearson Chi-squared and Fisher-exact tests; factors associated with perioperative respiratory adverse events among pediatric surgical patients underwent surgery under general anesthesia at UoGCSH and TGSH, Northwest Ethiopia; March 1–May 30, 2020 ($N = 210$).

Variables	Frequency *n* (%)	Desaturation *n* (%)	Breath holding n (%)	Coughing *n* (%)	Airway obstruction *n* (%)	Laryngospasm *n* (%)	Bronchospasm *n* (%)
Age							
≤ 1year	52 (24.8)	22 (44.0)[a]	8(50.0)	8 (53.3)[b]	5 (23.8)	5 (41.7)	1 (1.9)
> 1year	158 (75.2)	28 (56.0)	8 (50.0)	7 (46.7)	16 (76.2)	7 (58.3)	1 (0.6)
ASA							
≥ 3	21 (10)	14 (28.0)[a]	2 (12.5)	5 (33.3)	8 (38.1)	2 (16.7)	0
≤ 2	189 (90)	36 (72.0)	14 (87.5)	10 (66.7)	13 (61.9)	10 (83.3)	2 (1.1)
URTI							
Yes	23 (11)	17 (34.0)[a]	4 (25.0)	6 (40)[b]	6 (28.5)[b]	5 (41.7)[b]	0
No	187 (89)	33 (66.0)	12 (75.0)	9 (60)	15 (71.5)	7 (58.3)	2 (1.1)
Attempts							
≥3	9 (4.30)	7 (14.0)[b]	2 (12.5)	1 (6.7)	0	3 (25)[b]	1 (50)
≤2	201 (95.7)	38 (86.0)	14 (87.5)	14 (93.3)	21 (100)	9 (75)	1 (50)
Secretion							
Yes	26 (12.4)	15 (30.0)[a]	5 (31.2)[b]	8 (53.3)[b]	9 (42.8)[b]	5 (41.7)[b]	0
No	184 (87.6)	35 (70.0)	11 (68.8)	7 (46.7)	12 (57.2)	7 (58.3)	2 (1.1)
Procedures							
Airway	25 (11.9)	10 (20)[a]	3 (18.75)	4 (26.6)	7 (33.3)	4 (33.3)	0
Non-airway	185 (88.1)	40 (80)	13 (81.2)	11 (73.4)	14 (66.7)	8 (66.7)	2 (1.1)
Family history of Asthma							
Yes	4 (1.9)	4 (8.0)	0	0	1 (4.7)	0	2 (50.0)[b]
No	206 (98.1)	46 (92.0)	16 (100)	15 (100)	20 (95.3)	12 (100)	0

[a]*Significant in Pearson Chi-square test.*
[b]*Significant in Fisher-exact test.*

years. Most of the patients 189 (90%) were classified under ASA 1 and 2 while the rest were ASA 3 and above. The 23 (11%) patients had URTIs. Eighty-nine (42.4%) patients had low hemoglobin levels (< 11 g/dl) preoperative. The mean duration of surgery was 82 ± 41.5 min (**Table 2**).

Out of 210 pediatric patients, 55 (26.2%, CI: 20.5–30.9%) had developed PRAEs. We have observed 129 episodes of PRAEs and desaturation was the commonest adverse event which occurred 61 (47.3%) times; followed by partial upper airway obstruction 21 (16.3%), breath holding 17 (13.2%), persistent coughing 15 (11.6%), laryngospasm 11 (8.5%) and bronchospasm 2 (1.6%). Of 129 episodes of PRAEs, 89 (69.0%) occurred in the postoperative period while 23 (17.8) were occurred during induction of anesthesia, and 17 (13.2%) during the maintenance phase (**Figure 1**).

Among four pediatric surgical patients who had family history of asthma, bronchospasm occurred in the two of them. One was during induction of anesthesia and the other was after extubation. Fisher-exact test has showed the significant association between family history of asthma and per ioperative bronchospasm. However, none of the children had self-history of asthma. The relations of independent variables with outcome variables in Pearson's Chi-squared and Fisher-exact tests are presented (**Table 3**). Regarding severity of PRAEs, 10 (4.8%) patients had serious desaturation ($SpO_2 < 80\%$) and 1 (0.5%) patient had continuous coughing, 3 (1.4%) patients had complete airway obstruction which required muscle relaxant, and 9 (4.3%) patients had laryngospasm which was effectively managed by the applications of simple airway maneuvers and positive airway pressure (**Table 4**).

In bivariate binary logistic regression analysis, comorbidity, emergency surgery, multiple attempts of tracheal intubation (≥ 3 attempts), light anesthesia, perioperative opioid use and duration of surgery ≥ 60 min were found associated with PRAEs. The final multivariate binary logistic regression analysis demonstrated that age < 1 year, URTIs (recent or active), secretions in the upper airways, ASA ≥ 3 and airway related surgery were associated with PRAEs.

Among pediatric surgical patients, those who had URTIs were more than seven times likely to develop PRAEs (AOR: 7.6, CI: 1.9–30.2, p: 0.004). The likelihood of PRAEs to occur in infants was 3.6 times than older pediatric surgical patients (AOR: 3.6, CI: 1.3–10.0, p: 0.012). Interestingly, repeated attempts of tracheal intubation were noticed among infants (66.6 vs. 33.3%, p: 0.008). ASA physical status of three and above increases the occurrence of PRAEs by more than 5 folds (AOR: 5.2, CI: 1.9–22.9, *p*: 0.029). Pediatric surgical patients who underwent airway related procedures had developed PRAEs more frequently compared to their counterparts (AOR: 6.0, CI: 1.5–24.1, *p*: 0.012). Having moderate to copious oropharyngeal secretions was found associated with the occurrence of PRAEs (AOR: 4.8, CI: 1.4–15.9, *p*: 0.011). The results of this study claimed that prematurity,

TABLE 4 | Severity of perioperative respiratory adverse events among pediatric surgical patients underwent surgery under general anesthesia at UoGCSH and TGSH, Northwest Ethiopia; March 1–May 30, 2020 ($N = 210$).

Variables	Severity Score *n* (%)			
	1	2	3	4
SpO_2	160 (76.2)	22 (10.5)	18 (8.6)	10 (4.8)
Coughing (*n*)	194 (92.4)	2 (1)	14 (6.7)	0
Breath holding (seconds)	195 (92.9)	9 (4.3)	5 (2.4)	1 (0.5)
Laryngospasm	177 (84.2)	21 (10)	9 (4.3)	3 (1.4)
Bronchospasm	208 (99)	1 (0.5)	1 (0.5)	0
Secretions	184 (87.6)	0	15 (7.1)	11 (5.2)

premedication, induction agents, types of airway devices and experiences of the anesthetists were not associated with PRAEs (**Table 5**).

DISCUSSION

The overall prevalence of PRAEs among pediatric surgical patients who underwent surgery under general anesthesia at UoGCSH and TGCSH was high (26.2%). This result was congruent with a study done by Mamie et al. in which it was 21% (1). A systematic review also has revealed that the prevalence of PRAEs was in the ranges of 8–21% (2). Similarly, Ramgolam et al. concluded that the prevalence of PRAEs was 26–43% (7). The differences can be explained by the inclusion of only patients who had higher risk of developing PRAEs in the former study.

Prevalence of PRAEs was higher in our study compared to previous study in which it was 15% (15). The deviations could be due to inclusion of infants in our study as we noticed an increased occurrence of PRAEs in infants compared to older children. In addition, previous multiple studies verified lower prevalence of PRAEs compared to the current study (2.8, 5.7, and 17.8%) (27–29). Higher prevalence in our study might be due to the inclusion of patients with higher ASA physical status ($\geq$ 3), recovery of pediatrics patients at post-anesthesia care unit that were not staffed with professionals with special pediatric trainings and ill-equipped recovery area. A retrospective multicenter study done among 25,098 patients showed that the prevalence of PRAEs was 4.6%. The discrepancies might be explained by the incorporation of a large numbers of emergency patients in our study (54.3 vs. 27.4%) (12). In-addition, differences in the definitions of PRAEs, study design and sample sizes might explain it.

Oxygen desaturation was occurred in 50 (23.8%) patients which was the commonest PRAE, particularly among patients who had URTIs and airway secretions. This finding was similar with a multicenter study in terms of the overall occurrence. However, it was more frequent intraoperatively compared to emergence (12). In our study, desaturation was common after tracheal extubation. Anesthetic agents are known for diminishing respiratory drive that can results in hypoxemia in the postoperative period (30). Furthermore, almost all types of PRAEs can lead to desaturation.

Persistent coughing and upper airway obstruction were occurred in 15 (7.1%) and 21 (10%) patients respectively. In a previous study, the prevalence of upper airway obstruction was 3.6–9% (2). Budic and Simic have reported that persistent coughing was occurred only in three out of 682 patients (0.004%). The differences in definitions of persistent coughing might cause the inconsistencies. In the current study, persistent coughing was defined as coughing that sustained for 5 s; however, others have defined it as coughing that sustained for 5–10 s (28, 29).

Breathe holding was occurred in 16 (7.6%) patients and it was higher compared to a study done by Tait et al. (23). A large numbers of infant patients [52 (24.8%)] were included in our study. Younger children have a tidal volume that occurs at the same volume as a closing volume; therefore, the terminal bronchioles close easily causing apnea and desaturation (30). Furthermore, neuromuscular blocking agents were used extensively in 120 (57.1%) patients. This might contribute for higher incidence of breath holding among our patients (31). In our study areas, there was no any qualitative monitoring of residual neuromuscular blockade.

The prevalence of laryngospasm was 12 (5.7%) and consistent with a systematic review which claimed 0.1–16%. Particularly, it was 4% in general pediatric population (2). The commonest time of occurrence was extubation. Similarly to previous studies, laryngospasm was associated with presence of airway secretions and URTIs (22, 32). Family history of asthma was associated with perioperative bronchospasm. The phenomenon can be explained by bronchial hyper-responsiveness in children born from parents who have asthma (33).

Children that presented with recent or active sign and symptoms of URTIs were found to have increased risk of developing PRAEs (73.9%). The higher risk of PRAEs during URTIs can be justified by the morphologic damage to the epithelium and mucosa of the respiratory tract after infections and make the airway sensitive to potentially irritant anesthetic gases and secretions that result in activation of irritant receptors and contractions of airway smooth muscles (30). A study has showed that there was increased incidence of PRAEs in patients with an active URTIs than those who had recent URTIs (2–4 weeks before the procedure) (34). The effects of URTIs on the airway could last for several weeks (3). In our study there was no significant difference in the occurrence of PRAEs whether the URTI is recent or active (84.6 vs. 60%, p: 0.34). The occurrence of PRAEs was significantly higher immediately after tracheal extubation than induction and maintenance phases (30).

Infants were more vulnerable to develop PRAEs than older patients (8, 20). Desaturation occurs more frequently in infants (5, 8). Infants have higher oxygen demand and low oxygen reserves which make them risky to PRAEs such as hypoxia. Breath holding was common in this group of patients due to immature respiratory center. Additionally, we have noticed that multiple attempts of tracheal intubation in infants than older patients (66.7 vs. 33.3%, p: 0.008). A previous study concluded that multiple intubation attempts were associated with PRAEs (20).

There was higher occurrence of PRAEs among patients with higher ASA physical status ($\geq$ 3) and this is supported by

TABLE 5 | Bivariate and multivariate binary logistic regression analysis: factors associated with PRAEs in pediatric surgical patients underwent surgery under general anesthesia in UoGCSH and TGSH, Northwest Ethiopia; March 1–May 30, 2020 (*N* = 210).

Variables	PRAEs		Odds ratio (95% CI)		*p*-values
	Yes *n* (%)	No *n* (%)	Crude	Adjusted	
Age					
< 1 year	22 (42.3)	30 (57.7)	2.8 (1.4, 5.4)	3.6 (1.3, 10.0)	0.012
≥ 1 year	33 (20.9)	125 (79.1)	1	1	
ASA class					
≥ 3	15 (71.4)	6 (28.6)	9.31 (3.4, 25.8)	5.2 (1.2, 22.9)	0.029
≤ 2	40 (21.2)	149 (78.8)	1	1	
Urgency of the procedure					
Emergency	39 (34.2)	75 (65.8)	2.6 (1.3, 5.0)	1.41 (0.5, 3.7)	0.48
Elective	16 (16.7)	80 (83.3)	1	1	
URTIs					
Yes	17 (73.9)	6 (26.1)	11.1 (4.1, 30.1)	7.5 (1.9, 30.2)	0.004
No	38 (20.3)	149 (79.7)	1	1	
Surgical procedures					
Airway related	12 (48.0)	13 (52.0)	3.0 (1.3, 7.2)	6.0 (1.5, 24.1)	0.012
Non-airway related	43 (23.2)	142 (76.8)	1	1	
Secretions in the upper airway					
Moderate to copious	18 (69.2)	8 (30.8)	8.9 (3.6, 22.2)	4.78 (1.4, 18.8)	0.011
None to minimal	37 (20.1)	147 (79.9)	1	1	
Light anesthesia					
Yes	10 (41.7)	14 (58.3)	2.2 (0.9, 5.4)	2.6 (0.7, 9.8)	0.14
No	45 (24.2)	141 (75.8)	1	1	
Intubation attempts					
≥ 3	7 (77.8)	2 (22.2)	11 (2.2, 55.0)	3.9 (0.5, 28.0)	0.17
≤ 2	42 (24.1)	132 (75.9)	1	1	
Duration of surgery (hour)					
≥ 1	39 (37.7)	84 (68.3)	2 (1.1, 4.0)	2.0 (0.7, 5.9)	0.19
< 1	16 (18.4)	71 (81.6)	1	1	

NB: p-values are from multivariate binary logistic regression analysis.

previous studies (4, 11). In developing countries, anesthetists frequently encounter patients with poorly treated comorbidities which could lead to the occurrence of PRAEs (4, 5, 35). The majority of the patients were underwent emergency surgery 114 (54%); therefore, poor preoperative optimization might contribute for higher incidence of PRAEs (35).

The risk of developing PRAEs was increased by 6-folds when a surgical procedure involves the airway. Airway related procedures were associated with frequent desaturation and upper airway obstruction. Our finding was supported by previous multicenter prospective studies (3, 5, 36). Children who need airway related surgery commonly have chronic airway inflammation and bronchial hypersensitivity that could result in PRAEs. Surgical instrumentation and manipulation of the airway can lead to laryngeal reflex response (2). Moderate to copious airway secretions was found associated with PRAEs, particularly with desaturation and partial upper airway obstruction. Soiling of the airway which necessitate repeated suctioning can potentiate airway hyper-reactivity (23).

A multicenter study done by Habre et al. including 261 hospitals across Europe has concluded that the experience of the team of anesthesia providers was a very important factor that determines the safety and the rate of adverse events in the pediatric anesthesia practices (37). Our study have not showed this association. The discrepancy might be due to smaller sample size and setup differences as only two hospitals included in the current study done in a developing country.

The study was the first for its type in our country and we believe that it can be a foundation for future studies in the field; especially in resource-limited settings. Hypoventilation and residual neuromuscular blockade were not measured due to the lack of the devices in the post-anesthesia care units of the hospitals. Smaller sample size due to COVID-19 pandemic is another limitation of this study.

CONCLUSIONS

There was high prevalence of perioperative respiratory adverse events among pediatric surgical patients. The postoperative period was the most critical time for the occurrence of PRAEs and desaturation was the commonest adverse event. Age < 1 year, URTIs (recent or active), secretions in the upper airways, ASA $\geq$ 3 and airway surgery were significantly associated with adverse events. Clinicians should perform effective risk assessment, optimization and preparation for the management of perioperative respiratory adverse events.

AUTHOR CONTRIBUTIONS

DW and YWB have conceptualized the study, objectives, and manuscript preparation. DW has developed the proposal. YWB, WC, HA, and MW have criticized the proposal. All authors had participated in the data and statistical analyses and read and approved the final manuscript.

REFERENCES

1. Mamie C, Habre W, Delhumeau C, Barazzone Argiroffo C, Morabia A. Incidence and risk factors of perioperative respiratory adverse events in children undergoing elective surgery. *Pediatric Anesthesia.* (2004) 14:218–24. doi: 10.1111/j.1460-9592.2004.01169.x
2. Regli A, von-Ungern-Sternberg BS. Diagnosis and management of respiratory adverse events in the operating room. *Curr Anesthesiol Rep.* (2015) 5:156–67. doi: 10.1007/s40140-015-0103-z
3. von-Ungern-Sternberg BS, Davies K, Hegarty M, Erb TO, Habre W. The effect of deep vs. awake extubation on respiratory complications in high-risk children undergoing adenotonsillectomy: a randomised controlled trial. *Eur J Anaesthesiol.* (2013) 30:529–36. doi: 10.1097/EJA.0b013e32835df608
4. Lee S, Reddington E, Koutsogiannaki S, Hernandez MR, Odegard KC, DiNardo JA, et al. Incidence and risk factors for perioperative cardiovascular and respiratory adverse events in pediatric patients with congenital heart disease undergoing noncardiac procedures. *Anesth Analg.* (2018) 127:724–9. doi: 10.1213/ANE.0000000000003406
5. Murat I, Constant I, Maud'huy H. Perioperative anaesthetic morbidity in children: a database of 24 165 anaesthetics over a 30-month period. *Paediatr Anaesth.* (2004) 14:158–66. doi: 10.1111/j.1460-9592.2004.01167.x
6. Hackett S, Jones R, Kapila R. Anaesthesia for pneumonectomy. *BJA Education.* (2019) 19:297–304. doi: 10.1016/j.bjae.2019.04.004
7. Ramgolam A, Hall GL, Zhang G, Hegarty M, von-Ungern-Sternberg BS. Inhalational versus intravenous induction of anesthesia in children with a high risk of perioperative respiratory adverse events; a randomized controlled trial. *Anesthesiology.* (2018) 128:1065–74. doi: 10.1097/ALN.0000000000002152
8. Drake-Brockman TF, Ramgolam A, Zhang G, Hall GL, von Ungern-Sternberg BS. The effect of endotracheal tubes versus laryngeal mask airways on perioperative respiratory adverse events in infants: a randomised controlled trial. *Lancet.* (2017) 389:701–8. doi: 10.1016/S0140-6736(16)31719-6
9. Lerman J. Perioperative respiratory complications in children. *Lancet.* (2010) 376:745–6. doi: 10.1016/S0140-6736(10)61199-3
10. Najafi N, Veyckemans F, Vanhonacker D, Legrand C, Van de Velde A, Vandenplas Y, et al. Incidence and risk factors for adverse events during monitored anaesthesia care for gastrointestinal endoscopy in children: a prospective observational study. *Eur J Anaesthesiol.* (2019) 36:390–9. doi: 10.1097/EJA.0000000000000995
11. Charuluxananan S, Suraseranivongse S, Jantorn P, Sriraj W, Chanchayanon T, Tanudsintum S, et al. Multicentered study of model of anesthesia related adverse events in Thailand by incident report (The Thai Anesthesia Incidents Monitoring Study) results. *J Med Assoc Thai.* (2008) 91:1011.
12. Bunchungmongkol N, Somboonviboon W, Suraseranivongse S, Vasinanukorn M, Chau- in W, Hintong T. Pediatric anesthesia adverse events: the Thai Anesthesia Incidents Study (THAI Study) database of 25,098 cases. *J Med Assoc Thai.* (2007) 90:2072.
13. von-Ungern-Sternberg BS, Boda K, Schwab C, Sims C, Johnson C, Habre W. Laryngeal mask airway is associated with an increased incidence of adverse respiratory events in children with recent upper respiratory tract infections. *Anesthesiology.* (2007) 107:714–9. doi: 10.1097/01.anes.0000286925.25272.b5
14. Mir ghassemi A, Neira V, Ufholz LA, Barrowman N, Mulla J, Bradbury CL, et al. A systematic review and meta-analysis of acute severe complications of pediatric anesthesia. *Paediatr Anaesth.* (2015) 25:1093–102. doi: 10.1111/pan.12751
15. von-Ungern-Sternberg BS, Boda K, Chambers NA, Rebmann C, Johnson C, Sly PD, et al. Risk assessment for respiratory complications in paediatric anaesthesia: a prospective cohort study. *Lancet.* (2010) 376:773–83. doi: 10.1016/S0140-6736(10)61193-2
16. Li L, Zhang Z, Yao Z, Wang H, Wang H, An H, et al. The impact of laryngeal mask versus other airways on perioperative respiratory adverse events in children: a systematic review and meta-analysis of randomized controlled trials. *IJS.* (2019) 64:40–8. doi: 10.1016/j.ijsu.2019.02.020
17. Terry KL, Disabato J, Krajicek M. Snoring, trouble breathing, un-refreshed (STBUR) screening questionnaire to reduce perioperative respiratory adverse events in pediatric surgical patients: a quality improvement project. *AANA J.* (2015) 83:256–62.
18. Desalu I, Adeyemo W, Akintimoye M, Adepoju A. Airway and respiratory complications in children undergoing cleft lip and palate repair. *Ghana Med J.* (2010) 44:16–20. doi: 10.4314/gmj.v44i1.68851
19. Mason K, Green S, Piacevoli Q. Adverse event reporting tool to standardize the reporting and tracking of adverse events during procedural sedation: a consensus document from the World SIVA International Sedation Task Force. *BJA.* (2012) 108:13–20. doi: 10.1093/bja/aer407
20. Mandee S, Jitpakdee T, BNS TB, Aroonpruksakul N. The incidence of perioperative adverse events in neonates and infants undergoing non cardiac surgery with general anesthesia. *J Med Assoc Thai.* (2017) 100:44.
21. Group PALICC. Pediatric acute respiratory distress syndrome: consensus recommendations from the pediatric acute lung injury consensus conference. *Pediatr Crit Care Med.* (2015) 16:428. doi: 10.1097/PCC.0000000000000350
22. Birlie Chekol W, Yaregal Melesse D. Incidence and associated factors of laryngospasm among pediatric patients who underwent surgery under general anesthesia, in university of gondar compressive specialized hospital, Northwest Ethiopia, 2019: a cross-sectional study. *Anesthesiol Res Pract.* (2020) 2020:3706106. doi: 10.1155/2020/3706106
23. Tait AR, Malviya S, Voepel-Lewis T, Munro HM, Siewert M, Pandit UA. Risk factors for perioperative adverse respiratory events in children with upper respiratory tract infections. *Anesthesiology.* (2001) 95:299–306. doi: 10.1097/00000542-200108000-00008
24. Katz SL, Monsour A, Barrowman N, Hoey L, Bromwich M, Momoli F, et al. Predictors of postoperative respiratory complications in children undergoing adinotonsilectomy. *J Clin Sleep Med.* (2020) 16:41–8. doi: 10.5664/jcsm.8118
25. Luce V, Harkouk H, Brasher C, Michelet D, Hilly J, Maesani M, et al. Supraglottic airway devices vs tracheal intubation in children: a quantitative meta-analysis of respiratory complications. *Paediatr Anaesth.* (2014) 24:1088–98. doi: 10.1111/pan.12495
26. Kim SY, Kim JM, Lee JH, Kang YR, Jeong SH, Koo B-N. Perioperative respiratory adverse events in children with active upper respiratory tract infection who received general anesthesia through an orotracheal tube and inhalation agents. *KJA.* (2013) 65:136. doi: 10.4097/kjae.2013.65.2.136
27. Subramanyam R, Yeramaneni S, Hossain MM, Anneken AM, Varughese AM. Perioperative respiratory adverse events in pediatric ambulatory anesthesia: development and validation of a risk prediction tool. *Anesth Analg.* (2016) 122:1578–85. doi: 10.1213/ANE.0000000000001216
28. Gharaei B, Aghamohammadi H, Jafari A, Razavi S, Kamranmanesh M, Kermany ASP. Use of laryngeal mask airway in children with upper respiratory tract infection, compared with face mask: randomized

single blind clinical trial. *Acta Anaesthesiol Taiwan.* (2011) 49:136–40. doi: 10.1016/j.aat.2011.11.008

29. de Carvalho ALR, Vital RB, de Lira CCS, Magro IB, Sato PTS, Lima LHN, et al. Laryngeal mask airway versus other airway devices for anesthesia in children with an upper respiratory tract infection: a systematic review and meta-analysis of respiratory complications. *Anesth Analg.* (2018) 127:941–50. doi: 10.1213/ANE.0000000000003674
30. Budić I, Simić D. Risk factors for respiratory adverse events during general anesthesia in children. *Emergency.* (2004) 11:118–22.
31. Murphy GS, Szokol JW, Marymont JH, Greenberg SB, Avram MJ, Vender JS. Residual neuromuscular blockade and critical respiratory events in the post-anesthesia care unit. *Anesth Analg.* (2008) 107:130–7. doi: 10.1213/ane.0b013e31816d1268
32. Haile M, Legesse S, Miressa S, Desalegn N. Magnitude and associated risk factors of perioperative pediatrics laryngospasm under general anesthesia. *InternMed.* (2015) 5:2.
33. Jackson O, Basta M, Sonnad S, Stricker P, LaRossa D, Fiadjoe J. Perioperative risk factors for adverse airway events in patients undergoing cleft palate repair. *Cleft Palate Craniofac J.* (2013) 50:330–6. doi: 10.1597/12-134
34. Li C, Wang D, Cheng T, Zheng X. Effects of recent upper respiratory-tract infections on incidence of the perioperative respiratory adverse events in children: a prospective cohort study. *Journal of Peking University Health sciences.* (2017) 49:814–8.
35. Amucheazi AO, Ajuzieogu OV. Critical incidents during anesthesia in a developing country: A retrospective audit. *Anesth Essays Res.* (2010) 4:64–8. doi: 10.4103/0259-1162.73508
36. Virag K, Sabourdin N, Thomas M, Veyckemans F, Habre W. Epidemiology and incidence of severe respiratory critical events in ear, nose and throat surgery in children in Europe: a prospective multi-center observational study. *Eur J Anaesthesiol.* (2019) 36:185–93. doi: 10.1097/EJA.0000000000000951
37. Hebre W, Disma N, Virag K, Beck K, Hansen TG, Johr M, et al. Incidence of sever critical events in paediatric anaesthesia (APRICOT): a prospective multicentre observational study in 261 hospitals in Europe: Lancet. *Respir Med.* (2017) 5:412–25.

29

Congenital Pulmonary Airway Malformation in Children: Advantages of an Additional Trocar in the Lower Thorax for Pulmonary Lobectomy

Hiroyuki Koga [1], Takanori Ochi [1], Shunki Hirayama [2], Yukio Watanabe [2], Hiroyasu Ueno [2], Kota Imashimizu [2], Kazuhiro Suzuki [3], Ryohei Kuwatsuru [3], Kinya Nishimura [4], Geoffrey J. Lane [1], Kenji Suzuki [2] and Atsuyuki Yamataka [1]*

[1] Department of Pediatric General and Urogenital Surgery, Juntendo University School of Medicine, Tokyo, Japan, [2] Department of General Thoracic Surgery, Juntendo University School of Medicine, Tokyo, Japan, [3] Department of Radiology, Juntendo University School of Medicine, Tokyo, Japan, [4] Department of Anesthesiology and Pain Medicine, Juntendo University School of Medicine, Tokyo, Japan

***Correspondence:**
Hiroyuki Koga
h-koga@juntendo.ac.jp

Aim: To present the use of an additional trocar (AT) in the lower thorax during thoracoscopic pulmonary lobectomy (TPL) in children with congenital pulmonary airway malformation.

Methods: For a lower lobe TPL (LL), an AT is inserted in the 10th intercostal space (IS) in the posterior axillary line after trocars for a 5-mm 30° scope, and the surgeon's left and right hands are inserted conventionally in the 6th, 4th, and 8th IS in the anterior axillary line, respectively. For an upper lobe TPL (UL), the AT is inserted in the 9th IS, and trocars are inserted in the 5th, 3rd, and 7th IS, respectively. By switching between trocars (6th ⟷ 8th for the scope, 4th ⟷ 6th for the left hand, and 8th ⟷ 10th for the right hand during LL and 5th ⟷ 7th, 3rd ⟷ 5th, and 7th ⟷ 9th during UL, respectively), vital anatomic landmarks (pulmonary veins, bronchi, and feeding arteries) can be viewed posteriorly. The value of AT was assessed from blood loss, operative time, duration of chest tube insertion, requirement for post-operative analgesia, and incidence of perioperative complications.

Results: On comparing AT+ ($n = 28$) and AT– ($n = 27$), mean intraoperative blood loss (5.6 vs. 13.0 ml), operative time (3.9 vs. 5.1 h), and duration of chest tube insertion (2.2 vs. 3.4 days) were significantly decreased with AT ($p < 0.05$, respectively). Differences in post-operative analgesia were not significant. There were three complications requiring conversion to open/mini-thoracotomy: AT– ($n = 2$; bleeding), AT+: ($n = 1$; erroneous stapling).

Conclusions: An AT and switching facilitated posterior dissection during TPL in children with congenital pulmonary airway malformation enhancing safety and efficiency.

Keywords: thoracoscopic surgery, pulmonary lobectomy, congenital pulmonary airway malformation, child, anterior approach, posterior approach

INTRODUCTION

Thoracoscopic pulmonary lobectomy (TPL) is now an accepted, well-described procedure for treating congenital cystic lung disease. Reports of TPL being used for congenital pulmonary airway malformation (CPAM) are increasing, because of improvements in prenatal diagnosis and better understanding of its prognosis. In infants and children, TPL has the advantages of better cosmetic outcome, less musculoskeletal chest wall sequelae, better shoulder motility, and unimpaired future breast development compared with conventional open thoracotomy (1–3).

Being minimally invasive, TPL is associated with less post-operative pain, shorter hospitalization, and decreased long-term morbidity (4, 5); the general consensus is that while it is a safe, efficient procedure, it can be technically challenging in children because everything is physically smaller, the anatomy is often anomalous, and the working space is limited. In particular, in neonates, the distance a trocar can be inserted is limited which compromises maneuverability and the visual field. In other words, the ability to correctly identify vital structures (both normal and anomalous), assess what can be preserved or not, then safely secure the large pulmonary vessels can be so daunting, that even well-experienced pediatric surgeons with expertise have opted to wait until patients are larger if possible, rather than operate during the neonatal period.

In order to address these limitations, the concept of adding an additional trocar (AT) in the lower thorax to allow instruments and hands to be switched between trocars as required for comfort and effectiveness during a task was trialed during TPL. Here, a comparison of TPL performed with and without an AT was used to assess the impact of using an AT.

MATERIALS AND METHODS

The medical records of 55 consecutive CPAM cases treated by TPL at a single institution between June 2009 and November 2019 were reviewed retrospectively. All procedures were performed by one of two senior board-certified pediatric surgeons (AY or HK) under the direct supervision of one of five thoracic surgeons with extensive experience of TPL (KeS, YW, KI, HU, and SH).

Conventional TPL performed with an AT (AT+; five trocars) was compared with TPL performed without an AT (AT–; four trocars) for prenatal diagnosis, incidence of pre-operative infections, age and weight at surgery, blood loss, operative time, duration of chest tube insertion, requirement for post-operative analgesia, and incidence of perioperative complications.

Thoracoscopic Pulmonary Lobectomy

Essentially, TPL involves the same principles as open lobectomy, namely, isolation and division of the pulmonary artery, vein, and bronchus to the affected lobe, with separation of lung parenchyma using a combination of sharp and blunt dissection and electrocautery to define and isolate the pathologic lesion. All subjects were treated using the same equipment and devices. Details of the TPL performed in this series are described elsewhere (6–8). Briefly, after induction of general anesthesia and tracheal intubation, the patient is placed in the lateral decubitus position to allow access to the hilum both anteriorly and posteriorly. For thoracoscopy, the surgeon and assistant stand facing the patient while viewing a monitor positioned behind the patient (**Figure 1**). A closed technique is used to place the initial 5 mm optical trocar 1 cm below the inferior angle of the scapula to prevent leakage around the trocar site when an artificial pneumothorax is established to complete collapse of the lung. The initial trocar is used to define the position and status of the fissure and evaluate the general condition of the lung parenchyma and later for lung retraction. Carbon dioxide insufflated at low flow (0.5–1.0 L/min) and under low pressure (4–6 mmHg) is used to collapse the lung. A Fogarty catheter is used for single-lung ventilation. A chest tube is placed under direct vision in all cases.

Lower Lobe TPL

The initial trocar is used to retract the lung. For a left lower lobe TPL (LL), 5-mm trocars for a 5-mm 30° scope, the surgeon's left hand, and the surgeon's right hand are placed in the 6th, 4th, and 8th intercostal spaces (IS) in the anterior axillary line, respectively. The AT is placed in the 10th IS in the posterior axillary line to dissect or view vital structures, such as the pulmonary veins, bronchus, and feeding artery from a posterior perspective as well as observe the entire pulmonary artery, aortic arch, and course of the vagus nerve by switching the scope between the 6th and 8th IS trocars, the left hand between the 4th and 6th IS trocars, and the right hand between the 8th and 10th IS trocars (**Figure 2**). For a right LL, the procedure is the same, but the left and right hand trocars are reversed.

Upper Lobe TPL

For upper lobe TPL (UL), trocar positions on either side are one IS higher than for LL; i.e., 5th IS for the scope, 3rd IS for the left hand, 7th IS for the right hand, and 9th IS for the AT (**Figure 3**). The scope is switched between the 5th and 7th IS, the left hand between the 3rd and 5th IS trocars, and the right hand between the 7th and 9th IS trocars.

Middle Lobe TPL

Trocars for the scope, left hand, and right hand are placed in the 5th, 4th, and 7th IS in the anterior axillary line, respectively. To create more space between the scope trocar and the right-hand trocar, the scope trocar can be placed slightly more anteriorly than the right-hand trocar, which will prevent the scope and right-hand instruments from colliding.

Statistics/Ethics

Data were expressed as mean ± standard deviation. The Student's *t*-test and chi-square test were used for statistical analysis. A p-value <0.05 was considered to be statistically significant. This study was approved by the Juntendo University School of Medicine Institutional Review Board (IRB number: 17-209) and complies with the Helsinki Declaration of 1975 (revised1983).

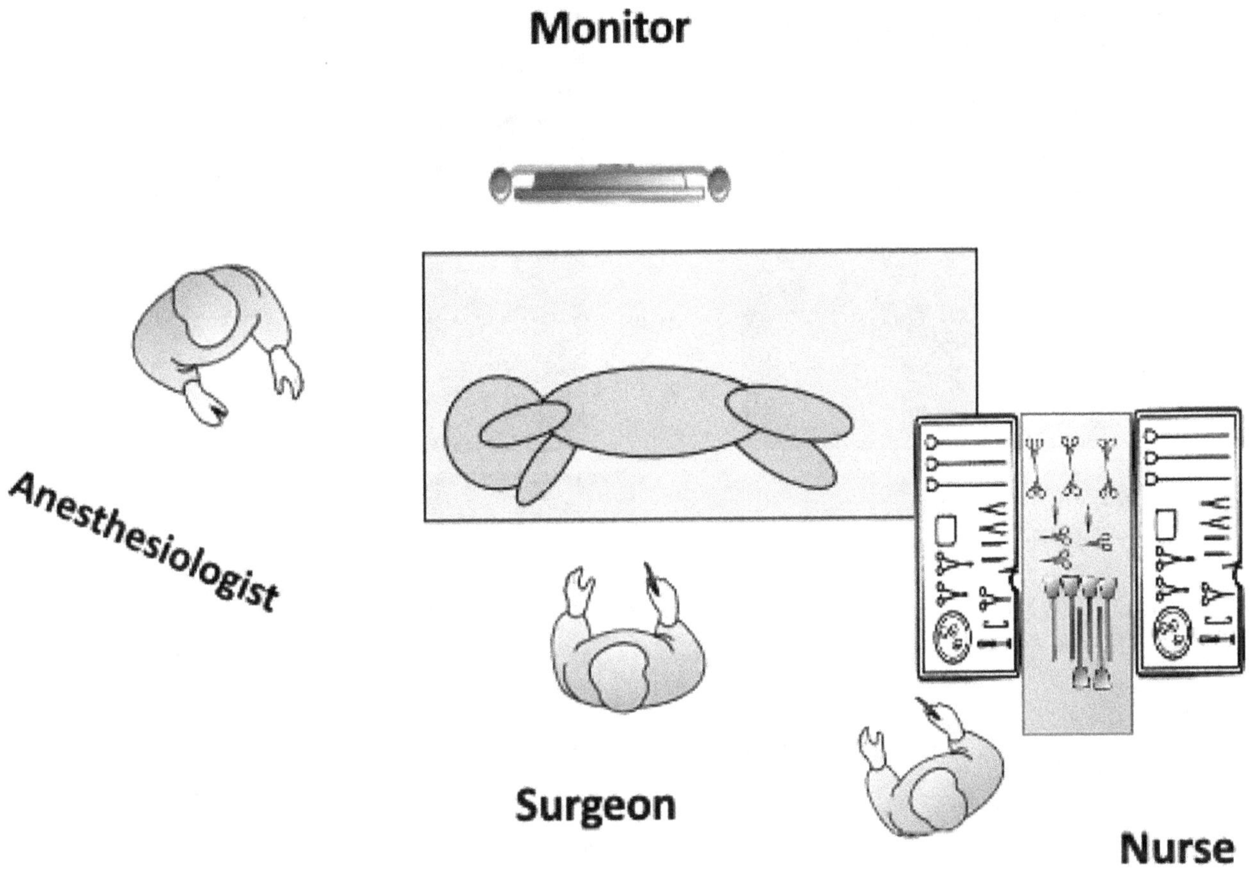

FIGURE 1 | Operating room layout and patient positioning for a left TPL. The patient is placed in the lateral decubitus position and should be placed toward the edge of the operating table in front of the operating surgeon to enhance maneuverability and prevent instruments from hitting the table. The operating surgeon stands facing the patient while viewing a monitor positioned behind the patient.

RESULTS

All 55 CPAM cases were Japanese. Groups were AT+ ($n = 28$) and AT− ($n = 27$). Both AT+ and AT− were similar for patient demographics and location of pathology. Prenatal diagnosis and incidence of pre-operative infections were not significantly different: 20 cases (71%) in AT+ vs. 20 cases (74%) in AT− for prenatal diagnosis ($p = 0.87$) and 7 cases (25%) in AT+ vs. 7 cases (28%) in AT− for pre-operative infections ($p = 0.93$), respectively. Mean ages and mean weights at TPL for AT+ and AT− were not significantly different (2.9 ± 2.3 vs. 2.6 ± 1.6 years old, $p = 0.57$, and 12.8 ± 5.1 vs. 12.0 ± 3.7 kg, $p = 0.80$, respectively). Pulmonary fissures were absent or incomplete in 13/28 (46%) cases in AT+ and 11/27 (41%) cases in AT−; these differences were not statistically significant ($p = 0.67$).

Types of TPL performed were the following: for AT+: left UL ($n = 4$), left LL ($n = 7$), right UL/right middle lobe TPL (ML) ($n = 1$), right ML/right LL ($n = 1$), right ML ($n = 2$), and right LL ($n = 13$); and for AT−: left UL ($n = 5$), left LL ($n = 10$), right UL ($n = 1$), right UL/right ML ($n = 1$), right ML ($n = 3$), and right LL ($n = 7$). There was no significant difference between AT+ and AT− for duration of post-operative analgesia (2.1 ± 1.1 vs. 2.6 ± 1.0 days; $p = 0.08$). However, differences for mean blood loss and mean operative time were significantly different between AT+ and AT− (5.6 ± 3.8 vs. 13.0 ± 5.6 ml, $p < 0.0001$ and 3.9 ± 1.5 vs. 5.1 ± 1.4 h, $p = 0.003$), respectively.

There were three intraoperative complications: bleeding from a bronchial artery during anterior-to-posterior dissection of a bronchus in AT− ($n = 2$) and accidental stapling of the Fogarty catheter used for single-lung ventilation in AT+ ($n = 1$). All three cases required conversion to open/mini-thoracotomy. Chest tubes were removed significantly earlier in AT+ than in AT− (2.2 ± 1.4 vs. 3.4 ± 2.0 days; $p = 0.01$). One case in AT− actually required a chest tube for 14 days post-operatively because of a persistent air leak from a sealed fissure.

DISCUSSION

To the best of our knowledge, this is the first report detailing the benefits of an AT in the lower thorax during TPL in children with CPAM. However, CPAM is rare (9–11), and the learning curve for TPL in children is steep. As with any surgical procedure, confidence comes from experience, and obtaining

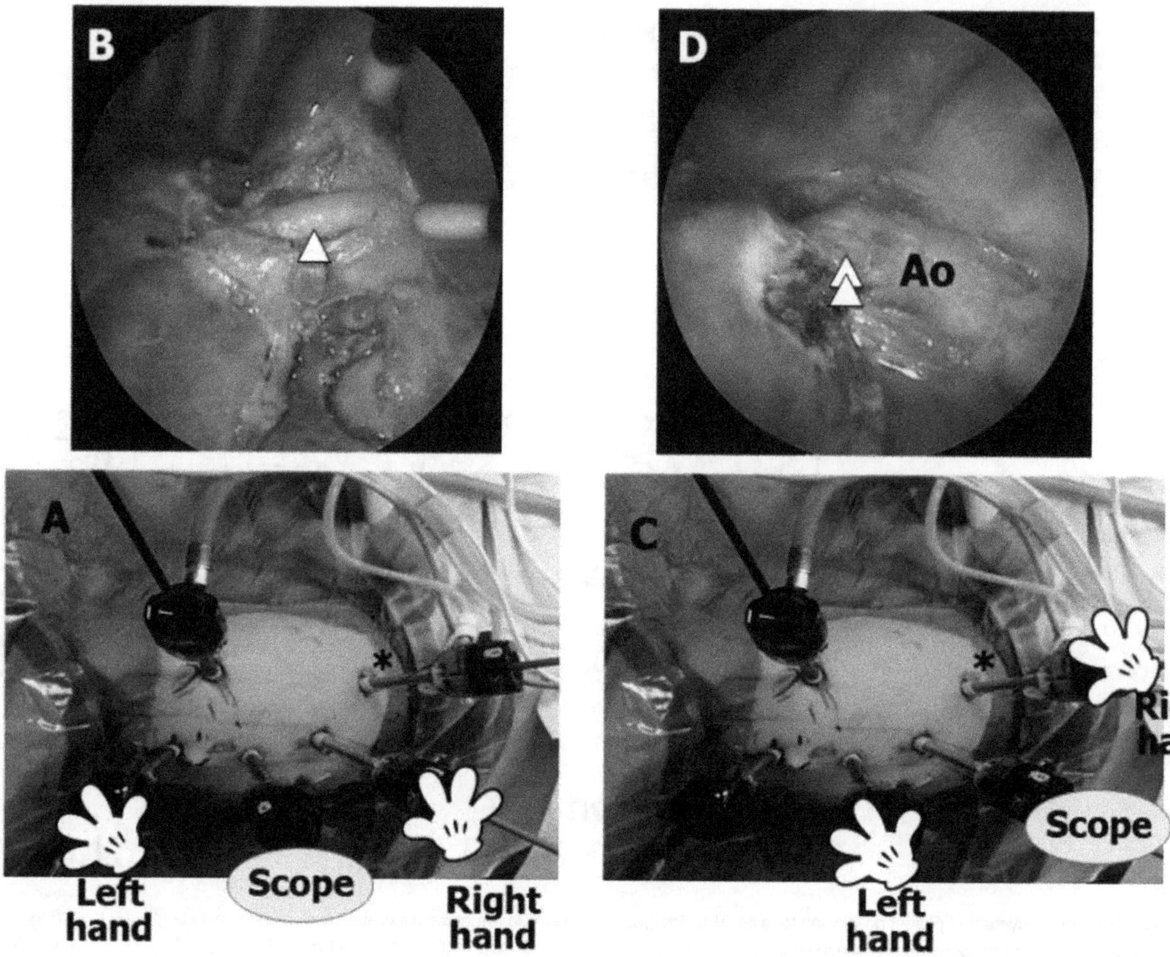

FIGURE 2 | Trocar positions for a left lower lobectomy TPL (left LL). **(A)** Most surgeons perform a LL with the scope in the 6th IS for the entire procedure without using an additional trocar (AT). **(B)** Anterior view using conventional trocar placement is adequate for dissecting the interlobar arteries, such as A8–10 (arrowhead), but dissection can only be viewed progressing in the anterior/posterior plane without viewing the posterior aspects of the bronchus and pulmonary vein and posterior mediastinum. By inserting an AT (asterisk) in the 10th IS, the same dissection can be observed from a different angle. **(C)** Asterisk shows the AT in the 10th IS. **(D)** Posterior view through the AT. The AT facilitates safe dissection of a feeding artery (double arrowhead) originating from the aorta (Ao) and visualization of the posterior aspects of the inferior pulmonary vein and left bronchus as well as the pulmonary artery, aortic arch, and course of the vagus nerve.

enough experience to perform TPL safely and efficiently is difficult. The literature reflects this, with most reports about TPL being from single specialist centers or, if they are from larger referral centers, involving few subjects. Despite improvements in technology and availability, TPL is generally considered too technically demanding for most pediatric surgeons to offer as a routine procedure. With this in mind, an AT in the lower thorax with switching between trocars as required was trialed during TPL in this series.

Conventional wisdom would dictate an anterior approach for TPL, particularly in children and especially in neonates because there is more space from the chest wall to the mediastinum where the pulmonary vessels arise. An anterior approach would also seem more logical because the visual field is easier to secure and allows hilar vascular structures to be viewed safely for orientation; dissection of bronchi and branches of pulmonary arteries could also be facilitated. However, an anterior approach is inadequate for viewing and understanding anatomic relationships in the mediastinum completely because the posterior aspects of bronchi and pulmonary veins, as well as the posterior mediastinum, cannot be viewed readily. AT trialed in this series expanded the visual field posteriorly to enable vital structures, such as the pulmonary veins, bronchi, and feeding vessels, to be inspected from a posterior perspective as well as allow the entire pulmonary artery, the aortic arch, and the vagus nerve to be viewed. Thus, by switching trocars using AT, the surgeon has access to the surgical field from all sides and can inspect and check progress from various angles, enhancing safety and reliability, especially during dissection of a feeding artery originating from the aorta and dissection of the posterior wall of the inferior pulmonary vein and bronchus during LL. During UL, A1+2, A3, and A6 branches located postero-lateral to the interlobar pulmonary artery can be

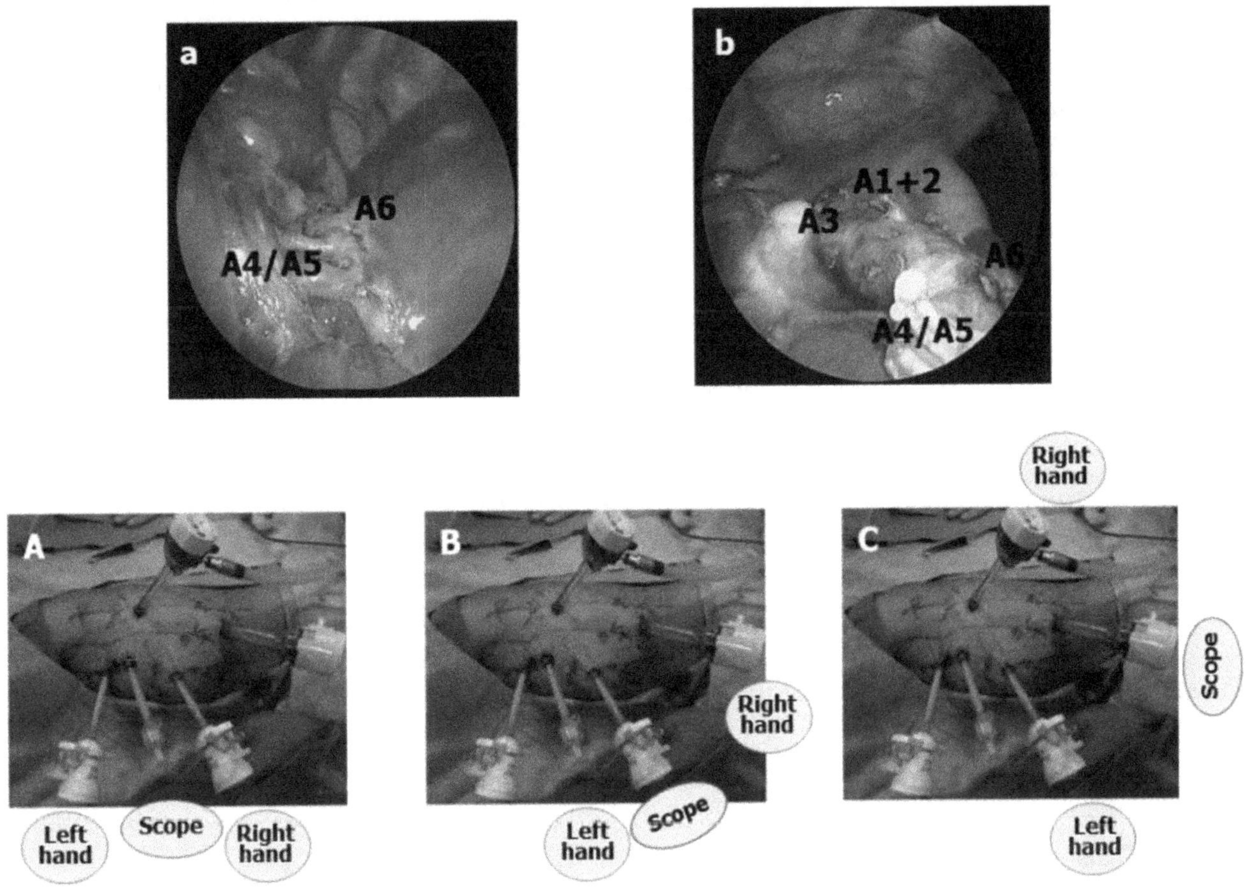

FIGURE 3 | Trocar positions for a left upper lobectomy TPL (left UL). **(A)** All trocar positions are one IS higher than for LL. By switching the scope from the 5th IS trocar to a trocar in the 7th or 9th IS, the entire course of the interlobar pulmonary artery can be visualized as well as the pulmonary hilum from the posterior mediastinum. **(B,C)** When the scope is switched from the trocar in the 5th IS to either one of the trocars in the 7th or 9th IS, interlobar pulmonary artery branches A1+2 and A3 can be observed more easily, enhancing the safety of TPL.

seen readily, ensuring added safety during TPL. In other words, without AT, the pulmonary hilum cannot be viewed from the posterior aspect throughout an entire TPL, with the result that a TPL can only be performed in the anterior–posterior plane which is stressful even for an experienced surgeon, because of the blind aspects, and further complicated if fissures are anomalous.

From experience, fissure cases can be handled with confidence by using an AT to switch instruments to view the same structures from a slightly different angle. In general, during TPL in infants and children, the view through the scope is from front to back and limited by the small size of the thorax, so treating an incomplete fissure located anteriorly, such as an incomplete fissure between S4+5 and S8 in the left lung, between the right UL and ML, or between the right ML and LL, is more difficult than treating an incomplete fissure located posteriorly, such as an incomplete fissure between S1+2 and S6 in the left lung or between the right UL and LL. Thus, by switching between trocars, there is less risk for injury because both anterior and posterior views are possible. As shown in this series, blood loss and operative time for AT+ were lower, although there were no significant differences in location or incidence of incomplete fissures between the two groups (AT+ and AT−). An AT with switching was crucial for preventing accidental injury to the pulmonary arterial wall during TPL with normal fissures but even more so when fissures were incomplete or absent.

Operator disorientation may also arise because of patient positioning during TPL. In conventional open thoracotomy, the surgeon and assistant usually stand behind the patient (5), but in TPL, they stand in front of the patient because the patient is in the lateral decubitus position. A thorough grasp of the anatomic relationships of each lobe cannot be overemphasized because intraoperatively, the three-dimensional relationships of vessels and bronchi to each lobe must be readily imaginable because the field of view through a scope is two-dimensional and everything may not be visible, so an operating surgeons must be completely comfortable with the anatomy of the lungs. In other words, anatomic relationships both normal and anomalous must be second nature, so the operating surgeon is always prepared and aware of the potential for the unexpected, especially important when no landmarks are present, for example, in cases of absent or incomplete fissure. In such patients, incising lung parenchyma that otherwise lacks superficial landmarks can cause air leakage which is one of the commonest complications of lung surgery and can require chest tube insertion if prolonged. Chest tube insertion extends hospitalization resulting in higher costs and greater risks for pleural infections. While an AT alone will not prevent air leakage absolutely, having a better grasp of the operative field from additional perspectives will provide more information about anatomic relationships (or lack thereof) and allow operating surgeons to make decisions with greater confidence.

In this series, there were three intraoperative complications. Of these, two were bleeding from bronchial arteries that occurred in AT– cases and have not occurred again since AT use became routine. The third, accidental stapling of the Fogarty catheter used for single-lung ventilation, was due to operator carelessness. Although subject numbers are limited, AT should be considered as improving safety of TPL in children.

Although there are limitations to this study because of its retrospective nature and the small number of cases, the results obtained attest to the value of using an AT, and as a result, TPL in children should really be considered a five-trocar procedure henceforth. While the concept of an AT may seem somewhat unconventional because skilled experienced surgeons can perform TPL with just three trocars, an AT with switching is a simple technique that effectively enhances safety by facilitating visualization and as shown in this series improves TPL in children with CPAM.

In conclusion, AT could be applied to any minimally invasive procedure that is challenging technically, anatomically, or logistically.

AUTHOR CONTRIBUTIONS

HK and AY designed the study. HK, TO, SH, YW, HU, KI, KaS, RK, KN, KeS, and AY were involved in clinical treatment. HK and TO collected and analyzed the data. HK and GL prepared and revised the manuscript. All authors contributed to the article and approved the submitted version.

ACKNOWLEDGMENTS

The authors would like to thank the nurses and surgeons from the Department of Pediatric General and Urogenital Surgery and Department of General Thoracic Surgery, anesthesiologists from the Department of Anesthesiology and Pain Medicine, radiologists from the Department of Radiology, operating room nursing staff, and Juntendo University Hospital administrative staff for their support and encouragement.

REFERENCES

1. Diamond IR, Herrera P, Langer JC, Kim PC. Thoracoscopic versus open resection of congenital lung lesions: a case-matched study. *J Pediatr Surg.* (2007) 42:1057–61. doi: 10.1016/j.jpedsurg.2007.01.043
2. Rothenberg SS. First decade's experience with thoracoscopic lobectomy in infants and children. *J Pediatr Surg.* (2008) 43:40–4. doi: 10.1016/j.jpedsurg.2007.09.015
3. Vu LT, Farmer DL, Nobuhara KK, Miniati D, Lee H. Thoracoscopic versus open resection for congenital cystic adenomatoid malformations of the lung. *J Pediatr Surg.* (2008) 43:35–9. doi: 10.1016/j.jpedsurg.2007.09.012
4. Lawal TA, Gosemann JH, Kuebler JF, Gluer S, Ure BM. Thoracoscopy versus thoracotomy improves midterm musculoskeletal status and cosmesis in infants and children. *Ann Thorac Surg.* (2009) 87:224–28. doi: 10.1016/j.athoracsur.2008.08.069
5. Rothenberg SS, Middlesworth W, Kadennhe-Chiweshe A, Aspelund G, Kuenzler K, Cowles R, et al. Two decades of experience with thoracoscopic lobectomy in infants and children: standardizing techniques for advanced thoracoscopic surgery. *J Laparoendosc Adv Surg Tech A.* (2015) 25:423–28. doi: 10.1089/lap.2014.0350
6. Koga H, Suzuki K, Nishimura K, Okazaki T, Lane GJ, Inada E, et al. Traction sutures allow endoscopic staples to be used safely during thoracoscopic pulmonary lobectomy in children weighing less than 15 kg. *J Laparoendosc Adv Surg Tech A.* (2013) 23:81–3. doi: 10.1089/lap.2012.0063
7. Sueyoshi R, Koga H, Suzuki K, Miyano G, Okawada M, Doi T, et al. Surgical intervention for congenital pulmonary airway malformation (CPAM) patients with preoperative pneumonia and abscess formation: "open versus thoracoscopic lobectomy". *Pediatr Surg Int.* (2016) 32:347–51. doi: 10.1007/s00383-015-3848-z
8. Yamataka A, Koga H, Ochi T, Imashimizu K, Suzuki K, Kuwatsuru R, et al. Pulmonary lobectomy techniques in infants and children. *Pediatr Surg Int.* (2017) 33:483–95. doi: 10.1007/s00383-016-4052-5
9. Duncombe GJ, Dickinson JE, Kikiros CS. Prenatal diagnosis and management of congenital cystic adenomatoid malformation of the lung. *Am J Obstet Gynecol.* (2002) 187:950–54. doi: 10.1067/mob.2002.127460
10. Laberge JM, Flageole H, Pugash D, Khalife S, Blair G, Filiatrault D, et al. Outcome of the prenatally diagnosed congenital cystic adenomatoid lung malformation: a Canadian experience. *Fetal Diagn Ther.* (2001) 16:178–86. doi: 10.1159/000053905
11. Park S, Kim ER, Hwang Y, Lee HJ, Park IK, Kim YT, et al. Serial improvement of quality metrics in pediatric thoracoscopic lobectomy for congenital lung malformation: an analysis of learning curve. *Surg Endosc.* (2017) 31:3932–38. doi: 10.1007/s00464-017-5425-0

30

The Role of Video-Assisted Thoracoscopic Surgery in Pediatric Oncology

Giovanna Riccipetitoni, Mirko Bertozzi, Marta Gazzaneo, Alessandro Raffaele and Fabrizio Vatta*

Department of Pediatric Surgery, Fondazione Istituti di Ricovero e Cura a Carattere Scientifico (IRCCS) Policlinico San Matteo, University of Pavia, Pavia, Italy

Correspondence:
Giovanna Riccipetitoni
g.riccipetitoni@gmail.com;
giovanna.riccipetitoni@unipv.it

Aim: Video-assisted thoracoscopic surgery (VATS) has been widely used in the last decades. Nevertheless, the pros and cons of thoracoscopy vs. open surgery in pediatric oncology are still under debate. In literature, VATS has been applied for both diagnostic and ablative surgery to treat neurogenic tumors, thymic neoplasms, lung tumors and metastases, germ cell tumors, lymphoproliferative diseases, and other rare tumors. Recent reviews described excellent outcomes in pediatric oncology as well as in the treatment of adult lung cancer, with a significantly higher rate of mortality and complication in thoracotomy compared to VATS. We reviewed our experience on thoracoscopy in pediatric malignancy and compared it to the literature.

Materials and Methods: This was a retrospective cohort-study of pediatric oncological patients who underwent VATS at our institution from 2007 to 2020, and a review of the recent literature on the topic.

Results: A total of 43 procedures were performed on 38 oncological patients (18 males, 20 females). Median age was years 7.72 (0.35–18.6). Diagnosis: 10 neurogenic tumors, nine hematological diseases, five metastases, four lypoblastomas, three thymic pathologies, three germ cell tumors, two pleuropneumoblastomas, two myofibroblastic tumors, one myoepithelial carcinoma, one liposarcoma, and three suspected oncological mass. In three cases, a 3D model was elaborated to better plan the surgical approach. Diagnostic biopsies were 22 (51.1%), and ablative surgeries, 21 (48.9%). One neurogenic tumor was resected with the Da Vinci Robot. Median operative time was 120 min (30–420). A drain was left in place in 20 (46.5%) for a median of 4 days. Median length of hospitalization was 5 days (1–18). One case (2.3%) was converted (intraoperative bleeding). There were three post-operative complications (7.0%): one pneumonia, one pleural effusion, and one diaphragmatic paralysis (need for plication). Results were compared to recent literature, and morbidity and conversion rate were comparable to reviewed publications.

Conclusion: VATS represents a valuable tool for diagnostic and therapeutic procedures in pediatric oncology. Nonetheless, it is a challenging technique that should be performed by expert surgeons on oncological and mini-invasive surgery. Three-dimensional reconstruction can optimize the pre-operative planning and guarantee a safer and more targeted treatment. Finally, the advent of robotics-assisted surgery represents a new challenge that may further implement the advantages of VATS.

Keywords: thoracoscopy, pediatrics, oncology, mini-invasive surgery, robotic-assisted thoracoscopic surgery

INTRODUCTION

Minimally invasive surgery (MIS), including thoracoscopy, has been widely applied in the last few decades and has now become the gold standard approach for a variety of procedures for both adults and children (1–3).

The advantages of MIS compared to the open approach are well-known, as it reduces tissue trauma, decreases post-operative pain, shortens hospital stay, and guarantees better cosmetic and long-term functional results (4, 5). Moreover, among of the most important benefits of thoracoscopy are the virtually non-existing musculoskeletal complications such as chest wall deformities, rib fusion, shoulder girdle weakness, and scoliosis, which can occur in up of 30% of pediatric patients undergoing thoracotomy (6, 7).

Nevertheless, video-assisted thoracoscopic surgery (VATS) still represents a challenge due to the limitation of working space, the smaller body size of children, reduced tactile feedback, and the lack of three-dimensional vision.

As far as it concerns pediatric oncology, in the last decades, many reports and experiences have been published on the use of thoracoscopy to diagnose and resect intrathoracic neoplasms. Nonetheless, the role of VATS is still considered a developing field and no consensus exists regarding the details of its application. Specific limitations are an even lower exposure in pediatric oncological cases compared to general thoracoscopic pathologies and the inability to perform digital palpation.

In the last years, robotics has been applied to perform a wide variety of procedures, including thoracic surgery (8). Nonetheless, very few reports describe the use of robotics in pediatric oncological thoracic surgery and its use is not yet validated.

The aim of this study is to review our experience in VATS and robotics-assisted thoracoscopy in pediatric malignancy and to compare it to the most recent literature.

MATERIALS AND METHODS

We performed a retrospective review of all pediatric oncological patients who underwent video-assisted thoracoscopic surgery (VATS) and robotics-assisted thoracoscopic surgery (RATS) at our Institution from 2007 to 2020.

Patients over 20 years old and/or with thoracic pathologies treated with thoracotomy or endoscopic procedures were excluded.

We analyzed demographic data, including age at surgery, sex, pathology, and possible comorbidities; operation time (OT); length of hospital stays (LHS); perioperative complications; and post-operative outcomes. All complications were classified according to the Clavien–Dindo classification and graded from I to V. If present, length of chest drain aspiration was evaluated.

A specific search was performed in scientific database (PUBMED, MEDLINE, and EMBASE) to compare our experience with the most recent literature on the field. We selected articles reporting thoracoscopy in oncological pediatric patients between 2014 and March 2021 using the following key-words: (pediatric) or (children) and (thoracoscopy) or (VATS) and (oncology) or (tumor).

Inclusion criteria were:

- Articles published between January 2014 and March 2021
- Articles written in English
- Articles focusing on VATS in pediatric oncology
- Median/mean age <18 years old
- Case series with more than 10 patients
- Articles where data concerning demographics, surgical indications, complication rate, and conversion rate were clearly deductible

All data were elaborated using the statistical software "R", version 3.4.1.

Descriptive statistics was used to present findings, and quantitative variables were expressed as median (range) to express our data. Data elaborated from the literature review were expressed as median (range) or mean ± standard deviations depending on the reference found in the original articles.

Surgical Methods

Under general anesthesia, lung collapse has been achieved by single-lung ventilation. We routinely used a double lumen endotracheal tube in adolescent patients, mainly for ablative procedures. In small children (more than 6 months of age), we adopted a standard endotracheal intubation associated to the use of an endobronchial blocker. Low-pressure CO_2 insufflation (4–5 mmHg; flow 0.5 L/min) was employed in infants <6 months or when a quick biopsy of anterior mediastinal tumors was required. NIRS and BIS brain-monitoring were applied according to the age of the patients.

Patients were placed in lateral decubitus, with an angle ranging from 60 and 90° to 120°, depending on the mass localization.

A 10-mm one-trocar operative optic was employed for biopsy in three cases (one germ cell tumor, one pleuropneumoblastoma, and one myofibroblastic inflammatory tumor).

A three-trocar technique was adopted in most of the remaining cases, positioned according to the characteristics of the lesion. The optic (5 or 10 mm) was placed in the typical mid-axillary position under the shoulder angle, whereas the operative trocars were placed in a triangulation fashion anteriorly or posteriorly depending on the site of the mass.

In small children, a 3-mm operative trocar technique with 5-mm optic was carried out to perform biopsies, whereas in ablative surgery, one 5-mm operative trocar was reserved for Ligasure® or other vessel sealers. In recent cases, a 3-mm vessel sealer has been used, allowing a 3-mm operative VATS also for ablative procedures.

Pulmonary resection was safely performed with staplers (5 or 12 mm), which required an additional trocar. Specimens were retrieved using a 5 mm Endobag.

Regarding the use of chest drain, we tried to avoid drainage placement in diagnostic biopsies, except in case of complications such as intraoperative bleeding. A drain was normally applied at the end of any ablative surgery.

When possible, an early extubation of the patients was made a few hours after the VATS procedure.

About RATS, we performed one procedure using the Da-Vinci SI® Robot for a mass located on the supero-posterior mediastinum. Optic trocar was positioned in the sixth intercostal space on the midaxillary line. Operative trocars were positioned 8 cm away from the optic, in the fifth intercostal space on the anterior axillary line, and in the seventh intercostal space on the paravertebral line, respectively. Finally, a 5-mm auxiliary trocar was placed in the fourth intercostal space on the anterior axillary line.

RESULTS

A total of 43 procedures were performed on 38 oncological patients (18 males, 20 females). Median age was 7.72 (0.35–18.6). Patients were grouped according to diagnosis, and we observed high prevalence of neurogenic tumors and hematologic diseases, as shown in **Table 1**.

We performed diagnostic biopsies in 22 cases (51.1%), compared to 21 cases of ablative surgeries (48.9%); 42 out of 43 procedures were completed by VATS technique (97.7%); only one patient required an open conversion (2.3%).

The procedures were carried out by single-lung ventilation using a double-lumen endotracheal tube in 14 adolescent patients, and standard endotracheal intubation associated to the use of an endobronchial blocker was adopted in 16 cases. In the remaining 13 cases, lung collapse was obtained with low-pressure CO_2 insufflation.

One patient with growing ganglioneuroblastoma intermixed of the supero-posterior mediastinum in a 7-years-old girl with Horner's syndrome and positive image-defined risk factor (IDRF) (symptomatic encased subclavian vessels) was operated with the Da-Vinci SI® Robot-assisted thoracoscopic surgery. The robotic approach was chosen to achieve a safer and more precise dissection.

In the whole series, median OT was 120 min (30–420): 90 for diagnostic biopsies, 190 for ablative surgery.

Overall, a thoracic drain was left in place in 20 cases, for a median length of 4 days.

Only three diagnostic procedures required chest drainage due to intraoperative bleeding (one germ cell tumor), pneumothorax (one pleuropneumoblastoma), and pleural effusion (one myofibroblastic inflammatory tumor). As for ablative surgeries, a chest tube was positioned in 17 out of 21 procedures.

Median LHS was 5 days (1–18).

In two cases, we observed intraoperative bleeding (4.7%): one biopsy of a germ cell tumor managed thoracoscopically and one lung resection for nephroblastoma metastasis which required conversion to open surgery. The conversion rate to open surgery was 2.3% in the whole series.

In our series, we observed three post-operative complications (7.0%): one pneumonia (Clavien Dindo: grade II) 2 weeks after biopsy for a germ cell tumor; one pleural effusion a week after resection of a posterior mediastinal ganglioneuroma, which required a re-insertion of a thoracic drain for a further 7 days (IIIb); and one persistent right diaphragmatic paralysis after the excision of a giant cystic lymphangioma, treated with a laparoscopic diaphragmatic plication (IVa) 1 year later, which required intensive care assistance.

No tumor upstaging or trocar site recurrences occurred.

An advanced 3D virtual reconstruction and printing technology was recently applied in three complex cases (multiple immature teratoma metastases, multiple cystic lesions after pleuro-pneumoblastoma excision, vessel encasement in IDRF-positive ganglioneuroblastoma intermixed).

A review of the most recent literature on the topic was performed. From a total of 229 articles, seven were included in the review according to the inclusion criteria (**Table 2**) (9–15).

All papers were retrospective reviews and analyzed VATS to perform either tumor biopsy, ablative surgery, or both. A total of 423 children were included in the review, with a median age of 8.8 years. Among pulmonary lesions, metastases resulted as the most common indication for surgery. On the other hand, in case of a mediastinal lesion, neurogenic tumor was the most represented group. Conversion rate ranged from 0 to 15.1%, most commonly due to intraoperative bleeding or difficult dissection of the mass due to strong adhesions. Complications occurred in 2.1–20% of cases, pneumothorax being the most common post-operative one. No articles reported port-site recurrences, intraoperative tumor rupture, or tumor upstaging. Average LHS ranged from 2 to 10 days.

DISCUSSION

VATS in pediatric oncological surgery represents a great surgical achievement but still faces many challenges. Alongside the limitations of the technique, there are no guidelines on the details of the use of VATS or its contraindications. However, its application is expanding, and the experience reported in literature is growing.

Our study presents a large cohort of oncological patients undergoing VATS and proves the feasibility and effectiveness of the use of MIS in pediatric oncology; 97.7% of cases in our series were successfully treated by thoracoscopy.

As far as it concerns the use of VATS for diagnostic procedures, MIS has been effectively used to perform mediastinal mass biopsies as well as pulmonary masses (10, 13, 16–18). Reported advantages of thoracoscopy are the possibility

TABLE 1 | Summarized data of all oncological patients undergoing VATS (in chronological order).

ID*	Sex	Year	Age (y)	Pre-op Imaging	Diagnosis	Localization	Side	Intervention	Operative Time (min)	Peri-op compli-cations	Conversion	Drain (days)	LHS (days)	Post-op complications	Type of complication (Clavien Dindo Classification)
JM	M	2007	14.00	TC	Germ cell tumor	Complete invasion of all hemithorax	R	Biopsy (1 trocar)	30	No	No	No	2	No	
VG	M	2007	14.00	TC	T-cell lymphoma	Anterior mediastinum	L	Biopsy	60	No	No	No	3	No	
BL	F	2008	3.00	TC	Germ cell tumor	Complete invasion of all hemithorax	L	Biopsy	90	Yes (bleeding)	No	Yes (4)	7	No	
GD	M	2009	1.00	TC	Pleuropulmonary blastoma	Superior and medium lobe	R	Biopsy (1 trocar)	60	No	No	Yes (3)	4	No	
AL	F	2010	8.07	TC	Suspicion of renal carcinoma metastasis (not confirmed at histology)	Inferior lobe	L	Biopsy	105	No	No	No	14	No	
BA	M	2010	3.94	TC	Nephroblastoma metastasis	Inferior lobe	L	Mass excision (atypical pulmonary excision)	155	No	No	No	2	No	
ML (1)	M	2010	18.16	TC	Casteman's disease	Anterior mediastinum	R	Biopsy	75	No	No	No	1	No	
PC	F	2010	4.79	TC	Ganglioneuroma metastasis	Costophrenic recess	L	Mass excision	180	No	No	No	3	No	
ML (2)	M	2011	18,65	TC	Casteman's disease	Anterior mediastinum	R	Mass excision	330	No	No	No	2	No	
CA	F	2012	0.50	TC MRI	Neuroblastoma	Superior mediastinum	L	Biopsy	90	No	No	No	3	No	
CS	F	2010	14.11	TC	Diffuse large B-cell lymphoma	Antero-Superior mediastinum	R	Biopsy	80	No	No	No	–**	No	
HL	M	2012	16.53	TC	Neuroblastoma	Posterior mediastinum	R	Biopsy	60	No	No	No	3	No	
DM	M	2012	11.04	TC	Precursor T-cell lymphoblastic lymphoma	Retrosternal region	R	Biopsy	150	No	No	No	–**	No	
PG	M	2012	0.35	TC	Cystic lymphangioma	Superior mediastinum	R	Mass excision	165	No	No	Yes (4)	2	Yes	Diaphragmatic paralysis, need for laparoscopic diaphragmatic plication (IVa) 1 year later
BL	M	2014	6.00	TC	Classical Hodgkin's lymphoma	Anterior mediastinum	R	Biopsy	70	No	No	No	3	No	

(Continued)

TABLE 1 | Continued

ID*	Sex	Year	Age (y)	Pre-op Imaging	Diagnosis	Localization	Side	Intervention	Operative Time (min)	Peri-op compli-cations	Conversion	Drain (days)	LHS (days)	Post-op complications	Type of complication (Clavien Dindo Classification)
BR	F	2014	10.00	MRI	Ganglioneuroblastoma	Posterior mediastinum	L	Mass excision	120	No	No	Yes (3)	5	No	
SR	F	2019	1.25	MRI	Lipoblastoma (recidive)	Lateral chest wall, medullar invasion	R	Mass excision	240	No	No	Yes (7)	–**	No	
FE (1)	F	2014	1.19	TC	Neuroblastoma	Antero-Superior mediastinum	R	Biopsy	180	No	No	No	5	No	
FE (2)	F	2014	1.84	TC MRI	Neuroblastoma	Antero-superior mediastinum	R	Biopsy	90	No	No	No	2	No	
GD	M	2014	13.61	TC	Osteosarcoma metastasis	Inferior lobe	L	Mass excision	90	No	No	No	2	No	
PI	F	2014	10.00	TC MRI	Ganglioneuroblastoma	Posterior mediastinum	L	Mass excision	120	No	No	Yes (3)	18	Yes	Pleural effusion after drain removal, need for thoracic drain re-insertion for 7 days (IIIb)
RG	F	2014	11.96	TC MRI	Myofibroblastic inflammatory tumor	Pulmonary hilum	R	Biopsy	250	No	No	Yes (4)	7	No	
VA	M	2014	16.13	TC	Germ cell tumor	Costophrenic recess	R	Biopsy	115	No	No	No	11	Yes	Post-op pneumonia (II)
AA (1)	F	2015	7.67	TC	Suspicion of neoplastic mass (not confirmed at histology)	Middle mediastinum	R	Biopsy	95	No	No	No	5	No	
AA (2)	F	2015	7.72	TC	Suspicion of neoplastic mass (not confirmed at histology)	Middle mediastinum	R	Biopsy	105	No	No	No	2	No	
AA (3)	F	2015	8.18	TC	Suspicion of neoplastic mass (not confirmed at histology)	Middle mediastinum	R	Biopsy + Culture test	110	No	No	No	3	No	
LAn	M	2015	15.77	TC	Classical Hodgkin's lymphoma	Costophrenic recess	L	Biopsy	160	No	No	No	2	No	
PB	M	2015	5.44	TC	Nephroblastoma metastasis	Superior lobe	R	Mass excision (atypical pulmonary excision)	350	Yes (bleeding)	Yes	Yes (4)	7	No	
RA	F	2015	10.00	MRI	Thymic teratoma	Anterior mediastinum	L	Mass excision (thymectomy)	200	No	No	Yes (5)	7	No	
ZS	M	2015	7.00	MRI	Thymic teratoma	Anterior mediastinum	R	Mass excision (thymectomy)	195	No	No	Yes (4)	6	No	
TM	F	2016	11.00	MRI	Thymoma	Anterior mediastinum	R	Mass excision (thymectomy)	220	No	No	Yes (5)	7	No	

(Continued)

TABLE 1 | Continued

ID*	Sex	Year	Age (y)	Pre-op Imaging	Diagnosis	Localization	Side	Intervention	Operative Time (min)	Peri-op compli-cations	Conversion	Drain (days)	LHS (days)	Post-op complications	Type of complication (Clavien Dindo Classification)
TL	F	2017	16.47	TC MRI	Pleomorphic liposarcoma	Costophrenic recess	R	Biopsy	110	No	No	No	3	No	
BB	F	2018	7.00	TC MRI	Neuroblastoma	Posterior mediastinum	L	Mass excision	190	No	No	Yes (3)	5	No	
BF	M	2018	12.00	MRI	Lipoblastoma	Lateral chest wall	R	Mass excision	180	No	No	Yes (5)	7	No	
EZ	F	2018	6.00	TC MRI	Myofibroblastic inflammatory tumor	Superior and medium lobe, trachea and heart invasion	R	Biopsy (1 trocar)	60	No	No	No	3	No	
LAr	M	2018	2.00	TC MRI	Neuroblastoma	Posterior mediastinum	L	Mass excision	119	No	No	Yes (4)	6	No	
LM	M	2018	7.00	TC MRI	Cystic lesions after pleuropulmonary blastoma excision	Superior, medium, and inferior lobe (3 different lesions)	R	Masses excision (atypical pulmonary excision)	190	No	No	Yes (2)	7	No	
LN	F	2018	7.00	TC MRI	Myoepithelial carcinoma	Superior and inferior lobe, heart invasion	L	Biopsy (with associated bronchoscopic biopsy)	80	No	No	No	7	No	
BG	F	2019	5.00	MRI	Lipoblastoma	Posterior mediastinum	L	Mass excision	150	No	No	Yes (4)	6	No	
BM	F	2020	13.28	TC MRI	Lipoblastoma	Superior mediastinum	R	Mass excision	305	No	No	Yes (7)	6	No	
FE (3)	F	2020	7.59	MRI	Ganglioneuroblastoma intermixed	Anterior mediastinum	R	Robot-Assisted mass excision	290	No	No	Yes (6)	7	No	
PD	M	2020	14.80	TC	Classical Hodgkin's lymphoma	Anterior mediastinum	R	Mass excision (thymectomy)	285	No	No	Yes (3)	5	No	
SL	F	2020	7.00	TC MRI	Immature teratoma metastases	Superior, medium and inferior lobe (6 different lesions)	R	Mass excision (multiple lesions)	420	No	No	Yes (7)	8	No	

*If in the same patient, a different number of procedures is specified within brackets.

**LHS was not considered as they started further therapy during the same hospitalization.

TABLE 2 | Review of the most recent literature.

References	Year	Study	Number	Indication*	Median age (y)	Types tumor*	LHS (days)	Conversion	Complications**	Port-Site metastases	Intraoperative rupture
Lautz et al. (9)	2021	Retrospective	48	AS	13.9 ± 4.5	Metastatic osteosarcoma	2	0%	2.1% SSI; 2.1%; DVT or PE 6.3%	0	0
Abdelhafeez et al. (10)	2019	Retrospective	179	B (81.6%) AS (18.5%)	NA	B: 113 Pulmonary lesions, 30 Mediastinal tumors, 3 Pleural lesions; AS: 21 Pulmonary metastases, 7 Neurogenic tumors, Other: 5	NA	15.1%	7.8% (B: 10 PNX, AS: 3 PNX, 2 bleeding, 1 SSI, 1 other)	0	0
Da et al. (12)	2019	Retrospective	43	AS	3.7 ± 2.9	13 Neurogenic tumors, 5 Cystic Teratoma, 4 Lymphangioma, Other: 21	10.0 ± 5.5	0%	4.7% (not precisely specified)	0	0
McDaniel et al. (15)	2018	Retrospective	35	AS	11.25 (0.67–23.50)	6 Osteosarcoma, 5 Ewing sarcoma, 5 Hepatoblastoma, 3 Rhabdomyosarcoma, 3 Synovial cell Sarcoma, Other: 13	NA	0%	17.0% (6 PNX)	0	0
Acker et al. (13)	2015	Retrospective	77	B (72.3%) AS (27.7%)	10.7 ± 6.3	B: Lymphoma 21, Metastases 29, Other: 6 AS: Neuroblastoma 11, Metastatic disease 9, schwannoma 1	5.9 (±8.1)	5.2%	11.0% (not precisely specified)	0	0
Sato et al. (11)	2016	Retrospective	21	AS	6.9 ± 4.6	11 Neurogenic tumors, 6 Germ Cell Tumors, Other: 4	8.0 ± 3.7	0%	20% (1 brachial plexus palsy, 1 Horner's syndrome, 1 atelectasis, 1 palsy of upper limb)	0	0
Irtan et al. (14)	2015	Retrospective	20	AS	3.3 (0.3–11.6)	Neuroblastic tumors	5.2 (2–10)	15%	20.0% (3 Chiyothorax, 1 Horner's syndrome)	0	0
Riccipetitoni et al. (2021)	2021	R	43	B (51.1%) AS (48.9%)	7.72 (0.35–18.6).	10 Neurogenic tumors, 9 Hematological diseases, 5 Metastases, 4 Lypoblastomas, 3 thymic pathologies, 3 germ-cell tumors, Other: 9 (see **Table 1**)	5 (1–18)	2.3%	7.0% (see **Table 1**)	0	0

**B, biopsy; AS, ablative surgery.*
***SSI, surgical site infection; DVT, deep venous thrombosis; PE, pulmonary embolism, PNX, pneumothorax.*

of exploring the entire surface of the lung and pleura, and performing multiple biopsies if required (e.g., germinal tumors). Morbidity, mortality, and length of hospitalization are lower when compared to open surgery (19). Success rate of thoracoscopic-assisted biopsies have been reported in literature ranging from 96.7 to 100% for both histological and/or bacteriological diagnosis (12, 19–28). Nonetheless, different techniques have been proposed to further enhance the accuracy of MIS, such as intraoperative ultrasound localization (both trans-pleural and endoscopic) (29), CT-guided needle localization with methylene blue staining, or micro-coil application (15, 30, 31).

Our experience confirms the feasibility of VATS for diagnostic procedures. Among our cases, we performed three one-trocar site procedures, without complications. Nevertheless, indication for this technique in pediatrics is limited to procedures with low risk of bleeding.

Thoracoscopic surgery has been largely applied to excise mediastinal malignancies, and its use has been extended in pediatrics as well. Although in our cohort we did not record conversion to open surgery, in the most recent literature, conversion rate has been reported in up to 15% of cases (10–14) (**Figure 1**).

When performing mediastinal mass excisions (n = 14), we positioned a chest drain in 85.7% of patients. Nonetheless, its use is not mandatory, and in literature, chest drainage is not performed in up to 35% of procedures (29–31). A recent review of 2021 by Yu-Wei Liu reported how eliminating chest drain placement after mediastinal tumor resection can decrease post-operative pain and hospital stay without increasing complications or compromising patient safety (32).

In pediatrics, the most common mediastinal neoplasms are neurogenic tumors (neuroblastoma, ganglioneuroblastoma, and ganglioneuroma). Surgical approach has been evolving, and their resection is now often performed thoracoscopically, guaranteeing the well-known advantages of MIS (30). Different studies have found similar oncological outcomes and comparable rates of complication between the MIS and open approaches (30, 31, 33). Nonetheless, at least one port-site dissemination has been described (34). To date, VATS for neurogenic tumors does not yet have specific guidelines, although there are no contraindications. Nonetheless, literature still reports the frequent use of open approach in case of a large mediastinal tumor (35). In our series, seven patients with neurogenic tumor underwent a total of 10 procedures (four biopsies and six mass excisions). Among the excision group, five patients were submitted to a thoracoscopic surgery and one patient to a robotics-assisted procedure. All children presented IDRF-negative tumors except the case treated by RATS.

Pre-operative diagnostic workup and identification of IDRFs obtained by computed tomography (CT) and/or magnetic resonance are essential to precisely localize the lesion and identify the extent of the disease. A recent systematic review conducted by the APSA Cancer Committee confirmed how a pre-operative objective assessment by IDRFs and size criteria are recommended to guide the approach, in order to follow oncologic principles of surgical resection of neuroblastic tumors with the least possible morbidity (36).

In recent years, 3D virtual reconstruction and printing technologies have been increasingly applied to further implement the possibility of a more precise surgical planning (37, 38). These technologies enable surgeons to simulate beforehand the surgical procedure, potentially reducing the risk of intraoperative complications and allowing a conservative surgery when indicated (39–41) (**Figures 2** and **3**). In our experience, these techniques were chosen in complex cases with multiple lesions and vessel encasement and allowed the formulation of a personalized surgical strategy.

VATS is largely used to perform segmentectomies and lobectomies for pulmonary lesions in oncological adult patients. A recent meta-analysis reviewed 34 studies (183,426 patients), comparing open-approach, VATS, and robotics-assisted surgery. Their results showed how MIS seemed safer compared to open surgery, with reduced 30-day mortality, pulmonary complications, and overall complications with equivalent oncologic outcomes and 5-year overall survival (42). Nevertheless, use of VATS in pediatric lung tumors is not yet validated, and only small case-series can be found.

As far as it concerns metastatic disease, osteosarcoma represents one of the most relevant causes of metastases in children. Surgical management of osteosarcoma is still strongly debated, knowing that the most important prognostic indicator for this disease is the complete resection of all lesions (43). One of the main disadvantages of VATS is the impossibility to perform digital palpation to detect possible lesions not identified at imaging. Compared to other neoplasia, the higher calcification of osteosarcoma metastases allows for manual palpation at sizes below the resolution of CT. Nonetheless, many centers have started using thoracoscopy for osteosarcoma metastases due to the acknowledged advantages of MIS compared to open thoracotomy. A recent collaborative study on 202 patients showed that, in patients with limited metastases, both mortality and risk of pulmonary recurrence were similar when comparing VATS and thoracotomy (44). The risk of possible port-site metastases should not be neglected, as it has already been reported in the case of an 18-year-old female who presented with port site metastases within 4 months of pulmonary metastasectomy for osteosarcoma (45).

In the last decades, robotics-assisted surgery (RAS) has been increasingly employed in several complex procedures, and its use is now standardized for many interventions. The known advantages are the 3D vision, seven degrees of freedom, tremor filtration, and precise camera control (46). In pediatrics, its usage has more limitations due to the mismatch between the robotic arms and trocar dimensions compared to small children, the absence of haptic feedback, and the potential risk of tumor rupture and spillage. No guidelines or recommendations have yet been proposed from the main association of pediatric surgery in this field (47). Despite this, RAS is starting to be implemented in this field as well. In a recent review of 2020 (48), a total of 13 thoracic oncological neoplasias were treated (thymoma, neuroblastoma, inflammatory myofibroblastic tumor, bronchial carcinoid tumor). No tumor recurrence or port-site metastases

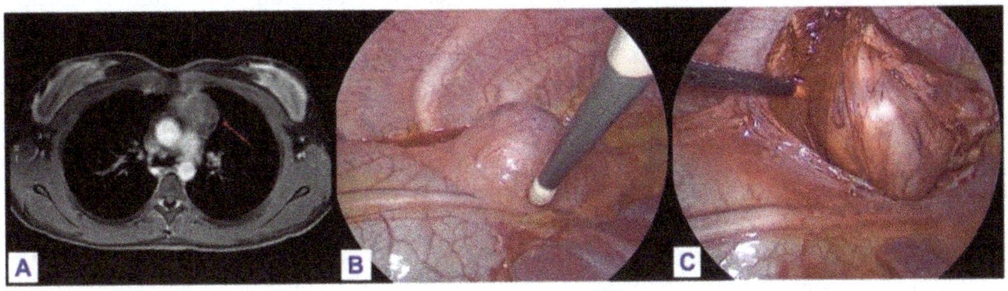

FIGURE 1 | Thymoma excision in an 11-year-old girl: **(A)** MRI pre operative imaging. **(B)** Identification and preservation of the phrenic nerve. **(C)** Dissection of the thymus from the pericardium.

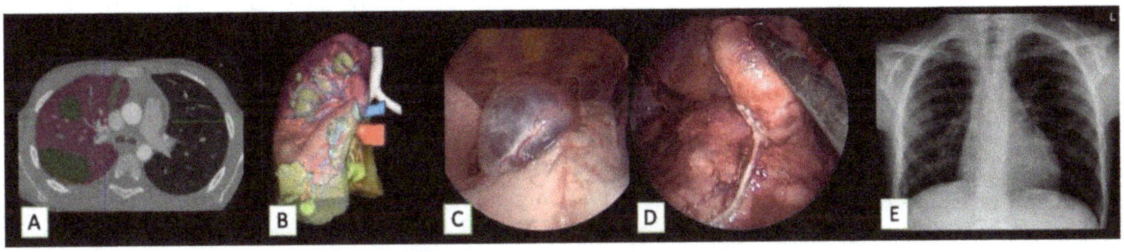

FIGURE 2 | Cystic lesions after surgery and chemotherapy for a pleuropulmonary blastoma in a 7-year-old boy, who then underwent MIS excision of multiple masses. **(A,B)** Reconstruction and 3D model of the lesions. **(C,D)** Intraoperative thoracoscopic view. **(E)** Post-operative X-ray.

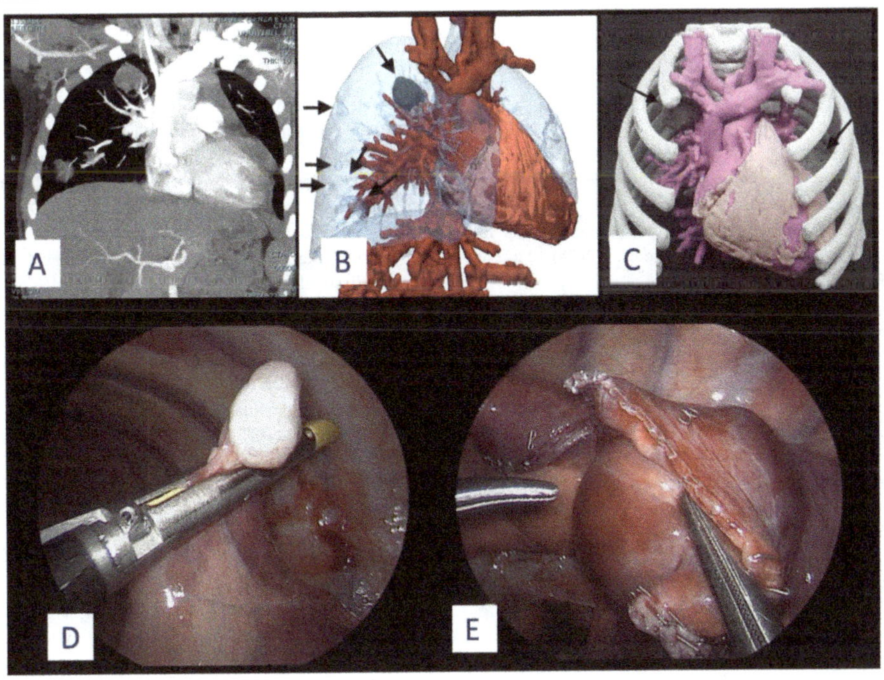

FIGURE 3 | Multiple metastases of immature teratoma in a 7-year-old girl. Left single metastasis was excised through an open procedure, due to dimension and site of the mass. The remaining lesions ($n = 6$, one solid, five cystic ones) on the right lobe were excised through VATS. **(A)** CT image. **(B)** 3D virtual reconstruction. **(C)** 3D printed model showing the two solid lesions (colored in gray). **(D,E)** Intraoperative view.

have been registered; two post-operative pneumothoraxes occurred, and one conversion due to difficult dissection of a neuroblastoma was recorded (48). In our single case, we did not observe any robot-related complications such as adjacent organ injury, positioning-related injury, or injury due to robotic arms. Despite some promising results of RAS reported in literature, its use should be reserved to highly selected cases and, due to lack of recommendations, surgical indication should be discussed by an expert multidisciplinary team (48–50).

LIMITATIONS OF THE STUDY

We should recognize some limitations of the study, related to the predictable low case-volume and heterogeneity of rare diseases that we treated. The analysis of the recent literature faces the same challenge. In addition, the comparison of MIS to open surgery may be problematic in ascertainment with observational studies due to potential unmeasured selection bias, difficulty of retrospective patient-level comparison, and lack of randomized trials (10, 51).

CONCLUSION

VATS has now become a standardized tool in pediatric surgery. From our experience, it may be applied effectively in thoracic pediatric oncology for both diagnostic and therapeutic purposes with low complication and conversion rate.

It is a challenging procedure that requires a dedicated multidisciplinary team with competencies in pediatric oncology, radiology, anesthesiology, and mini-invasive thoracic surgery.

Pre-operative patient selection requires a strict adherence to tumor protocols; IDRF evaluation; and assessment of biology, stage, and dimension of the tumor. Recent technologies such as 3D virtual reconstruction and 3D printing may optimize this selection and guarantee a safer and more targeted treatment. The role of robotics-assisted surgery needs to be defined.

ETHICS STATEMENT

Ethical review and approval was not required for the study on human participants in accordance with the local legislation and institutional requirements. Written informed consent to participate in this study was provided by the participants' legal guardian/next of kin. Written informed consent was obtained from the minor(s)' legal guardian/next of kin for the publication of any potentially identifiable images or data included in this article.

AUTHOR CONTRIBUTIONS

GR contributed to conception and design of the study. FV organized the database and performed the statistical analysis. FV, GR, and MB wrote the first draft of the manuscript. FV, MB, and GR wrote sections of the manuscript. MG and AR help the revision process and implemented sections of the manuscript. All authors contributed to manuscript revision, read, and approved the submitted version.

REFERENCES

1. Lacher M, Kuebler JF, Dingemann J, Ure BM. Minimal invasive surgery in the newborn: current status and evidence. *Semin Pediatr Surg.* (2014) 23:249–56. doi: 10.1053/j.sempedsurg.2014.09.004
2. Ponsky TA, Rothenberg SS. Minimally invasive surgery in infants less than 5 kg: experience of 649 cases. *Surg Endosc.* (2008) 22:2214–9. doi: 10.1007/s00464-008-0025-7
3. Ure BM, Schmidt AI, Jesch NK. Thoracoscopic surgery in infants and children. *Eur J Pediatr Surg.* (2005) 15:314–8. doi: 10.1055/s-2005-865793
4. Lawal TA, Gosemann JH, Kuebler JF, Glüer S, Ure BM. Thoracoscopy versus thoracotomy improves midterm musculoskeletal status and cosmesis in infants and children. *Ann Thorac Surg.* (2009) 87:224–8. doi: 10.1016/j.athoracsur.2008.08.069
5. Yang YF, Dong R, Zheng C, Jin Z, Chen G, Huang YL, et al. Outcomes of thoracoscopy versus thoracotomy for esophageal atresia with tracheoesophageal fistula repair. *Medicine.* (2016) 95:e4428. doi: 10.1097/MD.0000000000004428
6. Jaureguizar E, Vazquez J, Murcia J, Diez Pardo JA. Morbid musculoskeletal sequelae of thoracotomy for tracheoesophageal fistula. *J Pediatr Surg.* (1985) 20:511–4. doi: 10.1016/S0022-3468(85)80477-2
7. Korovessis P, Papanastasiou D, Dimas A, Karayannis A. Scoliosis by acquired rib fusion after thoracotomy in infancy. *Eur Spine J.* (1993) 2:53–5. doi: 10.1007/BF00301057
8. Durand M, Musleh L, Vatta F, Orofino G, Querciagrossa S, Jugie M, et al. Robotic lobectomy in children with severe bronchiectasis: a worthwhile new technology. *J Pediatr Surg.* (2021) 56:1606–10. doi: 10.1016/j.jpedsurg.2020.11.009
9. Lautz TB, Farooqui Z, Jenkins T, Heaton TE, Doski JJ, Cooke-Barber J, et al. Thoracoscopy vs thoracotomy for the management of metastatic osteosarcoma: a pediatric surgical oncology research collaborative study. *Int J Cancer.* (2021) 148:1164–71. doi: 10.1002/ijc.33264
10. Abdelhafeez A, Ortega-Laureano L, Murphy AJ, Davidoff AM, Fernandez-Pineda I, Sandoval JA. Minimally invasive surgery in pediatric surgical oncology: practice evolution at a contemporary single-center institution and a guideline proposal for a randomized controlled study. *J Laparoendosc Adv Surg Tech A.* (2019) 29:1046–51. doi: 10.1089/lap.2018.0467
11. Sato T, Kazama T, Fukuzawa T, Wada M, Sasaki H, Kudo H, et al. Mediastinal tumor resection via open or video-assisted surgery in 31 pediatric cases: experiences at a single institution. *J Pediatr Surg.* (2016) 51:530–3. doi: 10.1016/j.jpedsurg.2015.09.021
12. Da M, Peng W, Mo X, Fan M, Wu K, Sun J, et al. Comparison of efficacy between video-assisted thoracoscopic surgery and thoracotomy in children with mediastinal tumors: 6-year experience. *Ann Transl Med.* (2019) 7:653. doi: 10.21037/atm.2019.10.81
13. Acker SN, Bruny JL, Garrington TP, Partrick DA. Minimally invasive surgical techniques are safe in the diagnosis and treatment of pediatric malignancies. *Surg Endosc.* (2015) 29:1203–8. doi: 10.1007/s00464-014-3795-0
14. Irtan S, Brisse HJ, Minard-Colin V, Schleiermacher G, Canale S, Sarnacki S. Minimally invasive surgery of neuroblastic tumors in children: indications depend on anatomical location and image-defined risk factors. *Pediatr Blood Cancer.* (2015) 62:257–61. doi: 10.1002/pbc.25248
15. McDaniel JD, Racadio JM, Patel MN, Johnson ND, Kukreja K. CT-guided localization of pulmonary nodules in children prior to video-assisted thoracoscopic surgical resection utilizing a combination of two previously described techniques. *Pediatr Radiol.* (2018) 48:626–31. doi: 10.1007/s00247-018-4069-0
16. Smith TJ, Rothenberg SS, Brooks M, Bealer J, Chang J, Cook BA, et al. Thoracoscopic surgery in childhood cancer. *J Pediatr Hematol Oncol.* (2002) 24:429–35. doi: 10.1097/00043426-200208000-00004
17. Holcomb GW, Tomita SS, Haase GM, Dillon PW, Newman KD, Applebaum H, et al. Minimally invasive surgery in children with cancer. *Cancer.* (1995) 76:121–8.

18. Bassanezi BSB, Oliveira-Filho AG, Miranda ML, Soares L, Aguiar SS. Use of BiPAP for safe anesthesia in a child with a large anterior mediastinal mass. *Pediatr Anesth.* (2011) 21:985–7. doi: 10.1111/j.1460-9592.2011.03607.x
19. Rothenberg SS, Wagner JS, Chang JHT, Fan LL. The safety and efficacy of thoracoscopic lung biopsy for diagnosis and treatment in infants and children. *J Pediatr Surg.* (1996) 31:100–4. doi: 10.1016/S0022-3468(96)90328-0
20. Esposito C, Lima M, Mattioli G, Mastroianni L, Riccipetitoni G, Monguzzi G, et al. Thoracoscopic surgery in the management of pediatric malignancies: a multicentric survey of the Italian society of videosurgery in infancy. *Surg Endosc.* (2007) 21:1772–5. doi: 10.1007/s00464-007-9246-4
21. Sandoval C, Stringel G. Video-assisted thoracoscopy for the diagnosis of mediastinal masses in children. *JSLS.* (1997) 1:131–3.
22. Metzelder ML, Kuebler JF, Shimotakahara A, Glueer S, Grigull L, Ure BM. Role of diagnostic and ablative minimally invasive surgery for pediatric malignancies. *Cancer.* (2007) 109:2343–8. doi: 10.1002/cncr.22696
23. Spurbeck WW, Davidoff AM, Lobe TE, Rao BN, Schropp KP, Shochat SJ. Minimally invasive surgery in pediatric cancer patients. *Ann Surg Oncol.* (2004) 11:340–3. doi: 10.1245/ASO.2004.04.021
24. Iwanaka T, Arai M, Kawashima H, Kudou S, Fujishiro J, Imaizumi S, et al. Endosurgical procedures for pediatric solid tumors. *Pediatr Surg Int.* (2004) 20:39–42. doi: 10.1007/s00383-003-1078-2
25. Sailhamer E, Jackson CC, Vogel AM, Kang S, Wu Y, Chwals WJ, et al. Minimally invasive surgery for pediatric solid neoplasms. *Am Surg.* (2003) 69:566–8.
26. Holcomb GW. Minimally invasive surgery for solid tumors. *Semin Surg Oncol.* (1999) 16:184–92. doi: 10.3390/children5120158
27. Saenz NC, Conlon KC, Aronson DC, LaQuaglia MP. The application of minimal access procedures in infants, children, and young adults with pediatric malignancies. *J Laparoendosc Adv Surg Tech A.* (1997) 7:289–94. doi: 10.1089/lap.1997.7.289
28. Rodgers BM, Moazam F, Talbert JL. Thoracoscopy in children. *Ann Surg.* (1979) 189:176–80. doi: 10.1097/00000658-197902000-00008
29. Fraga JC, Aydogdu B, Aufieri R, Silva GVM, Schopf L, Takamatu E, et al. Surgical treatment for pediatric mediastinal neurogenic tumors. *Ann Thorac Surg.* (2010) 90:413–8. doi: 10.1016/j.athoracsur.2010.04.086
30. Fraga JC, Rothenberg S, Kiely E, Pierro A. Video-assisted thoracic surgery resection for pediatric mediastinal neurogenic tumors. *J Pediatr Surg.* (2012) 47:1349–53. doi: 10.1016/j.jpedsurg.2012.01.067
31. Malek MM, Mollen KP, Kane TD, Shah SR, Irwin C. Thoracic neuroblastoma: a retrospective review of our institutional experience with comparison of the thoracoscopic and open approaches to resection. *J Pediatr Surg.* (2010) 45:1622–6. doi: 10.1016/j.jpedsurg.2010.03.018
32. Liu YW, Chen HW, Lee JY, Chiang HH Li HP, Chang PC, et al. Is a chest tube necessary after video-assisted thoracoscopic mediastinal tumor resection? *Thorac Cardiovasc Surg.* (2019) 69:181–8. doi: 10.1055/s-0039-1683879
33. Malkan AD, Loh AHP, Fernandez-Pineda I, Sandoval JA. The role of thoracoscopic surgery in pediatric oncology. *J Laparoendosc Adv Surg Tech A.* (2014) 24:819–26. doi: 10.1089/lap.2014.0252
34. Pentek F, Schulte JH, Schweiger B, Metzelder M, Schündeln MM. Development of port-site metastases following thoracoscopic resection of a neuroblastoma. *Pediatr Blood Cancer.* (2015) 63:149–51. doi: 10.1002/pbc.25677
35. Christison-Lagay ER, Thomas D. Minimally invasive approaches to pediatric solid tumors. *Surg Oncol Clin N Am.* (2019) 28:129–46. doi: 10.1016/j.soc.2018.07.005
36. Gurria JP, Malek MM, Heaton TE, Gehred A, Lautz TB, Rhee DS, et al. Minimally invasive surgery for abdominal and thoracic neuroblastic tumors: a systematic review by the APSA cancer committee. *J Pediatr Surg.* (2020) 55:2260–72. doi: 10.1016/j.jpedsurg.2020.02.019
37. Sánchez-Sánchez Á, Girón-Vallejo Ó, Ruiz-Pruneda R, Fernandez-Ibieta M, García-Calderon D, Villamil V, et al. Three-Dimensional printed model and virtual reconstruction: an extra tool for pediatric solid tumors surgery. *European J Pediatr Surg Rep.* (2018) 06:e70–6. doi: 10.1055/s-0038-1672165
38. Smelt JLC, Suri T, Valencia O, Jahangiri M, Rhode K, Nair A, et al. Operative planning in thoracic surgery: a pilot study comparing imaging techniques and three-dimensional printing. *Ann Thorac Surg.* (2019) 107:401–6. doi: 10.1016/j.athoracsur.2018.08.052
39. Kiraly L, Tofeig M, Jha NK, Talo H. Three-dimensional printed prototypes refine the anatomy of post-modified Norwood-1 complex aortic arch obstruction and allow presurgical simulation of the repair. *Interact CardioVasc Thorac Surg.* (2015) 22:238–40. doi: 10.1093/icvts/ivv320
40. Barsness KA, Rooney DM, Davis LM. Collaboration in simulation: the development and initial validation of a novel thoracoscopic neonatal simulator. *J Pediatr Surg.* (2013) 48:1232–8. doi: 10.1016/j.jpedsurg.2013.03.015
41. Shiraishi I, Yamagishi M, Hamaoka K, Fukuzawa M, Yagihara, T. Simulative operation on congenital heart disease using rubber-like urethane stereolithographic biomodels based on 3D datasets of multislice computed tomography. *Eur J Cardiothorac Surg.* (2010) 37:302–6. doi: 10.1016/j.ejcts.2009.07.046
42. Aiolfi A, Nosotti M, Micheletto G, Khor D, Bonitta G, Perali C, et al. Pulmonary lobectomy for cancer: systematic review and network meta-analysis comparing open, video-assisted thoracic surgery, and robotic approach. *Surgery.* (2021) 169:436–46. doi: 10.1016/j.surg.2020.09.010
43. Tabone MD, Kalifa C, Rodary C, Raquin M, Valteau-Couanet D, Lemerle J. Osteosarcoma recurrences in pediatric patients previously treated with intensive chemotherapy. *J Clin Oncol.* (1994) 12:2614–20. doi: 10.1200/JCO.1994.12.12.2614
44. Lautz TB, Farooqui Z, Jenkins T, Heaton TE, Doski JJ, Cooke-Barber J, et al. Thoracoscopy vs thoracotomy for the management of metastatic osteosarcoma: a pediatric surgical oncology research collaborative study. *Int J Cancer.* (2020) 148:1164–71.
45. Sartorelli KH, Partrick D, Meagher DP Jr. Port-site recurrence after thoracoscopic resection of pulmonary metastasis owing to osteogenic sarcoma. *J Pediatr Surg.* (1996) 31:1443–4. doi: 10.1016/S0022-3468(96)90852-0
46. Meehan JJ. Robotic surgery for pediatric tumors. *Cancer.* (2013) 19:183–8. doi: 10.1097/PPO.0b013e318289486c
47. van Dalen EC, de Lijster MS, Leijssen LG, Michiels EM, Kremer LC, Caron HN, et al. Minimally invasive surgery versus open surgery for the treatment of solid abdominal and thoracic neoplasms in children. *Cochrane Database Syst Rev.* (2015) 1:CD008403. doi: 10.1002/14651858.CD008403.pub3
48. Blanc T, Meignan P, Vinit N, Ballouhey Q, Pio L, Capito C, et al. Robotic surgery in pediatric oncology: lessons learned from the first 100 tumours-A nationwide experience. *SSRN J [Preprint].* (2020). Available at: https://papers.ssrn.com/sol3/papers.cfm?abstract_id=3757404 (accessed September 5, 2021).
49. Blanc T, Pio L, Clermidi P, Muller C, Orbach D, Minard-Colin V, et al. Robotic-assisted laparoscopic management of renal tumors in children: preliminary results. *Pediatr Blood Cancer.* (2019) 66 (Suppl. 3):e28431. doi: 10.1002/pbc.27867
50. Mattioli G, Pini Prato A, Razore B, Leonelli L, Pio L, Avanzini S, et al. Da Vinci robotic surgery in a pediatric hospital. *J Laparoendosc Adv Surg Tech.* (2017) 27:539–45. doi: 10.1089/lap.2016.0390
51. Giordano SH, Kuo YF, Duan Z, Hortobagyi GN, Freeman J, Goodwin JS. Limits of observational data in determining outcomes from cancer therapy. *Cancer.* (2008) 112:2456–66. doi: 10.1002/cncr.23452

31

Management of Primary Spontaneous Pneumothorax in a Third-Level Pediatric Surgical Center

Giovanna Spezzotto[1], Alessandro Boscarelli[2†], Manuela Giangreco[3†], Giulia Ceschiutti[2], Daniela Codrich[2†], Maria-Grazia Scarpa[2], Marianna Iaquinto[2], Damiana Olenik[2], Edoardo Guida[2†] and Jürgen Schleef[2,4†]*

[1] Faculty of Medicine and Surgery, University of Trieste, Trieste, Italy, [2] Department of Pediatric Surgery and Urology, Institute for Maternal and Child Health - IRCCS "Burlo Garofolo", Trieste, Italy, [3] Clinical Epidemiology and Public Health Research Unit, Institute for Maternal and Child Health - IRCCS "Burlo Garofolo", Trieste, Italy, [4] Surgical Department, Institute for Maternal and Child Health - IRCCS "Burlo Garofolo", Trieste, Italy

***Correspondence:**
Alessandro Boscarelli
tboscar@hotmail.it

Introduction: The management of primary spontaneous pneumothorax (PSP) in pediatrics remains controversial. The aim of this study was to investigate the risk of recurrence after non-surgical treatment vs. surgery, the difference in the length of stay (LOS) between various treatment options, and the role of computed tomography (CT) in the management of PSP.

Materials and Methods: We retrospectively reviewed patients admitted to our Pediatric Surgery Unit for an episode of PSP between June 2009 and July 2020. Medical records including clinical presentation at admission, diagnostics, treatments, complications, and LOS were collected.

Results: Twenty-three patients (22 males and 1 female) were included in this study. Median age was 15.65 (range 9–18). Chest X-rays were performed in all patients and showed 5 small (22%) and 18 large (78%) PSP. Chest drain was used for large PSP ($\geq$2 cm) if the patient was clinically unstable. Eleven patients (48%) were managed non-operatively with observation alone and a recurrence rate of 18%, chest drain was used in 11 patients with a recurrence rate of 36%, and surgery was deemed necessary as a first treatment choice in one case. Six patients (27%) had an episode of relapse after non-operative management or chest drain placement. Following surgery, a relapse occurred in 2 of the 6 patients. Chest drain insertion was associated with a longer LOS than observation alone (6.36 vs. 2.4 days), and surgery resulted in a longer LOS than other types of treatment ($P = 0.001$).

Conclusion: According to our experience, small PSP or clinically stable larger PSP can be treated conservatively with observation alone. Operative management should be taken into consideration in children with large symptomatic PSP, persistent air leak, and/or relapse after chest drain insertion.

Keywords: primary spontaneous pneumothorax, children, management, conservative treatment, surgery

INTRODUCTION

Primary spontaneous pneumothorax (PSP) is defined as a spontaneously occurring pneumothorax in the absence of prior lung disease or trauma. The incidence of PSP has been reported to be around 3.4/100,000 in childhood, with a male to female ratio of 4:1 (1). Tall, thin boys with a below average body mass index (BMI) are typically affected (2). While it is widely accepted that blebs, bullae, or emphysema-like changes play a large role, the exact etiology remains to be elucidated (3).

The role of computed tomography (CT) is controversial. Some studies have noted that the risk of recurrence is much higher in patients with bullae and blebs visible at CT than in those without (4), while other studies have not found this match. Additionally, according to some authors, finding bullae and blebs at CT scan is not an indication for surgery (5). In the pediatric population, the high dose of radiation to which patients are subjected during CT should be taken into consideration.

The management of PSP in children remains debated and based on evidence from adult patients. Several studies have been published concerning the treatment of pneumothorax in children. However, their limitations include being largely retrospective and following a small number of patients. Initial management for small PSP is usually conservative, with observation alone and/or oxygen supplementation. By contrast, large PSP is typically treated with chest drain insertion, with surgery reserved for those cases presenting air leak or failure of the aforementioned strategies. Traditional thoracotomy surgery has been associated with a reduction of relapse but increased morbidity, LOS, and mortality. With the introduction of video-assisted thoracoscopic surgery (VATS), episodes of relapse have been significantly reduced. Some studies support that VATS is a safe treatment and should be considered if the air leak persists or in case of relapse (6–9).

The purpose of this study was to examine the best treatment strategy in terms of LOS and risk of relapse, and to establish the role of CT in the management of PSP.

MATERIALS AND METHODS

We retrospectively reviewed patients <18 years of age admitted to our Pediatric Surgery Unit for PSP from June 2009 to July 2020. Data were extrapolated from the departmental database and clinical notes were reviewed. Patients with traumatic or iatrogenic pneumothorax and underlying lung disease (asthma, pneumonia, cystic fibrosis, malignancy, connective diseases) were excluded. Demographic data (age and sex), clinical presentation at admission, diagnostics (X-ray and CT), primary and follow-up treatments (conservative, surgery), complications, and length of hospitalization were examined. X-ray study was performed in all patients and PSP size was calculated based on BTS guidelines. A "small" pneumothorax was defined as having a visible rim <2 cm between the lung margin and the chest wall (at the level of the hilum), while a "large" pneumothorax showed a rim ≥2 cm (10). CT scan was performed after a single episode of recurrence or in those patients with a history of spontaneous pneumothorax. Small pneumothorax was treated with observation alone, large pneumothorax was treated with chest drain, and surgery was performed in patients with relapse. Outcomes considered were recurrence rate post observation alone and post drain insertion, length of hospitalization related to a specific type of treatment, secondary treatments, and timing of CT scan.

Statistical Analysis

Fisher's exact test was used to analyze the relationship between categorial variables, and the Kruskal-Wallis test was used to analyze the relationship between continuous variables. A significance level of $P < 0.05$ was chosen.

RESULTS

Twenty-three patients, 22 males and 1 female, admitted to our Pediatric Surgery Unit with a first episode of PSP were included in this study. Mean age was 15.65 (range 9–18 years). One patient had a family history of pneumothorax, and one patient had a smoking habit. Twenty-one patients (92%) presented with a pneumothorax on the left side, one on the right side and one on both sides. Chest X-rays were performed in all patients and showed 5 small (22%) and 18 large (78%) PSP. None of the patients with small PSP relapsed. CT scan was performed in 9 cases (39%), 7 of them after a relapse (78%), and 6 of the 9 children (67%) presented apical blebs or bullae. All patients with blebs or bullae detected at CT scan had at least one episode of recurrence, but statistical analysis using Fisher's exact test showed this relationship was not significant ($P = 0.08$). Chest drain was used for large PSP (≥2 cm) if a patient was clinically unstable, presenting with dyspnea and significant hypoxia. Eleven patients (48%) were managed non-operatively with observation alone and a recurrence rate of 18%, chest drain was used in 11 patients with a recurrence rate of 36%, and surgery was deemed necessary as a first treatment choice in one case. Chest drain insertion was associated with a longer LOS than observation alone (6.36 vs. 2.4 days), and surgery resulted in a longer LOS than other types of treatment ($P = 0.001$). Six patients (27%) had an episode of relapse after non-operative management or chest drain placement in a median time of 12 months (range 1–24 months); 4 experienced an ipsilateral pneumothorax, one bilateral pneumothorax and one contralateral pneumothorax. Relapses were not related to the type of therapeutic strategy ($P = 0.24$). Thoracoscopic surgery was performed in 6 patients, in 5 cases after a relapse episode and in one case as a first therapeutic approach in a child with a history of recurrent pneumothorax. Indications for surgical intervention were recurrent ipsilateral pneumothorax (50%), contralateral pneumothorax (17%), and bilateral pneumothorax (33%). We performed a thoracoscopic procedure with a pulmonary wedge resection of the apical lung in 4 cases (67%), of which 2 were associated with mechanical pleurodesis and 2 with chemical pleurodesis. Two patients

Abbreviations: PSP, primary spontaneous pneumothorax; CT, computed tomography; LOS, length of stay; VATS, video-assisted thoracoscopic surgery.

TABLE 1 | Patient characteristics, management, and outcomes after recurrence.

Characteristics	Results
Age, median (IQR)	
	16 (15–17)
Sex, *n* (%)	
Female	1 (4)
Male	22 (96)
Smokers, *n* (%)	
	1 (4)
Familiarity, *n* (%)	
	1 (4)
Side, *n* (%)	
Left	21 (92)
Right	1 (4)
Bilateral	1 (4)
Size, *n* (%)	
Small (<2 cm)	5 (22)
Large (≥2 cm)	18 (78)
CT scan, *n* (%)	
	9 (39)
Bullae/blebs found at CT scan, *n* (%)	
	6 (67)
Management, *n* (%)	
Observation alone	11 (48)
Chest drain	11 (48)
Surgery	1 (4)
Relapse, *n* (%)	
After observation	2 (18)
After chest drain	4 (36)
After surgery	1 (100)
Management after relapse, *n* (%)	
Observation alone	1 (14)
Chest drain	0 (0)
Surgery, *n* (%)	6 (86)

IQR, interquartile range; n, number; CT, computed tomography.

TABLE 2 | Management-based results and CT-findings after recurrence.

Variables	Management			*P*-value
	Observation alone	Chest drain	Surgery	
Relapse, *n* (%)				
Yes	2 (18.2)	4 (36.4)	1 (100.0)	0.24*
No	9 (81.8)	7 (63.6)	0 (0.0)	
Lenght of stay, median (IQR)				
	2 (2–3)	5 (4–8)	10 (10–10)	0.001**
Variables				***P*-value**
Blebs/Bullae at CT scan after a relapse, *n* (%)				
Yes	6 (100.0)			0.08*
No	0 (0.0)			

**Fisher exact test.*
***Kruskall Wallis test.*
n, number; IQR, interquartile range; CT, computed tomography.

underwent apicectomy alone (33%). Following the surgical procedure, a relapse occurred in 2 of 6 patients (33%) with subsequent further relapses. In both cases, CT scan detected blebs or bullae, confirming that these lesions are involved in recurrence episodes. All variables analyzed are summarized in **Tables 1, 2**.

DISCUSSION

PSP is rarer in the pediatric population than in adults. It generally occurs in tall, thin males aged 10–30 (11). In our study, the mean age was approximately 16 years. Unfortunately, we do not routinely perform genetic workup and/or evaluation in patients admitted to our pediatric surgery unit for PSP, therefore we have not investigated any possible association with relapse rate in our study. Smoking is implicated in the development of PSP, and the dangerous effect of tobacco has been recognized. Some authors highlighted that most adult patients (up to 75%) (12) with PSP were smokers, but in our study only one patient reported a smoking habit.

The etiology of PSP remains unclear. It is well accepted that PSP occurs from the rupture of blebs and bullae on the apex of the lung. The formation of these lesions is most likely multifactorial, including physical characteristics, anatomic abnormalities of the bronchial tree, genetic factors, and growth (13, 14). Fujino et al. (15) suggested the hypothesis that growth during adolescence rapidly increases the vertical dimension of the thorax, causing an increase in negative pressure at the apex of the lung that may lead to formation of subpleural blebs or fluid-filled cysts with consequent pneumothorax upon rupturing. These lesions are not usually visible on X-ray but can often be detected using CT.

Diagnosis of PSP is generally clinical and confirmed by X-ray. In our study, like many others, CT was not usually performed at admission (16–18). Some authors argue that finding blebs at CT, even if performed for other indications, is a strong indication for surgery (19). In contrast, most authors state that CT evidence of bullae does not necessarily predict outcomes, even if they agree that CT is an effective method to delineate the anatomical status of the bullae and bleb formation (20, 21). Another consideration before undertaking CT scanning is the large amount of ionizing radiation involved.

In our study the biggest bleb size was 19 mm, while the average size was 4–5 mm. In all patients undergoing CT evaluation after a relapse, blebs and/or bullae were highlighted. However, the statistical analysis did not detect significance between recurrent episodes and lung injures ($P = 0.08$). Since the results showed no correlation between the presence of these lesions and the possibility of recurrence, there is no evidence that performing a CT scan on admission predicts future relapses. This supports our idea of reserving CT for cases of persistent air leak and relapse due to the high radiation dose involved in this imaging technique. Nonetheless, CT can assist in choosing the best therapeutic approach in selected cases.

The largest problem in PSP management is the lack of standardized guidelines. Consequently, PSP treatment is based on the experience of the individual surgery unit and evidence from the adult population. The main issues are choosing between observation alone with or without oxygen administration or chest drain insertion, and the correct timing for surgery. To date, the initial treatment approach is decided according to the size and symptoms at admission. The current management for small PSP is based on observation with oxygen administration in the majority of cases. By contrast, the presence of a large (≥2 cm) pneumothorax is the main indication for insertion of a chest drain. The therapeutic strategy used in our center for small PSP and clinically stable large PSP was simple observation. Despite this, the length of hospitalization of our patients was similar compared to patients treated with oxygen administration in other studies (1, 6, 9, 16). These patients generally underwent chest X-ray within 3 days of hospitalization to check if the pneumothorax had been reduced in size and to determine the possibly of discharge. In case of failure of conservative treatment (in terms of increase in size and/or exacerbation of symptoms such as dyspnea or hypoxia), we opted for the insertion of a chest drain. The LOS was longer in patients treated with chest drain insertion compared to those who were only observed (6.36 vs. 2.4 days), and this appears to be in keeping with other studies (8, 16). The longest LOS was related to surgery (10 days). Our statistical analysis showed that the LOS is linked to the therapeutic strategy ($P = 0.001$), confirming that it would be advisable to initially opt for a non-invasive treatment of observation alone in those patients with a small PSP and/or clinically stable to reduce the length of hospitalization.

Non-surgical management is still associated with a high failure rate. In our study, 27% of patients had an episode of relapse, but the incidence was even higher in other studies (1, 16). The statistical analysis showed that the possibility of relapse was not associated with the initial treatment chosen ($P = 0.24$). This confirms that patients with small and/or clinically stable larger PSP may be treated with observation alone, reserving more invasive treatments for any clinical exacerbation, persistent air leak and/or relapse. VATS was first reported by Rodgers in 1986 for the treatment of secondary pneumothorax in children with cystic fibrosis (22). This surgical advancement has completely changed the approach to surgery for the treatment of PSP. Prior to VATS, traditional surgery involved high morbidity and mortality. However, VATS is considered a safe method with significantly reduced morbidity and mortality (1, 16, 23, 24). In our study, surgery was required in 6 patients after an episode of relapse with a recurrence rate of 33%, slightly higher than reported by other studies (11–28%) (1, 14). A recent survey of pediatric surgeons found that most respondents preferred chest tube insertion in the

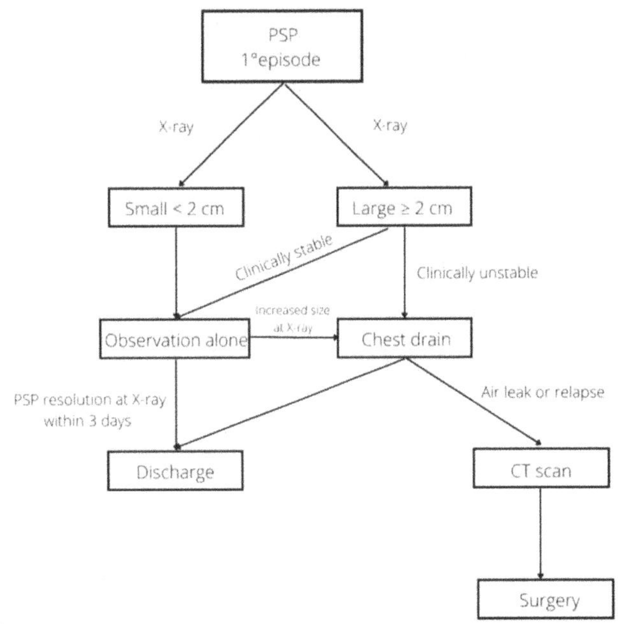

FIGURE 1 | Flow chart for management of pediatric patients with primary spontaneous pneumothorax at our institution.

management of a first episode of PSP and performed surgery for a second episode, in the presence of bullae more than 2 cm in diameter, or for recurrent pneumothorax (25). **Figure 1** shows the management flow-chart for PSP in our third level pediatric surgical ward.

Our study limitations include being retrospective and using a small cohort of patients. Prospective studies with a higher number of patients are encouraged to confirm our findings and establish evidence-based guidelines for the treatment of PSP in the pediatric population.

CONCLUSION

According to our experience, we recommend that small PSP or clinically stable larger PSP be treated conservatively with observation alone. An X-ray is advised within 3 days of starting observation; if it shows a reduction of the PSP the patient could be discharged home. If the PSP has not decreased in size, considering a chest drain insertion is appropriate. Persistent air leak or episodes of relapse should be investigated with a CT scan and considered a strong indication to proceed with surgery.

ETHICS STATEMENT

Ethical review and approval was not required for the study on human participants in accordance with the local legislation and institutional requirements. Written informed consent from the participants' legal guardian/next of kin was not required to participate in this study in accordance with the national legislation and the institutional requirements.

AUTHOR CONTRIBUTIONS

Conceptualization: AB, EG, and JS. Methodology: GS and GC. Investigation: GS, GC, and DO. Data curation: GS, AB, MG, and DC. Formal analysis: GS and MG. Validation: AB, DC, EG, and JS. Writing—original draft preparation: GS, M-GS, MI, and DO. Writing—review and editing: GS, AB, DC, M-GS, and MI. Supervision: JS. All authors approved the final version of the manuscript and attest that they meet the ICMJE criteria for authorship.

REFERENCES

1. Lopez ME, Fallon SC, Lee TC, Rodriguez JR, Brandt ML, Mazziotti MV. Management of the pediatric spontaneous pneumothorax: is primary surgery the treatment of choice? *Am J Surg.* (2014) 208:571–6. doi: 10.1016/j.amjsurg.2014.06.009
2. Poenaru D, Yazbeck S, Murphy S. Primary spontaneous pneumothorax in children. *J Pediatr Surg.* (1994) 29:1183–5. doi: 10.1016/0022-3468(94)90795-1
3. Noppen M, Baumann MH. Pathogenesis and treatment of primary spontaneous pneumothorax: an overview. *Respiration.* (2003) 70:431–8. doi: 10.1159/000072911
4. Sihoe ADL. Uniportal video-assisted thoracoscopic lobectomy. *Ann Cardiothorac Surg.* (2016) 5:133–44. doi: 10.21037/acs.2016.03.14
5. Martínez-Ramos D, Ángel-Yepes V, Escrig-Sos J, Miralles-Tena JM, Salvador-Sanchís JL. Utilidad de la tomografía computarizada para determinar el riesgo de recidiva tras un primer episodio de neumotórax espontáneo primario. *Implicaciones terapéuticas Arch Bronconeumol.* (2007) 43:304–8. doi: 10.1157/13106560
6. Seguier-Lipszyc E, Elizur A, Klin B, Vaiman M, Lotan G. Management of primary spontaneous pneumothorax in children. *Clin Pediatr.* (2011) 50:797–802. doi: 10.1177/0009922811404699
7. Lee LPY, Lai MHY, Chiu WK, Leung MW, Liu KK, Chan HB. Management of primary spontaneous pneumothorax in Chinese children. *Hong Kong Med J Xianggang Yi Xue Za Zhi.* (2010) 16:94–100.
8. Leys CM, Hirschl RB, Kohler JE, Cherney-Stafford L, Marka N, Fallat ME, et al. Changing the paradigm for management of pediatric primary spontaneous pneumothorax: a simple aspiration test predicts need for operation. *J Pediatr Surg.* (2020) 55:169–75. doi: 10.1016/j.jpedsurg.2019.09.043
9. Williams K, Oyetunji TA, Hsuing G, Hendrickson RJ, Lautz TB. Spontaneous pneumothorax in children: national management strategies and outcomes. *J Laparoendosc Adv Surg Tech.* (2018) 28:218–22. doi: 10.1089/lap.2017.0467
10. Henry M. BTS guidelines for the management of spontaneous pneumothorax. *Thorax.* (2003) 58:39ii–3952. doi: 10.1136/thorax.58.suppl_2.ii39
11. Sahn SA, Heffner JE. Spontaneous pneumothorax. *N Engl J Med.* (2000) 342:868–74. doi: 10.1056/NEJM200003233421207
12. Cheng Y-L, Huang T-W, Lin C-K, Lee SC, Tzao C, Chen JC, et al. The impact of smoking in primary spontaneous pneumothorax. *J Thorac Cardiovasc Surg.* (2009) 138:192–5. doi: 10.1016/j.jtcvs.2008.12.019
13. Shaw KS, Prasil P, Nguyen LT, Laberge JM. Pediatric spontaneous pneumothorax. *Semin Pediatr Surg.* (2003) 12:55–61. doi: 10.1053/spsu.2003.50006
14. Choi SY, Kim YH, Jo KH, Kim CK, Park JK, Cho DG, et al. Video-assisted thoracoscopic surgery for primary spontaneous pneumothorax in children. *Pediatr Surg Int.* (2013) 29:505–9. doi: 10.1007/s00383-013-3273-0
15. Fujino S, Inoue S, Tezuka N, Hanaoka J, Sawai S, Ichinose M, et al. Physical development of surgically treated patients with primary spontaneous pneumothorax. *Chest.* (1999) 116:899–902. doi: 10.1378/chest.116.4.899
16. Cerchia E, Conighi ML, Bleve C, Chiarenza SF, Sgrò A, Pini Prato A, et al. Feasibility of a standardized management for primary spontaneous pneumothorax in children and adolescents: a retrospective multicenter study and review of the literature. *J Laparoendosc Adv Surg Tech.* (2020) 30:841–6. doi: 10.1089/lap.2019.0493
17. Chiu C-Y, Chen T-P, Wang C-J, Tsai MH, Wong KS. Factors associated with proceeding to surgical intervention and recurrence of primary spontaneous pneumothorax in adolescent patients. *Eur J Pediatr.* (2014) 173:1483–90. doi: 10.1007/s00431-014-2352-0
18. Yeung F, Chung PHY, Hung ELY, Yuen CS, Tam PKH, Wong KKY. Surgical intervention for primary spontaneous pneumothorax in pediatric population: when and why? *J Laparoendosc Adv Surg Tech.* (2017) 27:841–4. doi: 10.1089/lap.2016.0163
19. Baumann MH. To bleb or not to bleb? *Chest.* (2007) 132:1110–2. doi: 10.1378/chest.07-1283
20. Laituri CA, Valusek PA, Rivard DC, Garey CL, Ostlie DJ, Snyder CL, et al. The utility of computed tomography in the management of patients with spontaneous pneumothorax. *J Pediatr Surg.* (2011) 46:1523–5. doi: 10.1016/j.jpedsurg.2011.01.002
21. Mitlehner W, Friedrich M, Dissmann W. Value of computer tomography in the detection of bullae and blebs in patients with primary spontaneous pneumothorax. *Respiration.* (1992) 59:221–7. doi: 10.1159/000196062
22. Tribble CG, Selden RF, Rodgers BM. Talc poudrage in the treatment of spontaneous pneumothoraces in patients with cystic fibrosis. *Ann Surg.* (1986) 204:677–80. doi: 10.1097/00000658-198612000-00010
23. Bialas RC, Weiner TM, Phillips JD. Video-assisted thoracic surgery for primary spontaneous pneumothorax in children: is there an optimal technique? *J Pediatr Surg.* (2008) 43:2151–5. doi: 10.1016/j.jpedsurg.2008.08.041
24. Zganjer M, Cizmić A, Pajić A, Cigit I, Zganjer V. Primary spontaneous pneumothorax in pediatric patients: our 7-year experience. *J Laparoendosc Adv Surg Tech A.* (2010) 20:195–8. doi: 10.1089/lap.2009.0070
25. Soyer T, Dariel A, Dingemann J, Martinez L, Pini-Prato A, Morini F, et al. European pediatric surgeons' association survey on the management of primary spontaneous pneumothorax in children. *Eur J Pediatr Surg.* (2021) s-0041-1739420. doi: 10.1055/s-0041-1739420

Individualized Analysis and Treatment of Difficult Weaning from Ventilation Following Open Cardiac Surgery in Young Children with Congenital Heart Disease

Xiaoming Wu [1], *Jinlan Chen* [1], *Chukwuemeka Daniel Iroegbu* [1], *Jian Liu* [2], *Ming Wu* [1,3], *Xia Xie* [1], *Kun Xiang* [1], *Xun Wu* [1], *Wangping Chen* [1], *Peng Huang* [2], *Wenwu Zhou* [3], *Chengming Fan* [1*] *and Jinfu Yang* [1*]

[1] *Department of Cardiovascular Surgery, The Second Xiangya Hospital, Central South University, Changsha, China,*
[2] *Department of Cardiothoracic Surgery, Hunan Children's Hospital, Changsha, China,* [3] *Department of the Cardiovascular Surgery of the Hunan Provincial People's Hospital, Changsha, China*

***Correspondence:**
Chengming Fan
fanchengming@csu.edu.cn
Jinfu Yang
yjf19682005@csu.edu.cn

Aims: The study explores the leading causes of postoperative extubation difficulties in pediatric patients (neonates and toddlers) with congenital heart diseases and establishes individualized treatment for different reasons.

Method: We retrospectively analyzed medical records of 4,971 pediatric patients with congenital heart defects treated in three tertiary Congenital Heart Disease Centres in China from January 2005 to December 2020, from whom we selected those with difficulty extubation but successful weaning during the postoperative period. Next, we performed an analysis of risk factors and reported the combined experience of individualized treatment for successful extubation.

Results: Seventy-five pediatric patients were identified in our database, among whom 23 had airway stenosis, 17 had diaphragmatic dysfunction, and 35 had pulmonary infection. The patients were all successfully weaned from the ventilator after an individualized treatment plan. In addition, the intubation time in the airway stenosis group was 17.7 ± 9.0, 33.6 ± 13.9 days in the diaphragmatic dysfunction group, and 11.9 ± 3.8 days in the pulmonary infection group.

Conclusion: Given the primary reasons for difficult weaning following open-heart surgery in pediatric patients with congenital heart diseases, an individualized treatment scheme can achieve the ideal therapeutic effect where patients can be weaned faster with a shorter intubation period.

Keywords: individualized treatment, difficult weaning, open cardiac surgery, pediatric patients, congenital heart disease, slide

INTRODUCTION

Mechanical ventilation, an effective treatment strategy used for most congenital heart disease following pediatric or adult cardiac surgery, is essential for post-operative recovery. In most cases, pediatric patients are post-operatively successfully weaned as planned; however, about 6–27% scenarios with weaning difficulties have been reported (1). Weaning difficulty is defined as the time required for the patient to pass the spontaneous breathing test SBT, or to successfully separate from the ventilator after the first SBT, which usually takes at least 24 h or longer (2, 3). Thus, in such cases, complications such as ventilator-associated lung injury, ventilator-dependency, malnutrition, and ventilator-associated pneumonia are frequently encountered (4–7), leading to higher extubation failure rates, longer hospital stays, and higher medical costs and consumption of medical resources (8).

Weaning difficulties after surgery for infants and children with congenital heart diseases are related to several factors, such as unstable hemodynamics following cardiac surgery, pulmonary hypertension, and delayed awakening (9, 10). In most cases, these patients often have accompanying structural health alignments such as tracheal or bronchial stenosis (11), lung infections, and acquired complications such as post-operative diaphragmatic dysfunctions (12), which have been identified as influencing factors of weaning difficulty in previous studies. Although there are some studies in the literature analyzing risk factors for extubation failure and how this affects patient outcomes, but there are few studies analyzing the treatment of failed weaning. In the study herein, we mainly explored the main causes of failure to wean from invasive mechanical ventilation following cardiac surgery in neonatal and pediatric patients. All hemodynamic causes were excluded, focusing on respiratory (congenital or acquired) causes. The three main causes identified are: airway stenosis (congenital or secondary), diaphragm dysfunction (partial or complete), and pneumonias. Although these factors can also be seen in ICU pediatric patients with non-cardiac surgery; however, the clinical characteristics after cardiac surgery are different, often accompanied by cardiac function inhibition, mediastinal and thoracic tissue destruction, organ damage, and systemic inflammation after cardiopulmonary bypass. Thus, the treatment is more complex, and the prognosis is less sanguine. It is extremely challenging as the combination conditions may require a change or alteration in conventional strategy. During the past 10 years, apart from simply extending mechanical ventilation or tracheotomy, some cardiac surgery centers pioneered many of the techniques that are currently used (13–15). However, a generally accepted individualized treatment plan is yet to be introduced or adopted.

Hence, in the study herein, we reviewed the surgical treatment of pediatric patients with congenital heart diseases from January 2005 to December 2020. Also, primary factors affecting weaning (except cardiac reasons including residual shunts) were statistically analyzed with proposed individualized treatment plans per cause or reasons.

METHODS

Study Population

This retrospective study was conducted in pediatric patients with congenital heart defects using the hospital information system. Records of congenital heart surgery cases performed at the Department of Cardiac Surgery of the Second Xiangya Hospital, Hunan Children's Hospital, and Hunan People's Hospital between January 2005 and December 2020 were reviewed. We selected cases from the database that met the following criteria: 1. Age <36 months, 2. diagnosed with congenital heart defects, 3. successfully wean after receiving invasive mechanical ventilation for more than 7 days, 4. no specialist conditions affecting weaning, such as postoperative cardiac hemodynamic instability, pulmonary hypertension, and delayed awakening. Exclusion criteria: 1. prolonged weaning due to incomplete correction of cardiac malformation, 2. postoperative hemodynamic instability or vasoactive-inotropic score (VIS) >15, 3. Postoperative delayed chest closure, 4. Postoperative ECMO assistance is required, 5. Short-term secondary surgery was performed. All patients were approved by the Ethics Committee of the Second Xiangya Hospital, Hunan Children's Hospital, and Hunan People's Hospital.

Variables

Demographic and clinical characteristics data were extracted from medical records for further details, including age, gender, weight, diagnoses according to International Classifications of Disease 10th revision, history and physical examination findings, ventilation settings, extubation attempts, various therapies, duration of mechanical ventilation in calendar days, etc.

Departmental criteria for weaning were: 1. good mental status, strong autonomic respiratory capacity; 2. hemodynamic stability, VIS <15, 3. ventilator parameters: CPAP/PS mode, oxygen concentration ≤0.5, PEEP ≤5 cmH2O, oxygenation index ≥150 mmHg, PS ≤14 cmH2O, tidal volume ≥7 ml/Kg; 4. No electrolyte disturbance and acid-base imbalance, arterial blood lactate ≤3 mmol/L, 5. No severe tissue edema.

Definition of weaning difficulty: the application of low-level CPAP/PS mode for the deextubation test, the child cannot meet the above withdrawal criteria, or the withdrawal of the ventilator 24 h autonomic breathing cannot maintain effective ventilation and/or oxygenation, the need for re-intubation for mechanical ventilation.

Statistics

All the data are presented as mean ± standard error of the mean (mean ± SE). For all the experimental data, statistical calculations were performed using the Statistical Product and Service Solutions 14.0 software (SPSS Institute). X^2 test was performed to determine differences between the groups. A p-value < 0.05 was considered statistically significant.

TABLE 1 | The profiles of the patients preoperatively.

	Stenotic tracheobronchial	Diaphragmatic dysmotility	Severe pneumonia	*P*-value
Case (*n*)	23	17	35	0.0847
Gender (male/female)	11/12	11/6	15/20	0.3303
Age (month)	7.09 ± 2.19	9.76 ± 4.78	3.51 ± 1.33	0.4661
Body weight (Kg)	7.67 ± 1.20	7.80 ± 1.94	5.58 ± 1.18	0.8968
Pulmonary sling (*n*)	17			<0.0001
Aortic ring (*n*)	3			0.0442
CAVSD (*n*)	1		4	0.3043
VSD (*n*)	1	2	21	0.0019
ASD (*n*)			2	0.3292
PDA (*n*)	1			0.3336
TAPVC (*n*)		6	5	0.0299
TOF (*n*)		4		0.003
TGA (*n*)		1	2	0.5206
PA (*n*)		2	1	0.1898
DORV (*n*)		2		0.0435

CAVSD complete atrioventricular septal defect, VSD ventricular septal defect, ASD atrial septal defect, PDA patent ductus arteriosus, TAPVC total anomalous pulmonary venous connection, TOF tetralogy of Fallot, TGA transposition of the great arteries, PA pulmonary atresia, DORV double outlet of right ventricular.

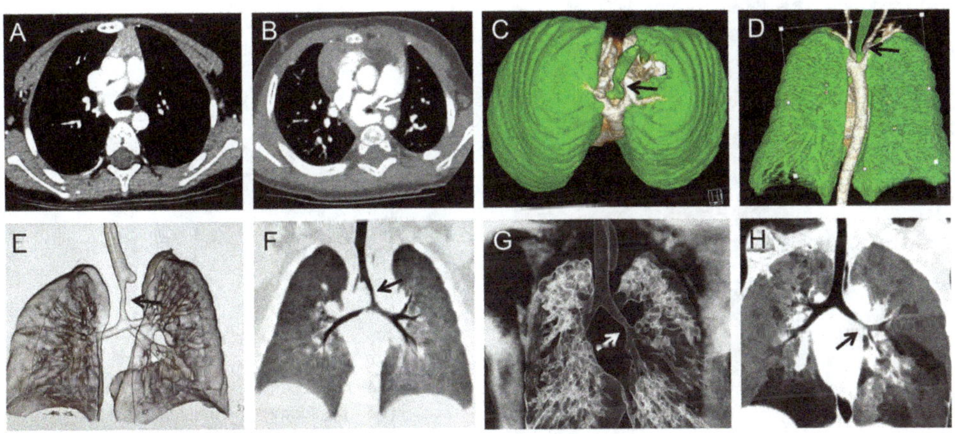

FIGURE 1 | Pulmonary CT and three-dimensional reconstruction of the airway, preoperatively showing the airway stenosis (arrows) was caused by pulmonary artery sling **(A,B)**, double aortic arch **(C,D)**, and a representative image of the stenosis (arrows) located in the trachea **(E,F)** and bronchus **(G,H)**.

RESULTS

Factors Associated With Weaning Difficulty

During the study period, a total of 4,971 pediatric patients underwent open heart surgery were retrieved from the hospital information database. After screening, there were 75 patients had weaning difficulties identified in our study.

- There were 23 stenotic tracheobronchial cases, (12 females and 11 males), with an age of 7.09 ± 2.19 months and a weight of 7.67 ± 1.20 Kg. Preoperative diagnosis included 17 pulmonary sling cases, 3 aortic ring cases, and 1 case of CAVSD, VSD, and PDA.
- There were 17 cases of diaphragmatic dysmotility (11 cases of bilateral and 6 cases of unilateral diaphragmatic dysmotility), including 6 females and 11 males, with an age of 9.76 ± 4.78 months and weight of 7.80 ± 1.94 Kg. Preoperative diagnosis included 6 TAPVC cases, 4 TOF cases, 1 TGA case, and 2 cases of DORV, PA, and VSD.
- There were 35 severe pneumonia cases, with an average age and weight of 3.51 ± 1.33 months and 5.58 ± 1.18 Kg. Preoperative diagnosis was VSD with pulmonary hypertension in 21 cases, ASD with pulmonary hypertension in 2 cases, TAPVC in 5 cases, CAVSD in 4 cases, TGA in 2 cases, and 1 PA case (**Table 1**).

Confirmation of the Diagnosis

In the airway stenosis group, 20 were identified concomitantly with the diagnosis of their heart defect (17 ulmonary artery sling, 3 aortic ring) due to routine preoperative examination

TABLE 2 | Confirmation of the diagnosis and mechanical ventilation duration.

	Check	Pre-operative confirmation	Postoperative confirmation	Band time (days)
Airway stenosis	CT	20	3	17.7
	Bronchoscopy	0	4	
Diaphragmatic dysfunction	CXR	0	17	33.6
Pulmonary infection	CT	22	0	11.9
	CXR	35	0	

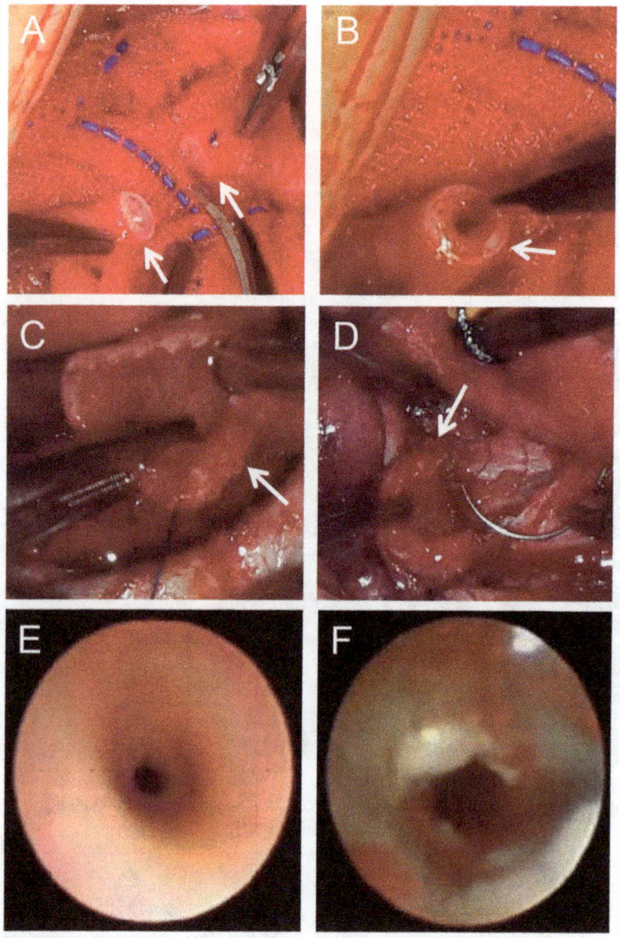

FIGURE 2 | Tracheal SLIDE operation **(A–D)**: Stenotic site was surgical resected (A, arrows), the upper (B, arrow) and lower part (C, arrow) were longitudinally extended and repaired by SLIDE anastomosis (D, arrow). Representative images of surgically treated trachea [before **(E)** and after **(F)**].

and 3 were identified subsequent to repair of their heart defects; compression stenosis of the left main bronchus was found by fiberoptic bronchoscopy in 4 cases. In the diaphragmatic dysfunction group, all cases were confirmed postoperatively by aside chest x-ray. In the pulmonary infection group, all cases had a history of multiple pediatric hospitalizations and underwent routine chest x-ray examination, and most of them were found to have pulmonary exudation; Twenty-two

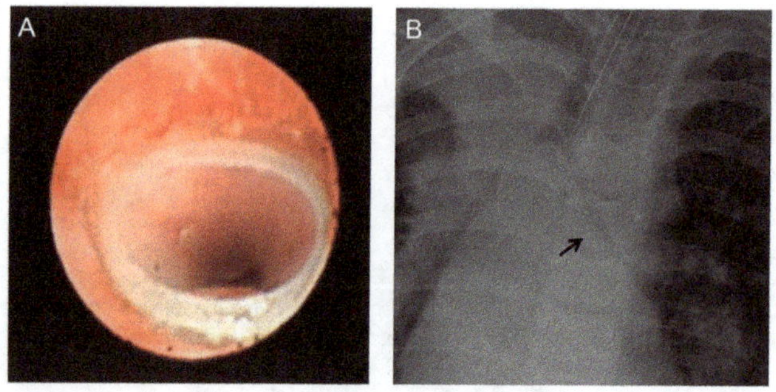

FIGURE 3 | Post-operative image of fiberoptic bronchoscopy stent implantation **(A)** and chest X-ray [**(B)**, arrow].

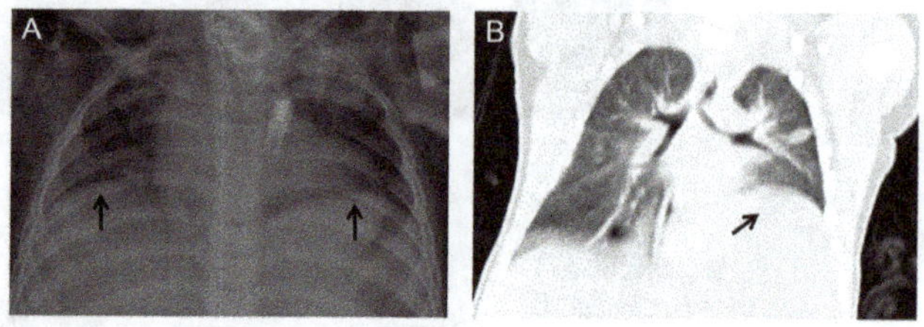

FIGURE 4 | Post-operative chest X-ray **(A)** and computed tomography in coronal view **(B)** showing the unilateral diaphragmatic elevation (arrows).

cases underwent lung CT examination before the surgery (**Figure 1**; **Table 2**).

Individualized Treatment

In addition to routine ICU treatment, we also adopted different treatment measures per different causes. In some cases, we integrated multiple treatment measures to establish an individualize treatment plan. More details are detailed below:

Airway Stenosis Group

In the airway stenosis group, most cases have no obvious clinical symptoms such as dyspnea before surgery. (i) Seven cases underwent SLIDE tracheoplasty concomitantly with primary surgery due to severe airway stenosis (**Figure 2**); (ii) four cases with tracheal stent implantation or bronchiectasis (**Figure 3**); (iii) four cases with tracheal intubation passing through the stenotic site to support softening collapse of the narrowed trachea; (iv) six cases with pure prolonged mechanical ventilation, fully discharge secretion and infection control; and (v) two cases with

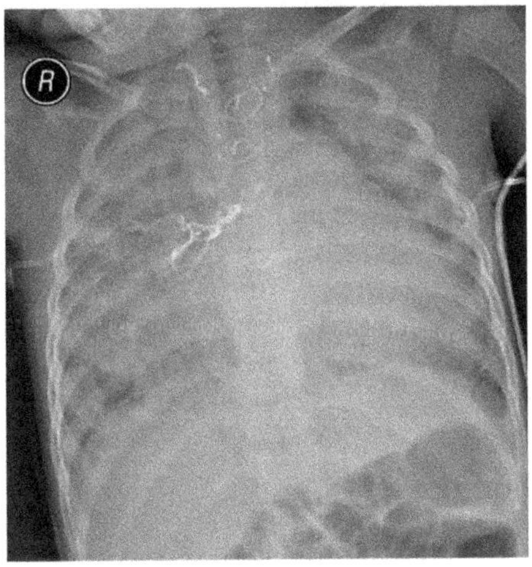

FIGURE 5 | Post-operative chest X-ray showing a representative image of severe pulmonary infection.

a tracheotomy to fully discharge secretions, control infection, and intermittently and gradually break away from the ventilator.

Diaphragm Dysfunction Group

In the diaphragm dysfunction group, clinical symptoms of phrenic nerve palsy after cardiac surgery varied in severity, ranging from asymptomatic conditions to life-threatening respiratory distress. Specific strategies for postoperative diaphragmatic dysfunction determined according to the specific situation: (i) Eight cases were controlled by prolonging mechanical ventilation time, using 45 degrees up semi-recumbent position, and eliminating secretions with infection control. (ii) Five cases were treated with the above method after tracheotomy, which was suitable for bilateral diaphragmatic paralysis and in patients with severe abnormal breathing. (iii) Four cases of diaphragm fold surgery, primarily for patients with unilateral septal muscle paralysis (**Figure 4**), significant elevation, with apparent abnormal breathing.

Severe Pulmonary Infection Group

In the pulmonary infection group (**Figure 5**), all cases were combined treated with postural drainage, prone ventilation, and full sputum discharge. According to the etiological examination, antibiotics were reasonably used to control infection. Combined with step-down weaning by raising the upper body position, high-frequency breathing apparatus was provided based on the clinical conditions following tracheal intubation removal, where the patients were all successfully weaned off.

Mechanical Ventilation Duration

The patients all recovered and were discharged from the hospital. The duration of wearing a ventilator ranged from 8 to 55 days (18.6 ± 12.1). Notably, diaphragmatic dysfunction had the longest time and was more challenging during weaning (33.6 ± 13.9 days). Even though severe lung infection is the most prevalent cause for difficult weaning, it was associated with shorter ventilator use (11.9 ± 3.8 days), while the intubation time in the airway stenosis group was 17.7 ± 9.0 days.

DISCUSSION

In this multicenter retrospective investigation, we examined the clinical characteristics and outcomes of congenital heart diseases patients with weaning difficulties, then identified the leading causes associated with this procedure and summarized individualized treatment experiences.

Weaning challenges in pediatric patients (neonates and toddlers) with congenital heart disease seriously affects recovery after surgery. After excluding the weaning failure caused by cardiac surgery, we found out the most critical reasons affecting the weaning failure in pediatric patients with congenital heart diseases, although we were unable to establish direct causality between any of these variables and the weaning procedure. Similar findings were previously identified in patients with diverse heart lesions (11, 12).

The novelty of our investigation is its specific focus on the individualized treatment strategies. An effective strategy to minimize weaning difficulty should include identification who has or may has a difficult weaning, preemptive recognition of situations at increased risk of weaning failure and appropriate individualized treatment planning. A flow chart of the three strategies adopted in the three situations was summarized in **Figure 6**. The following is a summary of individualized treatment experiences for three conditions:

Airway Stenosis

Airway stenosis can be divided into congenital and secondary stenosis. Congenital stenosis can exist alone and is accompanied by cardiac vascular malformation, such as double aortic arch, pulmonary artery sling, while secondary airway stenosis primarily has neoplastic obstruction and tracheobronchial compression. Approximately 0.15% of children with precordial disease have a combination of airway stenosis (16). The abnormal vascular structure and enlarged heart chamber in pediatric patients with congenital heart disease can easily mount pressure on the trachea or bronchus, causing tracheomalacia (17). The incidence of congenital heart disease combined with tracheomalacia is 4–12%. Stenosis near the glottis can be found during endotracheal intubation, while stenosis near the carina of the lower trachea is not easily found, and CT or bronchoscopy is often required to make such diagnosis (18). Although the pressure on the trachea is usually relieved after surgery and tracheal stenosis is relieved to some extent, it is not completely relieved in a short time. Narrow airway increases breathing in children, invariably increasing cardiac load, which is particularly significant in children whose cardiac function is yet to recover after surgery.

Narrow airways hinder the discharge of secretions, and increased secretions will increase airway resistance and increase the risk of lung infection. Therefore, trachea development should be carefully evaluated before surgery, and individualized measures, timely taken. However, the clinical manifestations of airway stenosis associated with congenital heart disease are easily

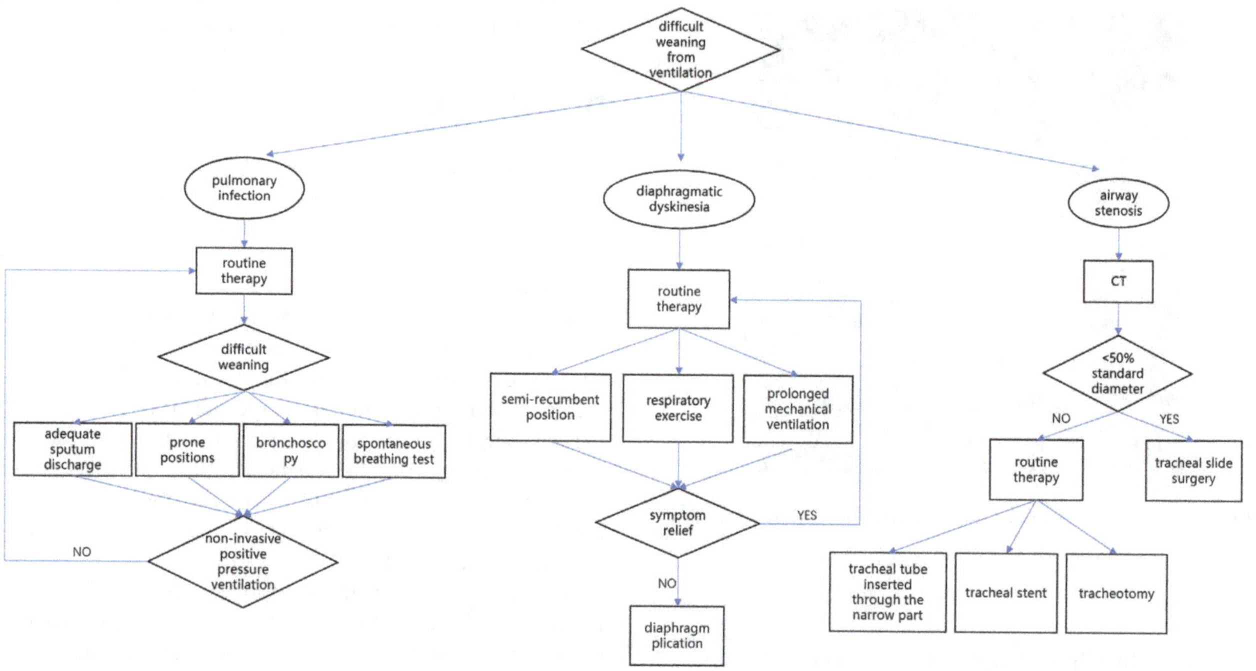

FIGURE 6 | The flow chart of the three strategies adopted in the three situations.

masked by the symptoms of the primary heart disease, and preoperative confirmation of the diagnosis relies heavily on CT and bronchoscopy Very few cases were confirmed preoperatively, but most cases were not noticed until they could not be taken offline or repeated endotracheal intubation. In this study, 20 of the 23 cases in this group were found to have different degrees of tracheal or bronchial stenosis on preoperative CT examination. Presently, we preoperationally anticipate that patients may have airway stenoses, such as pulmonary sling, vascular ring, and enlargement of the left atrium. Usually, pulmonary CTA and three-dimensional reconstruction of the airway are performed to evaluate the degree of airway stenosis (**Figure 1**). Tracheal SLIDE anastomosis technique was performed during surgery (**Figure 2**), given preoperative CT evaluation (**Figure 1**) showed that the diameter of the stenotic site was <50% standard diameter for age. In this study, 7 children who had difficulty in weaning after cardiac surgery with severe tracheal stenosis were extubated within 3 weeks after tracheal slide surgery and recovered well. Given the preoperative CT results, stenotic tracheal sites $\geq$50% standard diameter for age can be treated selectively per patient and conditions by: (1) Prolonging the ventilation time; and (2) Tracheotomy techniques for airway management and step-down weaning exercises if the patient is on a ventilator for over 3 weeks. Significantly, in the absence of inherent tracheal stenosis, relative stenosis (trachea softening or collapse) is thus caused by enlarged blood vessels or cardiomegaly. However, if the malformation is not severe, a tracheal tube can be inserted through the narrow part to support the softened trachea for $\sim$2 weeks. On the other hand, some cases can be treated by prolonging ventilator-assisted time; however, it might increase the risk of ventilator-associated pneumonia. If trachea collapse occurs following severe softening and is also challenging to gain recovery in a short time, a tracheal stent can be considered (**Figure 3**). Likewise, tracheal stents could also be considered for severe bronchomalacia collapse. If the trachea cannot be taken off the machine and a tracheal stent cannot be placed, we will consider tracheotomy after more than 3 weeks of mechanical ventilation.

Dysmotility of Diaphragm

Another reason for the difficulty of weaning in this study may be related to the diminished mobility of the diaphragm, and similar conclusions were reached in previous studies (19). Postoperative diaphragmatic dyskinesia is mainly due to phrenic nerve injury in the cardiac surgery (20), and postoperative chest radiographs often show one or both diaphragmatic elevations, with clinical manifestations of dyspnea and even paradoxical breathing. In children with low age, low body mass, and complex congenital heart disease, the possibility of diaphragmatic palsy should be considered first, and the diaphragm motor function should be evaluated by ultrasound and chest X-ray to clarify the diagnosis as soon as possible (21). In this study, the preoperative chest X-ray did not show diaphragm elevation in this group of children, and the postoperative chest X-ray showed unilateral diaphragm elevation in 6 cases and bilateral diaphragm elevation in 11 cases. We have found in clinical practice that the degree of bilateral diaphragmatic elevation is less than the degree of unilateral diaphragmatic elevation.

The measures we took for these children were: for patients with unilateral diaphragmatic elevation, we would first use conservative treatment with semi-recumbent position (22), postural drainage, simple prolonged mechanical ventilation, and adequate drainage of secretions, and in severe cases, we would also consider unilateral diaphragmatic folding surgery. For patients with bilateral diaphragm elevation, we will use semi-recumbent position, promote the diaphragm downward, strengthen respiratory exercise, and give some time to observe the possibility of self-recovery, if it obviously affects the respiratory status and is difficult to get off the ventilator, one side of the diaphragm will be folded first, and then exercise will be performed to gradually get off the machine, if after one side of the diaphragm is folded, the effect of getting off the machine is poor and the respiratory status does not improve significantly, then If one side of the diaphragm is folded and the breathing status does not improve significantly, the other side of the diaphragm is folded again. Among them, for those who have severe abdominal breathing, long recovery time and need longer mechanical ventilation (usually will exceed 30 days), we will consider performing tracheotomy around 3 weeks to facilitate sputum removal and airway management.

Severe Pulmonary Infection

The present study also found that severe preoperative pulmonary infection was one of the main causes of weaning difficulties in children after cardiac surgery, which is consistent with previous findings (12). A single-center, 2-year retrospective cohort study of critically ill pediatric patients by ChoiA et al. (23) showed that severe pulmonary infections were responsible for 74.1% of the disease factors influencing the occurrence of weaning difficulties in children, and a large cross-sectional survey of 40 comprehensive ICUs by Louise Rose et al. (24) found that severe pneumonia, acute lung injury, and severe systemic infections with sepsis were responsible for ~64% of the weaning difficulties. Children with incomplete treatment of preoperative pulmonary infection and increased postoperative pulmonary secretions are prone to ventilator-associated pneumonia, resulting in respiratory failure, difficulty in withdrawal, and prolonged mechanical ventilation. Concerning treatment with the routine use of sensitive antibiotics based on etiology and drug sensitivity tests, and regular oral care, we also emphasize using different postural drainage methods per the patients' conditions. In addition, we encourage adequate sputum discharge and suction of oral secretions, and intermittent prone positions during mechanical ventilation while using cuffed tracheal intubation (25), strict hand hygiene, disinfecting procedures, and tracheal intubation with a capsule to avoid secretions from the mouth and nose into the airway. Previous studies have shown that early fiberoptic bronchoscopy and bronchoalveolar lavage can effectively relieve clinical manifestations, pulmonary atelectasis, and airway obstruction (26). In the present study, 19 children had relief of symptoms after fiberoptic bronchoscopy due to severe pulmonary arthritis (27). In the absence of contraindications, the possibility of extubation was assessed with a daily spontaneous breathing test. Non-invasive positive pressure ventilation was selected per the patient's condition after extubation, which was helpful for early weaning. In the absence of contraindications, a daily spontaneous breathing test assesses the possibility of extubation. After extubation, non-invasive positive pressure ventilation is selected based on the patient's clinical condition, which is helpful for early weaning.

Limitations

Consideration of these findings should include acknowledgment of the limitations of our study design. First, this is a retrospective and non-randomized study, prospective intervention studies may be considered in the future. Second, there are some other factors that may affect weaning outcome and need to be verified in follow-up studies. Finally, as neonatal ventilation issues are often very different due to the congenital nature to infants, these results should be interpreted with caution.

CONCLUSIONS

In summary, airway stenosis, diaphragm dysfunction, and severe pulmonary infection are leading causes of postoperative meaning difficulties in pediatric patients with congenital heart diseases. These factors should be taken into consideration and individualized treatment decisions should be made when providing care for such patients.

AUTHOR CONTRIBUTIONS

XiaW and CF drafted the manuscript. CF and JY designed the study. JC, JL, CI, XX, PH, and WZ revised the manuscript. XiaW, MW, KX, XunW, and WC were responsible for the collection of data or analysis. All authors read and approved the final manuscript.

REFERENCES

1. Gupta P, Chow V, Gossett JM, Yeh JC, Roth SJ. Incidence, predictors, and outcomes of extubation failure in children after orthotopic heart transplantation: a single-center experience. *Pediatr Cardiol.* (2015) 36:300–7. doi: 10.1007/s00246-014-1003-6
2. Rose L, Schultz MJ, Cardwell CR, Jouvet P, McAuley DF, Blackwood B. Automated versus non-automated weaning for reducing the duration of mechanical ventilation for critically ill adults and children. *Cochrane Database Syst Rev.* (2013) 6:CD009235. doi: 10.1002/14651858.CD009235.pub2
3. Beduneau G, Pham T, Schortgen F, Piquilloud L, Zogheib E, Jonas M, et al. Epidemiology of weaning outcome according to a new definition. The WIND study. *Am J Respir Crit Care Med.* (2017) 195:772–83. doi: 10.1164/rccm.201602-0320OC
4. Francois B, Cariou A, Clere-Jehl R, Dequin PF, Renon-Carron F, Daix T, et al. Prevention of early ventilator-associated pneumonia after cardiac arrest. *N Engl J Med.* (2019) 381:1831–42. doi: 10.1056/NEJMoa1812379
5. Perkins GD, Mistry D, Gates S, Gao F, Snelson C, Hart N, et al. Effect of protocolized weaning with early extubation to noninvasive ventilation vs. invasive weaning on time to liberation from mechanical ventilation among

patients with respiratory failure: the breathe randomized clinical trial. *JAMA.* (2018) 320:1881–8. doi: 10.1001/jama.2018.13763
6. Kneyber MCJ, de Luca D, Calderini E, Jarreau PH, Javouhey E, Lopez-Herce J, et al. Recommendations for mechanical ventilation of critically ill children from the paediatric mechanical ventilation consensus conference (PEMVECC). *Intensive Care Med.* (2017) 43:1764–80. doi: 10.1007/s00134-017-4920-z
7. Khemani RG, Sekayan T, Hotz J, Flink RC, Rafferty GF, Iyer N, et al. Risk factors for pediatric extubation failure: the importance of respiratory muscle strength. *Crit Care Med.* (2017) 45:e798–805. doi: 10.1097/CCM.0000000000002433
8. Gaies M, Tabbutt S, Schwartz SM, Bird GL, Alten JA, Shekerdemian LS, et al. Clinical epidemiology of extubation failure in the pediatric cardiac ICU: a report from the pediatric cardiac critical care consortium. *Pediatr Crit Care Med.* (2015) 16:837–45. doi: 10.1097/PCC.0000000000000498
9. Winch P D, Staudt A M, Sebastian R, Corridore M, Tumin D, Simsic J, et al. Learning from experience: improving early tracheal extubation success after congenital cardiac surgery. *Pediatr Crit Care Med.* (2016) 17:630–7. doi: 10.1097/PCC.0000000000000789
10. Ip P, Chiu CS, Cheung YF. Risk factors prolonging ventilation in young children after cardiac surgery: impact of noninfectious pulmonary complications. *Pediatr Crit Care Med.* (2002) 3:269–74. doi: 10.1097/00130478-200207000-00013
11. Mainwaring RD, Shillingford M, Davies R, Koltai P, Navaratnam M, Reddy V M, et al. Surgical reconstruction of tracheal stenosis in conjunction with congenital heart defects. *Ann Thorac Surg.* (2012) 93:1266–72; discussion 72–3. doi: 10.1016/j.athoracsur.2011.12.063
12. Gerard-Castaing N, Perrin T, Ohlmann C, Mainguy C, Coutier L, Buchs C, et al. Diaphragmatic paralysis in young children: a literature review. *Pediatr Pulmonol.* (2019) 54:1367–73. doi: 10.1002/ppul.24383
13. Yang Y, Li X, Jiao A. Stent intervention for children with CHD and tracheal stenosis. *Cardiol Young.* (2020) 30:1532–4. doi: 10.1017/S1047951120002504
14. Arcieri L, Giordano R, Murzi B. To do or not to do? The management dilemma of congenital tracheal stenosis in the setting of the ring-sling complex. *J Thorac Dis.* (2017) 9:4896–8. doi: 10.21037/jtd.2017.11.79
15. Anton-Pacheco J L, Morante R. Operative or non-operative treatment of congenital tracheal stenosis: is there something new? *J Thorac Dis.* (2017) 9:4878–80. doi: 10.21037/jtd.2017.11.75
16. Xue B, Liang B, Wang S, Zhu L, Lu Z, Xu Z. One-stage surgical correction of congenital tracheal stenosis complicated with congenital heart disease in infants and young children. *J Card Surg.* (2015) 30:97–103. doi: 10.1111/jocs.12418
17. Singhal M, Gupta P, Singh RS, Rohit MK, Sodhi KS, Khandelwal N. Cardiovascular causes of pediatric airway compression: a pictorial review. *Curr Probl Diagn Radiol.* (2015) 44:505–10. doi: 10.1067/j.cpradiol.2015.04.005
18. Gupta P, McDonald R, Gossett JM, Butt W, Shinkawa T, Imamura M, et al. A single-center experience of extubation failure in infants undergoing the norwood operation. *Ann Thorac Surg.* (2012) 94:1262–8. doi: 10.1016/j.athoracsur.2012.05.033
19. Abdel Rahman DA, Saber S, El-Maghraby A. Diaphragm and lung ultrasound indices in prediction of outcome of weaning from mechanical ventilation in pediatric intensive care unit. *Indian J Pediatr.* (2020) 87:413–20. doi: 10.1007/s12098-019-03177-y
20. Serraf A, Planche C, Lacour Gayet F, Bruniaux J, Nottin R, Binet JP. Post cardiac surgery phrenic nerve palsy in pediatric patients. *Eur J Cardiothorac Surg.* (1990) 4:421–4. doi: 10.1016/1010-7940(90)90071-7
21. Akbariasbagh P, Mirzaghayan MR, Akbariasbagh N, Shariat M, Ebrahim B. Risk factors for post-cardiac surgery diaphragmatic paralysis in children with congenital heart disease. *J Tehran Heart Cent.* (2015) 10:134–9.
22. Zhuo X, Pan L, Zeng X. The effects of the 45 degrees semi-recumbent position on the clinical outcomes of mechanically ventilated patients: a systematic review and meta-analysis study. *Ann Palliat Med.* (2021) 10:10643–51. doi: 10.21037/apm-21-2359
23. Choi AY, Kim M, Park E, Son MH, Ryu JA, Cho J. Outcomes of mechanical ventilation according to WIND classification in pediatric patients. *Ann Intensive Care.* (2019) 9:72. doi: 10.1186/s13613-019-0547-2
24. Rose L, Fowler RA, Fan E, Fraser I, Leasa D, Mawdsley C, et al. Prolonged mechanical ventilation in Canadian intensive care units: a national survey. *J Crit Care.* (2015) 30:25–31. doi: 10.1016/j.jcrc.2014.07.023
25. Zhong QH, Duan J, Zhang CY, Feng YL, Qi ZY, He XY, et al. [Effect of prone positioning on respiratory function in very preterm infants undergoing mechanical ventilation]. *Zhongguo Dang Dai Er Ke Za Zhi.* (2018) 20:608–12. doi: 10.7499/j.issn.1008-8830.2018.08.002
26. Wang L, Wang W, Sun JM, Ni SW, Ding JL, Zhu YL, et al. Efficacy of fiberoptic bronchoscopy and bronchoalveolar lavage in childhood-onset, complicated plastic bronchitis. *Pediatr Pulmonol.* (2020) 55:3088–95. doi: 10.1002/ppul.25016
27. Ferguson KN, Roberts CT, Manley BJ, Davis PG. Interventions to improve rates of successful extubation in preterm infants: a systematic review and meta-analysis. *JAMA Pediatr.* (2017) 171:165–74. doi: 10.1001/jamapediatrics.2016.3015

Permissions

All chapters in this book were first published by Frontiers; hereby published with permission under the Creative Commons Attribution License or equivalent. Every chapter published in this book has been scrutinized by our experts. Their significance has been extensively debated. The topics covered herein carry significant findings which will fuel the growth of the discipline. They may even be implemented as practical applications or may be referred to as a beginning point for another development.

The contributors of this book come from diverse backgrounds, making this book a truly international effort. This book will bring forth new frontiers with its revolutionizing research information and detailed analysis of the nascent developments around the world.

We would like to thank all the contributing authors for lending their expertise to make the book truly unique. They have played a crucial role in the development of this book. Without their invaluable contributions this book wouldn't have been possible. They have made vital efforts to compile up to date information on the varied aspects of this subject to make this book a valuable addition to the collection of many professionals and students.

This book was conceptualized with the vision of imparting up-to-date information and advanced data in this field. To ensure the same, a matchless editorial board was set up. Every individual on the board went through rigorous rounds of assessment to prove their worth. After which they invested a large part of their time researching and compiling the most relevant data for our readers.

The editorial board has been involved in producing this book since its inception. They have spent rigorous hours researching and exploring the diverse topics which have resulted in the successful publishing of this book. They have passed on their knowledge of decades through this book. To expedite this challenging task, the publisher supported the team at every step. A small team of assistant editors was also appointed to further simplify the editing procedure and attain best results for the readers.

Apart from the editorial board, the designing team has also invested a significant amount of their time in understanding the subject and creating the most relevant covers. They scrutinized every image to scout for the most suitable representation of the subject and create an appropriate cover for the book.

The publishing team has been an ardent support to the editorial, designing and production team. Their endless efforts to recruit the best for this project, has resulted in the accomplishment of this book. They are a veteran in the field of academics and their pool of knowledge is as vast as their experience in printing. Their expertise and guidance has proved useful at every step. Their uncompromising quality standards have made this book an exceptional effort. Their encouragement from time to time has been an inspiration for everyone.

The publisher and the editorial board hope that this book will prove to be a valuable piece of knowledge for researchers, students, practitioners and scholars across the globe.

List of Contributors

Laura Antonia Ritz, Dietrich von Schweinitz and Jochen Hubertus
Department of Pediatric Surgery, Dr. von Hauner Children's Hospital, Ludwig-Maximilian-University of Munich, Munich, Germany

Mohammad Samer Hajji, Tobias Schwerd, Sibylle Koletzko and Eberhard Lurz
Department of Pediatric Gastroenterology, Dr. von Hauner Children's Hospital, Ludwig-Maximilian-University of Munich, Munich, Germany

Jinkui Wang, Xiaojun Tan, Chenghao Zhanghuang, Liming Jin, Mujie Li, Zhaoxia Zhang, Tao Mi and Dawei He
Department of Urology, Chongqing Key Laboratory of Children Urogenital Development and Tissue Engineering, Chongqing Key Laboratory of Pediatrics, Ministry of Education Key Laboratory of Child Development and Disorders, National Clinical Research Center for Child Health and Disorders, China International Science and Technology Cooperation Base of Child Development and Critical Disorders, Children's Hospital of Chongqing Medical University, Chongqing, China

Jie Tang
Department of Epidemiology, Public Health School, Shenyang Medical College, Shenyang, China

Tao Han, Buhao Sun, Weidong Wang, Jie Cui and Weimin Shen
Department of Burns and Plastic Surgery, Children's Hospital of Nanjing Medical University, Nanjing, China

Rui-jue Wang, Ming-man Zhang and Qiang Xiong
Chongqing Key Laboratory of Pediatrics, Department of Hepatobiliary Surgery, Children's Hospital of Chongqing Medical University, National Clinical Research Center for Child Health and Disorders, Ministry of Education Key Laboratory of Child Development and Disorders, Chongqing, China

Li Xiao and Xi-ming Xu
Department of Medical Record Statistics, Children's Hospital of Chongqing Medical University, National Clinical Research Center for Child Health and Disorders, Chongqing Higher Institution Engineering Research Center of Children's Medical Big Data Intelligent Application, Ministry of Education Key Laboratory of Child Development and Disorders, Chongqing, China

Junxiang Wang, Lixiang Zhao, Guiwen Feng and Wenjun Shang
The Department of Kidney Transplantation, The First Affiliated Hospital of Zhengzhou University, Zhengzhou, China

Riana Pauline Tamba and Yefta Moenadjat
Faculty of Medicine, Department of Surgery Cipto Mangunkusumo General Hospital, Universitas Indonesia, Jakarta, Indonesia

Zhibin Zhou, Yongqiang Yue, Ke Ma, Zhaohui Hua and Zhen Li
Department of Endovascular Surgery, The First Affiliated Hospital of Zhengzhou University, Zhengzhou, China

Wanbin Yin, Laian Li and Shuai Wang
Department of Anorectal Surgery, Affiliated Hospital of Jining Medical University, Jining, China

Lin Su
Department of Pediatric Surgery, Affiliated Hospital of Jining Medical University, Jining, China

Jin-Xi Huang, Qiang Chen, Song-Ming Hong, Jun-Jie Hong and Hua Cao
Department of Cardiothoracic Surgery, Fujian Branch of Shanghai Children's Medical Center, Fuzhou, China
Fujian Children's Hospital, Fuzhou, China
Fujian Maternity and Child Health Hospital, Affiliated Hospital of Fujian Medical University, Fuzhou, China
Fujian Key Laboratory of Women and Children's Critical Diseases Research, Fujian Maternity and Child Health Hospital, Fuzhou, China

Wing Ki Chan
Li Ka Shing Faculty of Medicine, The University of Hong Kong, Hong Kong, China

Patrick Ho Yu Chung and Kenneth Kak Yuen Wong
Department of Surgery, The University of Hong Kong, Hong Kong, China

Ge Sun and Monika Trzpis
Department of Surgery, Anorectal Physiology Laboratory, University of Groningen, University Medical Center Groningen, Groningen, Netherlands

Paul M. A. Broens
Department of Surgery, Anorectal Physiology Laboratory, University of Groningen, University Medical Center Groningen, Groningen, Netherlands
Department of Surgery, Division of Pediatric Surgery, University of Groningen, University Medical Center Groningen, Groningen, Netherlands

Yan Linhua, Jiang Linjun, Qu Xiangyang, Liu Xing, Li Ming and Wu Jun
Department of Orthopedics, Children's Hospital of Chongqing Medical University, Ministry of Education Key Laboratory of Child Development and Disorders, Chongqing Key Laboratory of Pediatrics, National Clinical Research Center for Child Health and Disorders, Chongqing, China

Weichao Zhu
Department of Pediatric Surgery, The Affiliated Hospital of Medical School, Ningbo University, Ningbo, China

Jie Sun
Department of Urology, Shanghai Children's Medical Center, Shanghai Jiao Tong University School of Medicine, Shanghai, China

Jianhua He
Department of Pediatric Surgery, The Affiliated Hospital of Medical School, Ningbo University, Ningbo, China
Diagnosis and Treatment Center of Pelvic Floor, The Affiliated Hospital of Medical School, Ningbo University, Ningbo, China

Wangping Zhang
Department of Anesthesiology, Women and Children's Hospital of Jiaxing University, Jiaxing, China

Meng Shi
Department of Anesthesiology, Xuzhou Medical University, Xuzhou, China

Andrew Hall and Michael T. Ashworth
Great Ormond Street Hospital for Children NHS Foundation Trust, London, United Kingdom

Claire Frauenfelder
Great Ormond Street Hospital for Children NHS Foundation Trust, London, United Kingdom
Discipline of Surgery, School of Medicine, University of Adelaide, Adelaide, SA, Australia

Colin R. Butler
Great Ormond Street Hospital for Children NHS Foundation Trust, London, United Kingdom
UCL Great Ormond Street Institute of Child Health, Great Ormond Street Hospital for Children, London, United Kingdom

Susan C. Shelmerdine, Ian C. Simcock and Owen J. Arthurs
Great Ormond Street Hospital for Children NHS Foundation Trust, London, United Kingdom
UCL Great Ormond Street Institute of Child Health, Great Ormond Street Hospital for Children, London, United Kingdom
National Institute for Health Research Great Ormond Street Hospital Biomedical Research Centre, London, United Kingdom

John Ciaran Hutchinson
Great Ormond Street Hospital for Children NHS Foundation Trust, London, United Kingdom
UCL Great Ormond Street Institute of Child Health, Great Ormond Street Hospital for Children, London, United Kingdom
National Institute for Health Research Great Ormond Street Hospital Biomedical Research Centre, London, United Kingdom
Department of Histopathology, St Thomas' Hospital, London, United Kingdom

Tao Qian, Zhong-Shi Wu, Ting Lu and Can Huang
Department of Cardiovascular Surgery, The Second Xiangya Hospital, Central South University, Changsha, China
Engineering Laboratory of Hunan Province for Cardiovascular Biomaterials, Changsha, China

Jian-Guo Hu, Yi-Feng Yang and Qin Wu
Department of Cardiovascular Surgery, The Second Xiangya Hospital, Central South University, Changsha, China

Jia Li
Clinical Physiology Laboratory, Guangzhou Women and Children's Medical Center, Institute of Pediatrics, Guangzhou Medical University, Guangzhou, China
Guangdong Provincial Key Laboratory of Research in Structural Birth Defect Disease, Guangzhou Women and Children's Medical Center, Guangzhou Medical University, Guangzhou, China

Christina Dalzell
School of Medicine, University of Virginia, Charlottesville, VA, United States

Paola A. Vargas, Frank Di Paola and Nicolas Goldaracena
Division of Transplant Surgery, Department of Surgery, University of Virginia Health System, Charlottesville, VA, United States

Kyle Soltys and George Mazariegos
Division of Transplant Surgery, Department of Surgery, University of Virginia Health System, Charlottesville, VA, United States
Department of Surgery, Hillman Center for Pediatric Transplantation, UPMC Children's Hospital of Pittsburgh, University of Pittsburgh School of Medicine, Pittsburgh, PA, United States

Sophie A. Costerus, Joen IJsselmuiden, René Wijnen and Dick Tibboel
Department of Paediatric Surgery, Erasmus Medical Center - Sophia Children's Hospital, Rotterdam, Netherlands

Dries Hendrikx, Sabine Van Huffel and Alexander Caicedo
ESAT-STADIUS Division, Department of Electrical Engineering, KU Leuven, Leuven, Belgium

Katrin Zahn and Lucas Wessel
Department of Paediatric Surgery, University Hospital Mannheim, Mannheim, Germany

Alba Perez-Ortiz
Neonatal Intensive Care Unit, University Hospital Mannheim, Mannheim, Germany

Robert B. Flint
Division of Neonatology, Department of Paediatrics, Erasmus Medical Center - Sophia Children's Hospital, Rotterdam, Netherlands
Department of Pharmacy, Erasmus Medical Center, Rotterdam, Netherlands

Jurgen C. de Graaff
Department of Anaesthesiology, Erasmus Medical Center, Rotterdam, Netherlands

Gunnar Naulaers
Department of Development and Regeneration, KU Leuven, Leuven, Belgium
Neonatal Intensive Care Unit, University Hospitals Leuven, Leuven, Belgium

Yanan Li, Xuepeng Zhang, Tong Qiu and Zhicheng Xu
Department of Pediatric Surgery, West China Hospital of Sichuan University, Chengdu, China

Siyuan Chen
Pediatric Intensive Care Unit, Department of Critical Care Medicine, West China Hospital of Sichuan University, Chengdu, China

Rufa Wang
Department of Orthopedic Surgery, Children's Hospital of Nanjing Medical University, Nanjing, China

Xiaoguang Zhou
Neonatal Medical Center, Children's Hospital of Nanjing Medical University, Nanjing, China

Elena Sophia Elekta Dilean Siahaan, Wahyudhy Adriansyah, Andika Purba Sasmita, Aditya Rifqi Fauzi, Andi Dwihantoro and Gunadi
Pediatric Surgery Division, Department of Surgery, Faculty of Medicine, Public Health and Nursing, Universitas Gadjah Mada/Dr. Sardjito Hospital, Yogyakarta, Indonesia

Weimo Zhou
Department of Pediatric Surgery, Guigang City People's Hospital, Eighth Affiliated Hospital of Guangxi Medical University, Guigang, China

Yingzuo Shi
Department of Pediatric Surgery, Wuxi People's Hospital, Wuxi, China

Ming Zhang
Clinical Laboratory, Zhucheng Maternal and Child Health Hospital, Zhucheng, China

Li Li
The Department of Pediatrics, Ganzhou People's Hospital, Ganzhou, China

Yi Ji
Department of Burns and Plastic Surgery, Children's Hospital of Nanjing Medical University, Nanjing, China
Department of Pediatric Surgery, West China Hospital of Sichuan University, Chengdu, China

Qiang Yuan, Xufei Duan and Xueqiang Yan
Department of Pediatric Surgery, Wuhan Children's Hospital (Wuhan Maternal and Child Healthcare Hospital), Tongji Medical College, Huazhong University of Science and Technology, Wuhan, China

Xiaolong Xie, Yang Wu, Kewei Li, Chengbo Ai, Qi Wang, Chuan Wang, Jing Chen and Bo Xiang
Department of Pediatric Surgery, West China Hospital, Sichuan University, Chengdu, China

Valeria Dipasquale, Laura Cannavò and Claudio Romano
Pediatric Gastroenterology and Cystic Fibrosis Unit, Department of Human Pathology in Adulthood and Childhood "G. Barresi", University of Messina, Messina, Italy

Enrica Antonelli, Giorgio Cavatoi and Carmelo Romeo
Pediatric Surgery Unit, Department of Human Pathology in Adulthood and Childhood "G. Barresi", University of Messina, Messina, Italy

Giuseppe Trimarchi
Department of Economy, University of Messina, Messina, Italy

Giuseppe Navarra
Surgical Oncology Division, Department of Human Pathology in Adulthood and Childhood "G. Barresi", University of Messina, Messina, Italy

Desalegn Muche Wudineh
Felege-Hiwot Referral Hospital, Bahirdar, Ethiopia

Yophtahe Woldegerima Berhe, Wubie Birlie Chekol, Habtu Adane and Misganaw Mengie Workie
Department of Anesthesia, University of Gondar, Gondar, Ethiopia

Hiroyuki Koga, Takanori Ochi, Geoffrey J. Lane and Atsuyuki Yamataka
Department of Pediatric General and Urogenital Surgery, Juntendo University School of Medicine, Tokyo, Japan

Shunki Hirayama, Yukio Watanabe, Hiroyasu Ueno, Kota Imashimizu and Kenji Suzuki
Department of General Thoracic Surgery, Juntendo University School of Medicine, Tokyo, Japan

Kazuhiro Suzuki and Ryohei Kuwatsuru
Department of Radiology, Juntendo University School of Medicine, Tokyo, Japan

Kinya Nishimura
Department of Anesthesiology and Pain Medicine, Juntendo University School of Medicine, Tokyo, Japan

Giovanna Riccipetitoni, Mirko Bertozzi, Marta Gazzaneo, Alessandro Raffaele and Fabrizio Vatta
Department of Pediatric Surgery, Fondazione Istituti di Ricovero e Cura a Carattere Scientifico (IRCCS) Policlinico San Matteo, University of Pavia, Pavia, Italy

Giovanna Spezzotto
Faculty of Medicine and Surgery, University of Trieste, Trieste, Italy

Alessandro Boscarelli, Giulia Ceschiutti, Daniela Codrich, Maria-Grazia Scarpa, Marianna Iaquinto, Damiana Olenik and Edoardo Guida
Department of Pediatric Surgery and Urology, Institute for Maternal and Child Health - IRCCS "Burlo Garofolo", Trieste, Italy

Manuela Giangreco
Clinical Epidemiology and Public Health Research Unit, Institute for Maternal and Child Health - IRCCS "Burlo Garofolo", Trieste, Italy

Jürgen Schleef
Department of Pediatric Surgery and Urology, Institute for Maternal and Child Health - IRCCS "Burlo Garofolo", Trieste, Italy
Surgical Department, Institute for Maternal and Child Health - IRCCS "Burlo Garofolo", Trieste, Italy

Xiaoming Wu, Jinlan Chen, Chukwuemeka Daniel Iroegbu, Xia Xie, Kun Xiang, Xun Wu, Wangping Chen, Chengming Fan and Jinfu Yang
Department of Cardiovascular Surgery, The Second Xiangya Hospital, Central South University, Changsha, China

Jian Liu and Peng Huang
Department of Cardiothoracic Surgery, Hunan Children's Hospital, Changsha, China

Ming Wu
Department of Cardiovascular Surgery, The Second Xiangya Hospital, Central South University, Changsha, China
Department of the Cardiovascular Surgery of the Hunan Provincial People's Hospital, Changsha, China

Wenwu Zhou
Department of the Cardiovascular Surgery of the Hunan Provincial People's Hospital, Changsha, China

Index

www.ingramcontent.com/pod-product-compliance
Lightning Source LLC
LaVergne TN
LVHW082207200926
848484LV00008B/2229